IMMEDIATE care of
the acutely ill and injured

D0861074

IMMEDIATE care of the acutely ill and injured

Edited by

HUGH E. STEPHENSON, Jr.

A.B., B.S., M.D., F.A.C.S.

Professor and Chief, Division of General Surgery,
University of Missouri School of Medicine, Columbia, Missouri

SECOND EDITION 119960

The C. V. Mosby Company

Saint Louis   1978

Second edition

Copyright © 1978 by The C. V. Mosby Company

Previous edition copyrighted 1974

Printed in the United States of America

The C. V. Mosby Company
11830 Westline Industrial Drive, St. Louis, Missouri 63141

Library of Congress Cataloging in Publication Data

Stephenson, Hugh E
    Immediate care of the acutely ill and injured.

    Bibliography: p.
    Includes index.
    1. Medical emergencies. 2. Care of the sick.
I. Title. [DNLM: 1. Emergencies. 2. Emergency
health services. WB100 I33]
RC86.7.S73 1978   616'.025   77-25939
ISBN 0-8016-4783-5

GW/M/M 9 8 7 6 5 4 3 2 1

Contributors

JOHN P. ADAMS, B.S., M.D., F.A.C.S.

Professor and Chairman, Department of Orthopaedic Surgery, George Washington University Medical Center, Washington, D.C.

JOHN T. BONNER, M.D.

Fresno, California; Formerly Assistant Professor of Surgery (Neurosurgery), University of Missouri, Columbia, Missouri

ELWYN L. CADY, Jr., J.D., B.S. (Medicine)

Medicolegal Consultant, Independence, Missouri; Guest Lecturer, Advanced Paramedic Training, Penn Valley Community College, Kansas City, Missouri

RICHARD O. COE, Jr., M.D.

Ophthalmology, Mission, Kansas

MARSHALL B. CONRAD, M.D., F.A.C.S.

Associate Professor of Clinical Orthopaedic Surgery, Washington University School of Medicine; Chief, Region VII, Committee on Trauma, American College of Surgeons, St. Louis, Missouri

JEFFERSON C. DAVIS, M.D., Colonel, U.S.A.F., M.C.

Chief, Hyperbaric Medicine Division, U.S.A.F. School of Aerospace Medicine, Brook Air Force Base, Texas

JEAN-RENÉ DUPONT, M.D., F.A.C.S.

Department of Surgery, Ferguson Medical Group and Missouri Delta Community Hospital, Sikeston, Missouri

JOHN A. FABRE, M.D.

Fellow, Pediatric Ophthalmology, University of Iowa, Iowa City, Iowa

CHARLES F. FREY, M.D., F.A.C.S.

Professor and Vice Chairman, Department of Surgery, University of California, Davis, California; Chief, Surgical Service, Veterans Administration Hospital, Martinez, California

WESLEY FURSTE, B.A., M.D., F.A.C.S.

Clinical Professor of Surgery, College of Medicine, Ohio State University, Columbus, Ohio

GEORGE R. GAY, M.D.

Hilo Medical Group, Hilo, Hawaii; Formerly Director, Clinical Activities, Haight-Ashbury Free Medical Clinic, San Francisco, California

DAVID G. HALL III, M.D.

Professor and Chairman, Department of Obstetrics and Gynecology, University of Missouri Medical Center, Columbia, Missouri

†RUSSELL E. HANLON, M.D.

Formerly Assistant Professor of Obstetrics and Gynecology, University of Missouri School of Medicine, Columbia, Missouri

JOHN H. HENZEL, M.D.

Associate Professor of Surgery, University of Missouri School of Medicine, Columbia, Missouri

---

†Deceased.

v

WALTER FORD KEITZER, M.D.

Professor of Surgery, University of Texas Southwestern Medical School; Chief of Surgical Services, Veterans Administration Hospital, Dallas, Texas

JAMES M. LANDEEN, M.D.

Fellow, Division of Plastic and Reconstructive Surgery, Department of Surgery, University of Florida, Gainesville, Florida

ALBERT B. LOWENFELS, M.D.

Associate Professor of Surgery, New York Medical College; Associate Director of Surgery, Westchester County Medical Center, Valhalla, New York

RICHARD H. MARTIN, M.D.

Professor of Medicine; Director, Division of Cardiology, University of Missouri School of Medicine, Columbia, Missouri

FRANKLIN L. MITCHELL, B.S., M.D., F.A.C.S.

Professor of Surgery; Director, Emergency Medical Services, University of Missouri School of Medicine, Columbia, Missouri

WALTER KIRT NICHOLS, M.D.

Assistant Professor of Surgery, University of Missouri School of Medicine, Columbia, Missouri

GEORGIA B. NOLPH, M.D.

Associate Professor of Family and Community Medicine, University of Missouri School of Medicine, Columbia, Missouri

GILBERT J. ROSS, Jr., M.D., F.A.C.S.

Professor and Chief of Urology, University of Missouri School of Medicine, Columbia, Missouri

HENRY M. PARRISH, M.D., Dr.P.H., F.A.C.P.

Ocala, Florida; Formerly Vice President of Health Affairs and Professor of Community Medicine, University of South Dakota, Vermillion, South Dakota

HUGH E. STEPHENSON, Jr., A.B., B.S., M.D., F.A.C.S.

Professor and Chief, Division of General Surgery, University of Missouri School of Medicine, Columbia, Missouri

†HUGH E. STEPHENSON, Sr., D.D.S.

Columbia, Missouri

BOYD E. TERRY, M.D., F.A.C.S.

Associate Professor of Surgery and Director, The George W. Peakton Memorial Burn Center, University of Missouri School of Medicine, Columbia, Missouri

GERARD J. VAN LEEUWEN, M.D.

Associate Medical Director, Missouri Division of Health, Jefferson City, Missouri

FRED A. WAPPEL, A.B., Trainer Certified

Athletic Trainer, Intercollegiate Athletics; Instructor in Physical Education, University of Missouri, Columbia, Missouri

JAMES M. A. WEISS, M.D., M.P.H., F.A.C.P.

Professor and Chairman, Department of Psychiatry, University of Missouri School of Medicine, Columbia, Missouri

EARL J. WIPFLER, Jr., B.S., M.D., F.A.C.S.

General Surgery, St. Charles, Missouri

With the editorial assistance of

ROBERT S. KIMPTON, A.B., B.S., M.Ed.

Journalistic Consultant, Columbia, Missouri

---

†Deceased.

TO

Students whose interest and enthusiasm
in this subject during the past 25 years have
stimulated the writing of this book.

Foreword

Change seems to be characteristic of the twentieth century. It may well be that people in each period have similar beliefs but historically we seem to have more direct evidence of change, such as the technological burst; the swing to urban living; the communications revolution as seen in telephone, radio, television, and satellite; transportation by railroad, motor car, airplane, and rocket. Congestion, speed, and use of mechanical devices have resulted in increased illness and injury.

The near defeat of contagion by scientific public health methods has also brought into prominence the increasing losses from stress and injury. The public has been taught to believe that good health is their right and they have concurred enthusiastically with the medical tenet that immediate care is a part of good treatment. Has the medical profession responded adequately?

Specialization, even in ever narrowing fields, has largely replaced general practice. The hospital, formerly a place to go to die, has become the primary physician to the majority in large cities. Outside of regular office hours the physician is not generally available in his office and does not make house calls. The disposition of the immediate care of the acutely ill and injured thereby becomes an unsettled problem.

While this load grows constantly, the medical profession, at least until quite recently, has shown little interest in the field. For more than 60 years the American Red Cross has been engaged in teaching first aid to laymen. Except in wartime this has rarely been widely popular. The Boy Scouts, Camp Fire Girls, Bureau of Mines, and public schools have also worked on this to a limited extent. Forty years ago an occasional medical school in this country and Canada conducted such a course for the first-year medical student. It seemed only fair, when he went home for his first Christmas vacation and his acquaintances called him "Doc," that he might know as much about first aid as a well-trained Boy Scout.

Dr. Stephenson recognized the need for such a course nearly 20 years ago and started one as an optional elective, which soon involved nearly 100% of the class. This has had sluggish adoption by medical schools in general. Dr. Stephenson circulated two medical school questionnaires on the subject and the majority of schools now seem to pay some attention to immediate care.

The circulation of these questionnaires was a major influence in adoption of such courses. Also the wide recommendation of mouth-to-mouth artificial respiration and, beginning in 1960, the acceptance of external cardiac compression brought home forcibly the great number of unnecessary deaths occurring each year from heart attacks and motor vehicle accidents because of lack of knowledge and training on the part of physicians and laymen in their use. In the past 10 years the brush fire of interest in immediate care has become a conflagration extending not only to doctors, but to nurses, ambulance personnel, and police and fire departments.

I have been interested in the field since World War I. To my knowledge no book covering immediate care has been written previously for the medical student. Dr. Stephenson has had this in mind for a number of years. It has come to fruition admirably as a result of his long period of dedicated teaching of this subject. He has gathered contributors who cover their subjects in similar fashion. His editing has succeeded in allowing few repetitions and making the book read like the composition of a single author. The coverage is broad and is up to the minute.

Quite uniformly, the text is limited to *immediate* care; otherwise the size of the book would have been impractical. Into whatever specialty the medical student enters, this material is basic to knowledge of his immediate care of a patient. He will put it to good use subconsciously when he may not even appreciate that he is doing so. This includes those who enter a life of teaching and research.

We are approaching the point where the medical profession will be adequately prepared to respond to the changes required in the quality of immediate care. This volume goes far toward filling the need of the medical and paramedical professions for learning and having ready reference assistance in the problems of immediate care.

Robert H. Kennedy, M.D., F.A.C.S.
1974

Preface to second edition

This new edition of *Immediate Care of the Acutely Ill and Injured,* which is an effort to update previous material as well as to include new chapters on subject matter not previously discussed, has been prepared because of the excellent response of the readers to the first edition.

Although the intent of the first edition was to present a book that could be used by students in the early part of the medical school curriculum, it soon became apparent that the book was receiving considerable attention from emergency medical training programs, nurses, and others. Nevertheless, this second edition is being written with the hope that the medical school curriculum will increase emphasis on preparing the medical student to approach a wide variety of medical emergencies with an acceptable pathophysiologic understanding of the problems at hand.

There are numerous texts and much available material for those interested in the definitive care of medical emergencies utilizing the sophistication of the intensive care unit and the operating room after the victim has reached the hospital. This little book, however, is concerned basically with what one should try to accomplish during the first few minutes after an emergency medical problem develops. Often it is in these moments of golden opportunity that the prognosis is determined.

At the end of many of the chapters readers will find questions that they should be able to answer that will serve to provide emphasis for areas of particular importance. In some instances key sources are suggested for additional reading.

The index is considerably more detailed than is often the case in this type of book, but this is done to provide the reader with more readily accessible information.

As always, the editor and publishers are appreciative of any criticisms or suggestions that the reader might have and welcome comments that may be applicable to this or future revisions.

Hugh E. Stephenson, Jr.

Preface to first edition

This book provides a "why and how" for immediate care and management of acutely ill and injured persons by utilizing a rational approach based on anatomic and physiologic considerations. Despite adequate definitive care in hospitals and clinics, the eventual outcome of a medical emergency is frequently determined by the care rendered immediately following the initial insult to the patient. The quality of immediate care is a major determinant of the degree of permanent disability.

The major impetus for this book stems from a belief in the increasing urgency to provide students with formal instruction in the pathophysiology and management of one of the major health problems of our time. The need for adequate emergency care is obvious when we consider that the principal cause of death until age 39 in the United States is trauma. For the population as a whole, accidents rank behind only cardiovascular disease and cancer as a leading cause of death. During the past decade 450,000 persons have died from accidents on our highways.

Of even greater impact, however, is the realization that the principal health problem is the high incidence of sudden cardiac death occurring outside of the hospital. It is estimated that as many as 365,000 such deaths occur each year in the United States. It is no longer debatable that large numbers of these victims, mostly with malignant cardiac arrhythmias, can be saved.

How effectively are students being trained for the delivery of emergency care efforts? In an effort to determine curriculum commitments by the medical schools to the teaching of emergency care for the acutely ill and injured, I conducted two national surveys at 5-year intervals in my role as State Trauma Chairman of the American College of Surgeons Trauma Committee. It seems quite apparent that medical school curriculum committees, mindful of or committed to this current trend, are accelerating efforts to revise and reshape curriculum content to include formalized instruction in the management of emergency care, including that of the trauma victim. Slightly more than half of all of the medical schools now provide such formal instruction. Whereas the teaching of emergency medical care of the acutely ill and injured patient has too often in the past been relegated to an insignificant role in the undergraduate medical curriculum, there now appears to be a trend toward a sophisticated and organized presentation to the student.

With regard specifically to the matter of trauma, the spectrum of instruction is becoming increasingly broad to provide the necessary exposure to the ecologic patterns of injury, to the pathogenesis of injury, and to the psychologic and economic ramifications of injury. The Trauma Committee has expressed strong recommendations for an increased tempo of instruction in the care of the injured patient as an integral part of the medical curriculum. From their survey it is apparent that a wide variety of approaches is currently in use. These vary from elective courses for freshman and sophomore students in emergency care to specific surgical and medical clerkship periods devoted to the subject. Student assignment to the emergency unit of the hospital is commonly employed. The potential benefits of effectively administered emergency care are greater than at any previous time. It is high time that curriculum priorities recognize this potential.

Nurses and paramedical personnel also have a growing role in the delivery of immediate care. The emergency room personnel, perhaps more than any others, must work well as a team. So it is hoped, and intended, that this book will be used by these people as well as by medical students.

In an effort not to overlap with other areas of the medical curriculum, we have avoided inclusion of material concerning definitive care beyond the immediate or emergency stage or concerning emergencies of a medical and surgical nature occurring primarily within the hospital.

Medical students interested in the subject of immediate care of the acutely ill and injured have been the major stimulus to the writing of this book and to them I am grateful. Over a period of 20 years the subject has been presented to the freshmen or sophomore class, either as an elective or required course. Several medical students at the University of Missouri have served as journalistic consultants during the writing of the book, and I am indebted to them for their help. They were Glenn H. Bock, Eric Jan Carlson, Donald Clayton Patterson, Linda Pauline Boch, John W. Williams, Jr., John Dale Yeast, Donna Conard, Sanford J. Greenberg, David G. Hof, Martha J. Holt, John J. Krautman, and James E. Remkus.

Several years of contact with Dr. Robert H. Kennedy while at Bellevue and University Hospital in New York City served as an initial stimulus to my interest in this field. Dr. Kennedy has been a source of continued personal encouragement and enthusiastic support in efforts to initiate or accentuate the teaching of emergency care in the medical schools of the United States. Like so many others whom he has influenced, I, too, am grateful. His legacy to the Trauma Committee of the American College of Surgeons can hardly be fully appreciated. Dr. Wilbur P. McDonald, as Regional Chairman of the Trauma Committee, has always strongly supported our efforts on trauma here at the University of Missouri.

Through a long gestational period this book has changed form as new trends and developments emerged in emergency medical care. I am grateful to the contributors, whose efforts have been outstanding. Mr. Robert S. Kimpton has struggled with the manuscript and its many revisions. His suggestions and contributions to the book over a period of 10 years are greatly appreciated. The friendly prodding and continued assistance of my secretary, Miss Ruth McCown, who finally brought the book to fruition, are appreciated.

A special thanks should go to the faculty members of the medical schools of this country and Canada who kindly cooperated in both of our surveys of the teaching of emergency care in the medical schools. Drs. Oscar P. Hampton, Jr., Curtis P. Artz, J. Cuthbert Owens, and a host of others on the Trauma Committee of the American College of Surgeons have given their support and encouragement. These studies added much insight into the various approaches being used and the subject matter being presented.

Finally, I wish to thank my wife, Sally, as well as Ted and Ann, for their patience, tolerance, and sharing of many weekends and evenings with this effort.

Hugh E. Stephenson, Jr.

Contents

PART FOUR

Cardiorespiratory emergencies

PART FIVE

Emergencies involving environmental excess

PART SIX

Emergencies involving pharmacologic excesses

PART SEVEN

Emergencies resulting from physical trauma

PART EIGHT

Special considerations

PART NINE

Psychiatric emergencies

IMMEDIATE care of the acutely ill and injured

INTRODUCTION

Accidents and emergency medical services

CHARLES F. FREY

Accidents are the fourth leading cause of death in the United States, after heart disease, cancer, and stroke. Because of the magnitude of the problem, one would think that accidents would deserve attention by the public and by the medical profession. Yet accidents have not been called the neglected disease of modern society by the National Research Council without reason.

Why do government and the private sector give millions of dollars for medical research and clinical care for the study of diseases much less lethal or disabling and affecting far fewer people than do motor vehicle accidents alone? Why are funds available for care of patients who are often old and who are victims of chronic, malignant, and often incurable diseases. Why in the same institution is there not an intensive care or shock unit for victims of trauma, for patients who are usually young, with their future still before them? In contrast to many diseases on which funds are lavished, the etiology of accidents, methods for prevention, and technology to improve the treatment of the injured and effect a reduction in mortality are all known and available. Why is it that an occasional homicide arouses a community to a frenzy? Newspaper and television editorials are felt necessary, police leaves are canceled, and the public is aroused. On the other hand, deaths from motor vehicle accidents are most likely to occur among young people and are far more frequent than homicides, yet they evoke no more than a mention from the newspapers, are seldom mentioned on television, and stir no break in routine for the police. Apparently, the manner in which one is killed is crucially important to arousing the sensibilities of vocal, seemingly pavlovian-reflexed groups in our society.

Perhaps some cultural anthropologist from another planet might have the objectivity to understand why customs and taboos inhibit members of our society from examining the problem of accidents so that measures can be taken to protect society from the accident epidemic.

Unfortunately, medical school curriculum planners are subject to the same taboos, fads, and foibles as the remainder of society. For the most part they have chosen not to include the study of accidents in their curricula, although in the United

1

States in 1969 accidents claimed 115,000 lives, disabled 11 million persons, were the leading cause of death between ages 1 and 39, cost the nation $22 billion, and took up 22 million bed days a year, or 12% of the total general hospital space. Past neglect of the accident problem by medical school curriculum planners might be understandable if the etiology of the disease were unknown or if treatment were impossible, but this is not the case.

There are many paradoxes and inconsistencies in the public attitude toward accidents and their sequelae. Perhaps it is understandable that the public believes accidents to be "inevitable" or to result from carelessness that is an "inevitable trait of human nature." Then why does the public, having seemingly accepted the "inevitability of accidents," not also accept the need and responsibility for good emergency medical services to care for the accident victim? Why do they not accept the definition of emergency medical services as including the care the patient receives at the scene of the accident and in transit to the hospital, as well as the care received after hospital arrival? Unfortunately, the public has accepted no more responsibility for emergency medical services than it has for accident prevention. Both the medical community and the public would be shocked if a child in the community died from diphtheria or smallpox. Because of the availability of immunization, these diseases are preventable. Yet it is estimated that over half the deaths resulting from motor vehicle accidents can be preventable if shoulder and lap belts are always worn. Perhaps the public feels that those careless enough to cause accidents are not deserving of good emergency medical service. However, this hardly seems a satisfactory solution for those innocent victims of someone else's carelessness.

There is now much talk about the need to reestablish the priorities of society. Medical school curricula are no exception. Subjects and diseases to be included in the curriculum should be reexamined. How can the medical schools any longer ignore accidents, a disease that is the fourth most common cause of death and the leading cause of death between ages 1 and 37 years in the United States? The medical schools must help future physicians and health care leaders understand the causes and prognosis of the accident epidemic, not just the treatment of specific injuries. Let us then look at the major causes of accident epidemic.

During the 5-year period from 1964 through 1968, in spite of increases in population, there was little change in the total number of deaths from work or home accidents.

	Work	Home
1964	14,200	28,000
1968	14,300	28,500

However, in spite of efforts by motor companies, road designers, and law enforcement agencies to prevent accidents and reduce injury occurring during accidents, the deaths from motor vehicle accidents rose from 47,700 to 1965 to 56,600 in 1972 in the United States. It now seems probable that death and injury from motor vehicle accidents will continue to be an appreciable problem for some time.

Therefore the medical profession must prepare itself and the public to treat, rehabilitate, and return to society large numbers of injured patients. To meet this responsibility the medical profession must actively participate in and initiate training programs for emergency medical technicians, establish ordinances, support efforts for a communications network between hospital and ambulance, and see that hospital emergency departments are adequately staffed and equipped to meet the needs of acutely ill and injured individuals. The medical profession, through advance planning on an areawide basis, must make provisions so that the injured patient can always be delivered to an emergency department equipped to cope with his injuries.

For the physician to fulfill these responsibilities, he will have to step outside the ivory tower of his hospital to deal with police, firemen, ambulance drivers, hospital administrators, public health officials, businessmen, labor unions, and politicians in his community. Establishment of emergency services health councils with wide representation in the community is one technique physicians may employ to influence community action to improve emergency medical services. If the medical profession does not provide leadership in the effort to improve emergency medical service, it is my conviction that the government, because of the seriousness of the problem, may eventually tell the medical profession what it must do.

The medical profession needs to arouse the social conscience of medical school curriculum planners to the necessity of educating medical students about the accident epidemic. The accident problem should be presented to the students in a wide, overall view that includes its etiology in terms of human factors and road or vehicle design, the pattern of injury, the physiologic and metabolic responses of the body and its tissues to injury, heart-lung resuscitation, and the physical and emotional reactions of the patient and his family to injury and economic loss.

It is the medical schools' duty to help medical students recognize their responsibility for improving emergency medical services in the local community, in the state, and in the nation. It is also the medical schools' responsibility to help the medical student realize that implementation of improved emergency medical service requires him to step outside the hospital to communicate and work with nonmedical groups and politicians within his community. Accidents are more than just another disease; they are an epidemic.

●   ●   ●

Since this chapter appeared in the first edition of this text in 1974, there has been a rapid evolution in the care available to the acutely ill and injured in the United States.

PREHOSPITAL

Most improvements in emergency medical care have occurred in the prehospital phase of emergency medical services whose components consist of *access* to the emergency medical service ambulance, hospital and central dispatch, *training* of emergency medical technicians and paramedics, and *ambulances* designed and equipped to standards recommended by the American College of Surgeons.

HOSPITAL

The hospital phase includes the care the patient receives after hospital arrival. This care involves the staffing and equipment available in the emergency department and the hospital.

The emergency department is the first stop in hospital care. It is a sorting area or center for triage activity where patients requiring specialized services are sent as rapidly as possible from the emergency department to the intensive care unit, the burn center, the coronary care unit, or the operating room. It may be a surprise to some medical students and house officers that the time spent in evaluating and preparing an injured patient after hospital arrival for emergency surgery far exceeds by three or four times the average interval between accident and pickup and delivery to the hospital in most suburban and urban communities. Not all hospitals have the staff, particularly those with special skills for caring for the injured, that is, general, vascular, thoracic, and orthopedic surgeons and neurosurgeons. Not all hospitals can afford the expense of keeping x-ray and blood bank technicians, operating room staff, and physicians available in the hospital 24 hours a day including weekends. An enormous amount of preplanning is required to integrate and coordinate the activities of many people within the hospital to provide expeditious care for the injured. Because each injured patient's problem is different and has different priorities, only a surgeon experienced in trauma care has the judgment and expertise to treat the severely injured patient. Few hospitals have done the planning, have the specialty physicians on staff, or keep an experienced trauma surgeon and operating room team available in the hospital at all hours to cope with the severely injured patient. Hospital care of the injured patient requires more than a well-equipped and staffed emergency department.

COORDINATION OF PREHOSPITAL AND HOSPITAL COMPONENTS

To coordinate and integrate the prehospital and hospital components of emergency medical services into an operational system requires regional planning and funding. Those regions (defined by geographic and political jurisdictions) that have progressed most rapidly in developing and funding emergency medical care systems have had input and impetus for improved emergency care provided by energetic, concerned individuals and professional organizations. These organizations include the Committee on Trauma of the American College of Surgeons, the University Association for Emergency Medical Services, the American College of Emergency Physicians, the Emergency Department Nurses' Association, and the American Academy of Orthopaedic Surgeons among others.

PROCESS OF DEVELOPING EMERGENCY MEDICAL CARE SYSTEMS

Emergency medical services (EMS) have undergone a very rapid evolution, and like any other sudden evolution there is a predictable pattern of events. First, there are the crusaders and consciousness raisers who make people aware of the problem. Then there are the organizers and fund raisers who develop and integrate systems to solve the problem; then there is the institutionalization of these new concepts in some governmental bureaucracy, such as the health department.

Emergency medical service systems in the United States have not progressed in all regions at the same rate. When the 1974 edition of *Immediate Care of the Acutely Ill and Injured* was being written, this chapter exhorted medical and lay personnel to support the development of emergency medical care systems to save the lives of those dying unnecessarily from accidents and acute illness. At that time there were virtually no emergency medical care systems in existence. Today many emergency medical care systems have been developed, covering perhaps two thirds of the land area and population of the United States. The regions still lacking an emergency medical care system still need the crusaders to exhort the public and community leaders to improve emergency medical care. Therefore the original text has been presented as in the first edition not only because the deficiencies in emergency medical care it decries still exist in many areas of the country but also the perspective it represents serves as a benchmark to measure and marvel at the rapid progress that has occurred in two thirds of the United States during the last 5 years.

The crusaders and missionaries in emergency medical services performed a great service in defining the deficiencies and needs of emergency medical services and creating the dynamics that made change possible.

In regions in which the emergency medical services message has been heard and emergency medical services systems have been planned, new types of problems require different personnel. Organizers, fund raisers, planners and technical experts are needed to make the system operational. While further progress and refinements are needed in most regions that have implemented emergency medical services systems, the improvements needed are often of a technical nature and are not always solved by public pressure and appeals to community leaders.

THE GOVERNMENT AND EMERGENCY MEDICAL SERVICES

A whole new system of planning councils and advisory bodies to state governors and comprehensive A and B planning agencies evolved during the early 1970's. A new bureaucracy was created to administer the new emergency medical care system. Through 1975 the emergency medical services development in most states consisted of a statewide planning effort through a subcommittee or task force of the comprehensive health planning agency or the governor's council on health and medical affairs. Implementation of statewide planning was usually delegated to an emergency medical service subdivision of the state health department. Activities likely to be made the responsibility of the emergency medical service division of the health department were licensing of ambulances, certification of emergency medical technicians, and publication of guidelines for regional emergency medical service systems (including definition of the emergency medical service regions within the state and establishment of guidelines for the regions). This statewide planning prevented duplication and overlapping of services and communications between regions.

Since 1975 regional planning and implementation of emergency medical services have become the responsibility of the newly formed health services agencies which have supplanted the comprehensive health care agencies and regional medical plans. The emergency medical service councils of the health services agencies require that 51% of their membership be consumers and 49% be producers. The definitions of "producer" and "consumer" may sometimes seem questionable to those uninitiated in bureaucratic thinking. However, the important net effect of these regulations regarding membership on the council is to delete the much-needed medical and technical expertise important to the operation of an emergency system whose emphasis is on medical services. Often on a 12- or 21-member council, there may be no more than one or two physicians. Therefore some of the individuals and professional organizations who exhorted, organized, planned, and helped obtain funding to improve emergency medical services are being excluded from any meaningful role in these new regional and state emergency medical service systems.

Exclusion of individuals or groups knowledgeable in emergency medical services systems development in the course of institutionalizing and bureaucratizing emergency medical services should be a cause for concern. The problems of developing emergency medical services are sufficiently large and diverse to require the talents of all interested and concerned individuals and groups. The interest and expertise of these groups and individuals in improving emergency medical services should be welcomed and utilized by the public agencies having operational control of emergency medical services.

SCOPE OF THE ACCIDENT PROBLEM

In one of the great ironies of our time some good came from the oil crisis in 1973. We learned that speed does kill. Consequent to the reduction in speed limits the accident toll was reduced in subsequent years from the high levels of 1972. During the same years the incidence of home and industrial accidents remained stable. However, the mortality and morbidity associated with motor vehicle accidents and other accidents are still excessive even though the epidemic has abated. In 1975, 103,320 people died from accidents, 45,060 from motor vehicle accidents. Accidents are still enormously wasteful of our resources in the United States. The accident problem should be viewed as a public health responsibility, and efforts to control accidents should be mounted on two fronts: One effort has been directed at accident prevention and another at reducing the extent of injuries and the mortality of those injured. These efforts are supported by the American Trauma Society.

FUNDING ACCIDENT PREVENTION
AND EMERGENCY MEDICAL SERVICE SYSTEM
COMPONENTS

The American Trauma Society, composed of both lay and professional leaders, is a rapidly growing organization dedicated to developing the financial support and foundation necessary to provide programs in public education and research designed to reduce the morbidity and mortality from injuries and accidents. The development of this society is patterned after the financially successful American Heart Association.

State and local emergency medical service programs designed to improve the care of the injured after an accident were stimulated at the national level through funding based on Standard 11 of the Highway Safety Act of 1968. These Department of Transportation funds were distributed at state levels through the governors' representatives. The Emergency Medical Services Act passed in 1973 as PL 93154, involved the Department of Health, Education, and Welfare in emergency medical services. This new act created the Emergency Medical Services Program through the Department of Health, Education, and Welfare that was funded for $26,600,000 during 1974. This program has been ably administered by Dr. David Boyd, one of the pioneers of the Illinois statewide emergency medical service program. Dr. Boyd's department provided funding for planning, implementing, or expanding regional and state emergency medical services systems.

In 1972, The Robert Wood Johnson Foundation, in an effort to improve emergency medical services, solicited grant proposals for emergency medical services communication systems. These grants were to be awarded only to those regions demonstrating evidence of planning a complete emergency medical service system. This program stimulated tremendous activity at the regional and state levels in the planning of emergency medical care systems. Proposals were received from regions that covered approximately half of the population and geographic area of the United States. Forty-four grants totaling $15,000,000 were awarded in 1973. No single grant effort has done more to stimulate improvements in emergency health services and regional planning than this act by the Robert Wood Johnson Foundation.

Emergency medical care systems are for both the acutely ill and injured. Conceptual changes about ways to improve the organization of emergency medical service systems have also occurred during the last 5 years. Initially, planning and funding for emergency medical service systems separated the care of the acutely ill patient from the care of the injured patient. Planners now recognize that the best system of emergency medical care is a totally integrated service that simultaneously provides life support for victims of both accidents and disease. The emergency medical care system is composed of a number of clearly defined components: communication, training, transportation, hospitals, and regional planning. Within the last 5 years the components of the emergency medical service system have been developed with remarkable rapidity.

COMMUNICATIONS

Emergency medical service communications, which include the elements of central dispatch of ambulances, linkage of ambulances to hospitals, and linkage of hospitals to hospitals, has proceeded at an astounding pace. The development of telemetry now makes it possible for physicians working in the emergency department to communicate with and to assist the emergency medical technician in the diagnosis and treatment of disease or injury at the scene of the accident or illness.

TRAINING

Training programs for emergency medical technicians have been improved and are now widely available, thanks to the volunteer efforts of many dedicated physicians. The courses have been standardized and training aids developed, no mean feat in the short time of 5 years. The Dunlop Emergency Medical Technician Course— Basic is now available for training ambulance personnel. The course consists of 81 hours of instruction, 10 of which are in the hospital. More recently, the emergency medical technician paramedic course has been implemented. It consists of 240 hours of instruction qualifying the individuals to perform such acts as endotracheal intubation, intravenous fluid therapy, and cardiac monitoring and defibrillation. Licensure programs for emergency medical technicians now exist in many states. Also, a national registry has been developed for emergency medical technicians that should aid in the career development of these new professionals.

TRANSPORTATION: STANDARDIZATION OF EQUIPMENT

Licensing programs for ambulances and their equipment are now a part of many state programs in emergency medical services.

HOSPITALS

While the prehospital phase of emergency medical care has improved markedly in the last 5 years, there has been no corresponding improvement in the hospital phase of care. In 1977 four reports from different urban and rural areas showed that many patients are continuing to die unnecessarily from inadequate, poorly planned hospital care after reaching a hospital alive. While improved training of the emergency department physician in the care of the trauma patient is surely needed, much of the difficulty arises from patients being delivered to the nearest hospital rather than to a hospital capable of caring for their injuries. Categorization of a hospital's ability to provide care for victims of burns, perinatal illness, spinal cord injury, cardiac conditions, and trauma is a necessary step in the regionalization of emergency medical care. Categorization permits regional emergency medical service planners to match patient needs with hospital resources so that the victim of injury or illness can be delivered to a hospital staffed and equipped to take care of his needs. Categorization and regionalization of emergency medical care in urban and suburban areas has great appeal to emergency medical service planners as duplication of costly facilities and staffing can be avoided while at the same time patient care is improved.

Categorization and regionalization of care have been well accepted for burn, perinatal, and spinal cord injury patients, as well as the patient with acute psychiatric illness. These patients all require care that is costly to the hospital and onerous to most physicians.

However, categorization of the injured patient has not been popular with many hospital administrators and physicians. They are concerned that categorization may be used to divert the injured patients from their hospital with a resultant decline in bed census and revenue. Much of this concern is unwarranted as only the most severely injured patients require specialized care and this concept would probably not affect the diversion of more than 5% of the victims of trauma. There is a tremendous need for leadership, innovation, tact, and diplomacy to develop alternative trade-offs for those hospitals that will be bypassed by the trauma patient to compensate them for any loss of patients. Such trade-offs might include reciprocal transfer of obstetric and gynecologic facilities or evening and weekend walk-in clinics.

The care provided in emergency departments in the United States has markedly improved in the last 5 years because of the presence of skilled professional staffs working full time in the emergency departments. The explosively rapid development of this new career and professional discipline, a remarkable phenomenon in itself, is a reflection of the tremendous resourcefulness and flexibility of our voluntary medical care system to meet new needs without governmental edicts. There are now approximately 5,000 full-time emergency department physicians and 15,000 part-time emergency department physicians in the United States.

TRAINING AND EDUCATION OF PERSONNEL

Many of the developments and improvements in the areas of training, transportation, and communication in components of the emergency medical care system have been facilitated by the publication of curricular standards and guidelines, standard texts, and visual aids. Organizations that have assisted in the development of standards, guidelines, and visual aids include the American College of Surgeons' Committee on Trauma, American Academy of Orthopaedic Surgeons, American Medical Association, American College of Emergency Physicians, University Association for Emergency Medical Services, as well as governmental agencies: the Department of Health, Education, and Welfare, the Department of Transportation, and the National Academy of Science Research Councils on Emergency Services.

Medical school curriculum planners have kept pace with development in emergency medical services in other areas. Required courses in emergency medical care systems are now available in two thirds of the medical schools in the United States. Additionally, there are now 34 residency training programs that train physicians to provide emergency medical care in the emergency department. Standards and curricula have been developed and published by the University Association for Emergency Medical Services and the American College of Emergency Physicians to train and to educate medical students and house officers in emergency department medicine.

To improve emergency medical services the medical student or physician must be willing to step outside the hospital and communicate and work with nonmedical groups and politicians within the community. Participation by medical students and house officers in Department of Health, Education, and Welfare and emergency medical service activities would, I believe, be welcomed. It would serve a most useful apprenticeship in preparing a medical student or a physician for a meaningful role in emergency medical services planning, funding, and implementation.

PART ONE

Diagnostic challenges

CHAPTER 1

Examination and evaluation

Initial evaluation is the crux of successful immediate care. One cannot too frequently ask, "How capable, reliable, knowledgeable, and observant are the initial evaluation efforts?" The first person who gives immediate aid to the acutely ill and injured victim obviously has a major responsibility. These initial efforts may not only be lifesaving but may well determine the degree and extent of any future disability.

Unlike the careful, methodic, and all-inclusive examination one would perform under well-controlled situations—for example, in the office or hospital examination room—the evaluation of the patient at the scene of an accident, in a near-drowning situation, or under other such chaotic conditions requires a much quicker appraisal of the nature of the victim's problem and, indeed, may be a most demanding situation even for the most experienced practitioner. Frequently, without any medical equipment and with an uncooperative or even a comatose patient, the physician may lack even the bare essentials desirable for the usual rendering of medical care. The medical history may be impossible to obtain. Any knowledge of previous illnesses or prior treatment may be lacking. The disruptive influence of a crowd or the sense of panic experienced by the patient or the family adds to the difficulties of making calm and objective decisions. Nevertheless, the need for lifesaving measures may be obvious.

Throughout the initial evaluation and establishment of immediate priorities of care one should display an attitude of confidence, reassurance, and optimism. Other individuals immediately available should be properly utilized to seek aid and to call for an ambulance, if available. Traffic may need to be controlled until the police arrive.

CARDIORESPIRATORY PRIORITIES

First attention is directed to the victim's cardiorespiratory system. Is the patient breathing? Is the airway open? Are palpable pulses present? Are the pupils dilated? The priority of maintaining adequate tissue perfusion to the vital organs of the body, most importantly the brain, tops the list. The usually emphasized "ABCD's" (airway, breathing, cardiac massage, and definitive therapy) of emergency care may vary somewhat in that external cardiac massage may need be the first in the order of activities, given almost simultaneously with artificial ventilation efforts. In an emergency situation one usually assumes an optimistic view as to the probability of successful cardiopulmonary resuscitation. Obvious exceptions exist and will be discussed in Chapter 12.

When the patient's pulse is still present but when he is in a comatose or uncon-scious state, one quickly makes a judgment regarding need for artificial ventilation. Are respiratory efforts labored? Is the patient cyanotic? Is there evidence of acute hypoxia, asphyxia, and cyanosis? Is obstruction of the airway by the patient's tongue, vomitus, or hemorrhage a possibility? Obviously, immediate measures are indicated to remove any upper airway obstruction and to keep the patient's head and neck in the proper position for maintaining an adequate airway. Regardless of the elected method of artificial ventilation, whether it be mouth-to-mouth, expired air, or bag-compression ventilation, delay cannot be tolerated.

The establishment of an adequate airway and the maintenance of artificial ventila-tion and assisted circulation by external cardiac compression are extremely basic to present-day immediate care needs and should be a part of the armamentarium of even the freshman medical student. These techniques are outlined in detail else-where in the book and are referred to throughout much of the text.

The presence of blood on the patient's body and clothing may present a dismaying sight. Control of hemorrhage and the prevention of exsanguination require prompt and decisive efforts. Clothing should be removed as needed to identify the area of hemorrhage. Most sources of external bleeding can be quickly controlled or stopped by direct application of pressure over the bleeding area; only infrequently will a tourniquet be required. The assessment of internal hemorrhage is, of course, much more difficult. Active intra-abdominal or intrathoracic bleeding represents one of the few indications for unusually rapid transportation to the hospital.

STATE OF CONSCIOUSNESS

One should make a quick assessment of the state of consciousness of the patient. Does the patient respond to stimuli? What is the response to verbal stimulation? If he is responsive to pain but not to verbal stimulation the patient is often regarded as being in a stupor. If the patient is unresponsive to both verbal and painful stimuli, then a status of coma is commonly designated. Not only is the immediate appraisal of the state of consciousness important, but one should also make frequent and serial notations because of their bearing on future diagnostic efforts when definitive care is reached. Similarly, one should note the patient's affect. Does it appear ap-propriate to the situation? Is the patient hallucinating and out of touch with reality?

IMPORTANCE OF PATIENT HISTORY

Concurrently with the examination and evaluation of the patient, a history of events leading to the emergency may be elicited from family, friends, or bystanders. When time is available one should make careful note of the circumstances surround-ing the event, since a definitive description of the emergency may be unavailable to physicians in the emergency room or hospital at a later date.

This importance of a precise, inclusive history should be obvious in such emer-gencies as poisoning, drug abuse, and animal bites, but at least an equal factual need is referred to throughout much of the text in situations in which this need may not be as readily apparent. For example, Dr. Adams in discussing treatment of hand injuries makes an excellent case for careful initial observation.

Some patients carry emergency medical tags signifying their predisposition to allergic reactions or such conditions as diabetes or the presence of a particular cardiac problem, including an implanted pacemaker.

MISTAKES OF COMMISSION

The person giving immediate care must be cognizant of not only the things that need doing but also of the many "don't's" of immediate care. The mistakes of commission as well as omission will be emphasized throughout the text. For example, serious harm may be done by the well-intentioned person providing emergency care at the time of a burn, an eye injury, or an injury to the hand. Unfortunately, improper emergency measures may seriously jeopardize future definitive care in such situations.

Although one is prone to focus attention on the obvious, one should conscientiously "touch all bases" so as not to overlook the less obvious but equally important conditions amenable to immediate care. While it may not be feasible to completely disrobe the patient to fully examine him, one can observe precautions. For example, as outlined in detail in Chapter 25, special care must be taken to avoid movement of the patient with back and neck injuries because he may possibly have associated damage to the spinal cord. Any areas of deformity, tenderness, or swelling should be particularly noted. Pressure over the scalp, rib cage, and cervical spine is important, as is pressure over the anterior superior iliac spine and pubic symphysis. As discussed in Chapter 29, one needs to immediately tamponade an open chest wound. One should pay particular attention to the highly important principle of immediate and proper splinting of fractures, which has been properly discussed by Dr. Conrad (Chapter 24). Open wounds should be protected and covered with sterile dressings prior to transportation of the patient to the hospital.

Once again, it should be emphasized how important comparative observations can be relative to the patient's vital signs. For example, once the patient arrives in the emergency room it is significant to note whether there has been a recent increase in the pulse rate, whether the skin has become cool and clammy, and if the patient's alertness has decreased.

One's ability to examine and evaluate the patient who requires immediate care is largely dependent on awareness of the many pathophysiologic changes encountered in emergency care of patients. Many portions of this book are devoted to a logical extension of this chapter as it involves specific emergency type problems largely outside the hospital.

QUESTIONS

1. Explain what is meant by "mistakes of commission" in giving immediate care.
2. "How much time shall we waste?" in writing down notes about the patient history in a true emergency situation?
3. Discuss the criteria for deciding the need for artificial ventilation in the comatose or unconscious patient.
4. What is the importance of frequent and serial notations of the patient's state of consciousness?
5. How important is initial evaluation in the total emergency care picture?

CHAPTER 2

The unconscious patient

It is not surprising that medical students react with considerable interest to a discussion of the unconscious patient. Not only does the evaluation of the unconscious patient present an unusual challenge in the delegating of the immediate priorities but also finding a denouement of the etiologic possibilities brings forth the best of diagnostic acumen.

Often without any history relating to the patient, one is required to make the best possible use of one's observatory capacities, including the sense of smell. It is in the management of the undiagnosed, unconscious patient that the real "medical detective" emerges. Comatose patients are found in all types of situations with innumerable unknowns. The duration of their unconscious state may be unknown. They are found by complete strangers, police, or individuals with only fragmentary knowledge of the patient. Positive revealing physical signs may be virtually absent or misleading.

Unfortunately medical personnel are seldom schooled in the diagnosis and management of the unconscious patient. It is not surprising that each year personnel in emergency rooms inadvertently release alcoholics who die a few hours later on the streets or in jail from an undiagnosed head injury. Unfortunately too many unconscious patients are initially given poor or inadequate treatment by bystanders, ambulance attendants, or emergency-room personnel. The unconscious patient may be shaken, doused with cold water, given smelling salts, or have various liquids including alcohol poured into his mouth. In the emergency room, further examination of the patient by ill-advised flexion or positioning of the head and neck may convert a simple cervical fracture into one associated with quadriplegia.

A consideration of the unconscious patient does excite one's attention as much as or more than any other topic in the area of immediate care and first aid. When suddenly faced with an unconscious patient, how does one proceed, particularly in view of the multitude of possibilities as to the etiology of the unconsciousness?

In lectures I usually select a patient who, along with some special prompting, may provide an ideal "unconscious patient." One of the best such "patients" was a 65-year-old physician who had had a bilateral below-knee amputation for vascular insufficiency. I properly "prepared" the patient with intravenous administration of a vasopressor, placing clotted blood in the external auditory canal, bandaging a simulated laceration of the scalp, dilating the pupils with 10% phenylephrine (Neo-Synephrine), and adding a strong odor of ethyl alcohol. One of the members of the class was instructed to go to the emergency room and help a resident bring up the "victim" who had just been admitted to the emergency room. On arrival in the classroom the patient's controlled respirations were of a Cheyne-Stokes nature, and he could barely be aroused. The patient had an emergency medical identification tag around his neck indicating that he was a diabetic.

At this point one of the members of the class volunteered to examine the patient and, with the help of the rest of the class, explored the whole range of possible explanations of unconsciousness. During one lecture on the unconscious patient, the doctor mentioned was brought in on a stretcher with a prosthesis on one leg and the other leg stump exposed. It was a source of much good-natured amusement to the class when one of their number affirmed that there were good peripheral pulses over the prosthesis!

On one occasion, a student became quite agitated, believing that the patient's condition was rapidly deteriorating in the classroom. In addition, several students have admitted to being somewhat irritated that such a severely ill patient should be used for teaching purposes in the classroom.

This type of demonstration provides an excellent opportunity to show the uninitiated medical student the importance of careful observation simply by using one's sense of sight, touch, hearing, and even smell.

INITIAL PRIORITIES

Keeping in mind the don't's of caring for the unconscious patient, one should turn first to the problem usually requiring immediate attention: the matter of the airway and adequate ventilation. Although this aspect is covered in detail in Chapters 10 and 12, emphasis is again given to the need to maintain an open airway—whether this requires manual maintenance of an extended head in relationship to the neck, an oral airway, an endotracheal airway, or rarely a tracheostomy. Oral-pharyngeal suctioning may be urgently required. Whenever doubt exists about the adequacy of ventilation, mouth-to-mouth breathing should be instituted.

Obvious hemorrhage should be controlled by the means outlined in Chapter 34.

If clinical features of shock are evident—such as a faint thready pulse, cool moist skin, and hypotension—initial efforts should be directed toward improved tissue perfusion. After an intravenous route is established, 5% dextrose and water to which 10 mg of phenylephrine (Neo-Synephrine) has been added can be used to provide mild support in raising the level of blood pressure.

RESPIRATION

Once the initial priorities have been met, attention is turned to a more thorough examination to accurately pinpoint the reason for unconsciousness. The patient must be disrobed. The respiratory excursions are observed. Are they thoracic or abdominal in origin? Do the ala nasi move excessively? Are accessory muscles of respiration in play? How regular are the excursions?

There is often significance in noting the various types of respiration. For example, Cheyne-Stokes respirations are deep and somewhat labored excursions alternating with periods of absent respiration (apnea). Whereas Cheyne-Stokes respirations often indicate a poor prognosis such as is associated with severe head injuries or brain damage, this is not always true.

Patients in diabetic coma may have respiratory activity increased in both depth and rate. Although many laboratory procedures require sophisticated techniques and a certain amount of time, one can usually get an immediate urinalysis, which may confirm a diagnosis of diabetic acidosis. A hemoglobin determination and white cell count can give almost immediate worthwhile information.

The tendency of one cheek to puff out each time the patient exhales is indicative of partial facial paralysis.

Sighing respirations may make one suspect "unconsciousness" of a psychosomatic nature. Respirations are generally slow in the uremic patient, the diabetic individual, the patient with morphine intoxication, the acute alcoholic individual, and the patient with intracranial bleeding.

Are there *breath odors* that should be noted? Perhaps the odor of alcohol is the most frequently encountered, but again caution is urged lest the observation serve as a red herring. Diabetic acidosis may produce a fruity odor such as from overripe apples. The foul, uriniferous odor of uremia may be present, in which instance the patient may also have "uremic frost" about the upper lip and face. Some instances of poisoning are associated with characteristic odors, for example, the garlicky odor of phosphorus poisoning. If one knows the odor of bitter almonds or peach kernels, one may recognize prussic acid (hydrocyanic acid) poisoning.

Listen. In addition to the stertorous stridor of respirations, less obvious auditory clues may be present. With the stethoscope one should carefully auscultate the heart, noting any abnormalities in rate or rhythm. Occasionally a markedly slow heartbeat may lead one to suspect digitalis intoxication, and, of course, syncope resulting from heart block may be detected. The heart may be beating so fast that output is insufficient to provide the necessary brain perfusion to maintain cerebration. Listen carefully to the lungs for any area of obviously absent breath sounds or rales. The possibility of unconsciousness caused by inadequate ventilation may be detected by findings suggestive of bronchial obstruction.

Feel the pulse. Palpate large vessels. Is it a bounding pulse, a weak thready pulse, or a paradoxic pulse?

SKIN CONDITION

The *color* of the skin and mucous membranes is a significant observation. If the patient is obviously pale, the possibility of blood loss anemia or shock is suggested. A plethoric red appearance may mean either a hypertensive encephalopathy or a cerebrovascular accident or both (or even a state of septic shock). Drug reactions or a febrile illness will give the skin a reddish color, as will a sunburn. The tell-tale bright cherry red color of carbon monoxide poisoning should immediately prompt one to institute resuscitative measures as outlined in Chapter 12.

Localized discolorations are also important because they suggest blunt trauma. Icteric sclera prompt one to think of hepatic failure. Most importantly, generalized cyanosis must be detected early so that means for adequate tissue perfusion may be employed.

Touch the patient. Pinch the skin. Is there dehydration? Is the skin warm and dry, suggesting heat stroke? A cold, clammy skin—indicative of peripheral vasoconstriction—often means shock or impending shock, including insulin shock and blood loss or hemorrhagic shock. Palpation of abdominal viscera may give clues. A posterior penetrating abdominal aortic aneurysm as a cause of intra-abdominal hemorrhage and shock may be detected. More rarely, an enlarged spleen or liver will indicate hepatic failure or some hematologic disorder.

Look for needle marks indicating an intravenous injection. If there is strong evidence that unconsciousness is caused by poisoning or drug overdosage, then measures outlined in Chapter 20 should be followed.

A note of warning: Do not touch the unconscious patient at the scene of an accident until the possibility of electrocution is excluded. Many would-be rescuers have themselves been electrocuted.

EYES

Examination of the eyes may be especially revealing in the unconscious patient. Are the eyes sunken within the orbits, indicating marked dehydration or severe wasting? Pupillary inequality (anisocoria) suggests a subdural hematoma on the side opposite the dilated pupil. Bilaterally dilated pupils may mean barbiturate intoxication. Dilated pupils may also be seen in the highly emotional patient and in the patient with glaucoma or with fever. A constricted pupil is often present in old age, after pilocarpine injection, or with Horner's syndrome.

Bilaterally dilated pupils may indicate severe brain damage. Completely dilated pupils are present when cerebral circulation has ceased. Failure of the pupils to respond to light is especially ominous. Pinpoint pupils classically suggest morphine or a similar drug intoxication. Do not forget the possibility of a glass eye!

Look at the eyegrounds. Papilledema of the fundus generally indicates brain tumor or subarachnoid hemorrhage or even hypertensive encephalopathy. Marked arteriovenous nicking supports the likelihood of cerebral arteriosclerosis. The luetic Argyll Robertson pupil accommodates, but not to light. The patient with epilepsy may have fixed and staring eyes. Cotton wool exudates are seen with uremic coma.

STATE OF CONSCIOUSNESS

The matter of *terminology* may prove disturbing but it is important, particularly as one records any changing levels of consciousness or responsiveness to the environment, providing that one notes the mode of stimulation along with the subsequent response.

Syncope refers to a brief loss of consciousness. Other terms including drowsiness, stupor, lethargy, coma, and semicoma have been used to describe varying levels of unconsciousness; however, their usage has varied among physicians and today it may be preferable to note merely the means of stimulation and the manner of response.

What is the depth of consciousness? Can the patient be aroused? Stimuli likely to arouse patients in a semicomatose state may be provided by pressure on the supraorbital nerve at its foramen. Rubbing the knuckles on the sternum with pressure may arouse the patient, or even a simple pinprick may do the job.

Unlike many other medical situations, the patient in coma may need certain types of treatment even before a diagnosis is made. It should not be difficult to note that throughout much of this book there is repeated emphasis on the establishment of an adequate airway and ventilation in addition to the need for an accurate assessment of circulatory status.

Finally, there may be more than one reason for the unconscious state of the patient. As a result of a systemic disturbance of some type, the patient may have suddenly lost consciousness and in falling he may have hit his head with sufficient force to cause a significant intracranial hemorrhage. Throughout the duration of the patient's unconscious state, changes are taking place, and the importance of continually monitoring the patient's vital signs should be obvious.

There are many ways of grouping unconscious patients. Some authors prefer to group them according to signs and symptoms. One possible grouping would include a broad categorization under central nervous sytem pathology:

1. Cerebral strokes caused by embolism, hemorrhage, or thrombosis
2. Intracranial tumor
3. Subarachnoid hemorrhage
4. Cerebral anemia (This would include the patient who is briefly unconscious from fainting caused by general cerebral anemia of a temporary nature. Also included in this group would be unconscious states that accompany shock, cardiac output failure, arrhythmias, and general morbid states.)
5. Cerebral edema most commonly resulting from hypertensive encephalopathy
6. Head injuries most commonly associated with intracranial hematomas, concussions, and the like
7. Psychogenic factors, psychosis and hysteria being the most common
8. Poisonings from alcohol, narcotics, and other drugs
9. Metabolic disorders, including a broad group of unconscious states caused by uremia, hepatic failure, hypoglycemia, and diabetic acidosis
10. Infections including meningitis, encephalitis, and septic shock

Persons subject to recurrent medical emergencies may wear medical *wristbands* or *necklaces* and pertinent information may be found in their pocketbooks or in their clothing. Diabetic, hemophiliac, or cardiac patients or those subject to convulsive episodes often carry some sort of medallion. Some patients may have certain drug sensitivities. Pills found in the possession of the patient must be properly identified since the patient may be on steroid therapy.

• • •

Throughout the examination, maintain a watch on the vital signs. Whenever possible, turn the patient's head to the side to prevent aspiration if he vomits. Save any specimen of vomitus for analysis. Has involuntary defecation or urination occurred? Is there drainage from any body orifice? Blood from the ear alerts one to the possibility of basal skull fracture. Clear fluid drainage from the nose may indicate fracture of the cribriform plate.

Check for any apparent stiffness or rigidity of the patient's neck as a possible indication of meningeal irritation.

Obviously, the many aspects of diagnosis and management of the unconscious patient go beyond the problems of immediate care with which this text is concerned. Until definitive care is given, the unconscious patient should be watched closely and, of course, should never be left alone. Tracheal suctioning may be required. Oxygen administration may be indicated on the way to the hospital in the ambulance.

If marked hyperthermia or temperature elevation is present, one should immediately make efforts to reduce the temperature. This can be accomplished by rubbing ice over the surface of the body or sponging the patient with water or rubbing alcohol. When the patient reaches the hospital, a cooled oxygen tent, tapwater enemas, or a hypothermic blanket can be applied. Although the etiology of the patient's hyperthermia may not be known, one should not delay in trying to control excessive temperature elevation.

When the patient is unable to communicate, much valuable history may be neglected if all details of the patient's state prior to unconsciousness are not explored. The family may be able to provide much of this information. The ambulance attendant should be questioned as to the circumstances surrounding the patient when first seen by him.

A grand mal seizure or epileptic convulsion may be a source of great alarm to those viewing the seizure, but the immediate care required is relatively simple. There is little one can do to prevent the seizure from running its course; hence an air of calmness is essential to reassure bystanders. One should not interfere with the movements of the patient during convulsions but should obviously make an effort to prevent him from injuring his body during the convulsive activity. The victim may stop breathing momentarily during the seizure but as jerking motions decrease, the patient should resume breathing provided that the airway is unobstructed. One should use the techniques discussed in the chapter on airway obstruction to ensure a patent airway. It is unwise to force an airway between the patient's teeth during the seizure. At the conclusion of the convulsion as the patient regains consciousness, one should maintain an air of reassurance to the patient.

Although not a part of the immediate evaluation of the unconscious patient, a number of definitive studies is often required as soon as the patient reaches a medical facility capable of providing definitive care. Certainly, laboratory studies should be done and should include determination of the blood glucose level to ascertain if hypoglycemia is present. A complete blood count should be done along with typing, and cross-matching of blood for transfusion if the signs of hypoglycemia are present. A number of urinalysis tests may be helpful, including those for determination of acetone and sugar levels as well as for the phenothiazines. Toxicologic studies should be started early including tests for levels of various drugs such as barbiturates and bromides. Blood gases are also an important determination.

In some instances skull films will be ordered, but they are not usually of a first priority. Obviously a spinal tap should be performed as soon as possible if there is evidence of meningeal irritation secondary to infection or subarachnoid hemorrhage. These tests should be delayed, however, until an adequate neurologic examination has ruled out the presence of increased intracranial pressure. The spinal tap should not be a part of the immediate activity concerned with the unconscious patient but becomes a later action if indicated. It should not, of course, be an indiscriminate diagnostic procedure, but one made with a great deal of judgment on the basis of careful neurologic studies and, oftentimes, only after consultation with a neurologist and a neurosurgeon, if they are available. Electroencephalography may also be ordered.

It must again be emphasized that certain aspects of the management of the unconscious patient often cannot await definitive diagnosis. Attention to airway obstruction or respiratory difficulties obviously requires immediate priority.

QUESTIONS

1. Discuss the particular challenge presented to the medical practitioner by the unconscious patient.
2. What major clues to condition of the patient are provided by coloring of the skin?
3. Describe several important diagnostic aids provided by examining the eyegrounds of the unconscious patient.
4. Evaluate the use of efforts to lower hyperthermic body temperatures as a part of immediate care.
5. Which special aspects of management of the unconscious patient cannot always await definitive diagnosis?
6. Explain the importance to the patient of evaluating the state of consciousness as a part of emergency medical care.
7. What is the place of auscultation in evaluating the status of the unconscious patient?
8. Discuss clinical shock as a factor in diagnosis of the unconscious patient.

PART TWO

Pathophysiology of trauma

CHAPTER 3

Metabolic response to trauma

WALTER FORD KEITZER and WALTER KIRT NICHOLS

Acute trauma calls into play a number of homeostatic mechanisms perfected during eons of biologic evolution. Our role in caring for the acutely injured patient is to aid and support these vital mechanisms and not to block, overload, or reverse them.

One should remember that trauma has been a part of all life and that many trauma victims survived long before the invention of the hollow needle. We do not mean to advocate therapeutic nihilism with regard to trauma; instead, we suggest that we can learn much by understanding how the organism can survive without support and by knowing the limits of its inherent mechanisms.

The very mechanism important to survival in uncomplicated trauma can turn on the organism and become the principal mediator of one of the organ system failures. For example, the intense sympathetic-mediated vasoconstriction that aids in hemostasis, maintains cardiac output, and redistributes the cardiac output to vital cardiac and cerebral circulation is also the mechanism that can set the stage in the microcirculation for the development of irreversible shock or acute renal failure.

We need to recognize that overzealous or inappropriate therapeutic efforts can compound the problem and can convert a vital defense mechanism to one lethal to the patient. As in the example cited previously, it took many years to recognize the antisurvival effect of norepinephrine as a therapeutic agent for shock.

Our purpose in this chapter will be to outline the principal alterations in the metabolic balance associated with any trauma, to define the associated mechanism, and to discuss the therapeutic implications.

VARIOUS IMBALANCES

Trauma initiates several alterations of the metabolic balance. Principally these involve the balance of water, of protein (the chief constituent of protoplasm), of sodium (the chief cation of the extracellular fluid), and of potassium (the chief cation of the intracellular fluid). The degree of alteration of these constituents can be a measure of the magnitude of the trauma. These elements represent the "visible" part of complex metabolic mechanisms for establishing homeostasis and ensuring survival of the injured organism. The purpose of these alterations is not only to

25

promote survival but also to reorient the body's metabolic priorities for initiation of wound healing.

FUNDAMENTAL RESPONSE—CONSERVATION OF ENERGY OF THE CIRCULATORY SYSTEM

One of the most fundamental responses of the injured organism is the tendency to maintain and conserve energy in the circulatory system, the principal function of which is to deliver to the tissue sufficient hydraulic energy to maintain function: kinetic energy of flow to transport nutrients, wastes, and humoral agents to and from tissues, and potential energy to direct the fluids of the blood through the nutrient and non-nutrient circuits of the microcirculation. For the heart to produce sufficient hydraulic energy, it must have sufficient mass to act on, which means that the blood volume must be maintained. This tendency to maintain volume is one of the strongest responses of the injured organism.

MAINTAINING BLOOD VOLUME

The blood volume is a part of the extracellular fluid (ECF) space, and changes in the ECF tend to parallel changes in the blood volume. Changes in the ECF are intimately related to the metabolic balance of sodium, potassium, and body water. Under ordinary conditions the volume of the ECF is largely a function of the total amount of sodium present. External losses, and thus the balance of sodium and water, are controlled primarily by the kidney. Trauma initiates two principal mechanisms that cause almost complete reabsorption of sodium and maximum reabsorption of water in the kidney and thus maintain the ECF volume. These mechanisms are the antidiuretic hormone (ADH) effect and the aldosterone effect. (We prefer using the term *effect* because volume regulation is not entirely the result of ADH nor is sodium conservation a result of aldosterone alone. Although these hormones are the principal mediators of these mechanisms, both are more complex than can be explained by the physiologic action of each hormone alone.)

In addition to renal conservation of water and sodium by the ADH and aldosterone effects, trauma initiates a general redistribution of body water from intracellular fluid (ICF) to the compartments of the ECF in response to ECF losses. Trauma can cause a loss of blood volume not only through hemorrhage but also by sequestration of extracellular fluid into the so-called third space. Sequestered ECF, although not fluid lost from the body, is fluid that is no longer functional in the sense of supporting or replacing blood volume. For all practical purposes the ionic content of sequestered fluid is the same as that of the ECF. Examples of sequestered fluid include vast accumulation of fluid in the gastrointestinal tract secondary to ileus associated with trauma, fluids in edematous regions of traumatized tissue, and transudates associated with pleural or peritoneal inflammation. In disease states other than trauma, fluid from the ECF can also be lost from the body during vomiting, diarrhea, or fistulization.*

The contraction of the ECF, resulting from either sequestration or fistulization, is rapidly corrected by redistribution of ICF to ECF. At the same time the intra-

---

*Any abnormal loss of isotonic fluids from the gastrointestinal tract through intubation or fistulas.

vascular compartment of the ECF is rapidly replaced by movement of interstitial fluid across the capillary membranes to reestablish the blood volume. Water entering the ECF from the ICF is termed endogenous water. This water is sodium free but rich in potassium and amino acids. Endogenous water is derived not only from intracellular water but also from catabolism of fat, carbohydrate, and protein. The largest source is fat; approximately 1,050 ml of water per kg of fat is utilized as opposed to about 575 ml from each kg of protein. In general, approximately 750 ml of endogenous water is obtained from each kg of lean body mass metabolized. The rest of the water is obtained from reduction of cell volume without loss of cell integrity.

Following injury a large amount of albumin is liberated by the liver into the intravascular compartment, maintaining the oncotic pressure of the intravascular fluid. With an associated decrease in hydrostatic pressure at the capillary level there is a positive movement of water from the interstitial space to the intravascular space of the ECF. Thus the primacy of the blood volume is maintained.

Dilution of extracellular fluid space

The redistribution of body water is characterized by dilution. The dilution of the greatest magnitude is in the blood volume by reduction of erythrocyte concentration. Because endogenous water is sodium free, there is a strong tendency to dilute the ECF sodium concentration. Thus in the trauma patient one characteristically sees a drop in hematocrit and serum sodium concentration. The change in hematocrit is always greater than the decrease in serum sodium. On the average the hematocrit will change 3% for each unit of blood lost from the body. This equilibration begins immediately after trauma and becomes fairly well established in a matter of a few hours. On the other hand, the maximum decrease in serum sodium is not seen for several days. The addition of exogenous blood and sodium will influence the final concentrations; however, even with adequate replacement of blood by transfusion and isotonic replacement of sodium, one should still anticipate some degree of dilution. Thus after an injury or operation one can expect a continued drop in hematocrit that does not necessarily mean continued blood loss.

Independent of hemodynamic factors controlling the filtration rate, there will be a reduction in water and sodium excretion from the ADH and aldosterone effects despite adequate exogenous water and sodium loading. In fact, with excessive loads of water and sodium, dilution of the red cell mass and extracellular sodium can be greater than that which is usually seen or that which would be anticipated. On the other hand, severely deficient isotonic replacement (caused by decreasing renal blood flow) will be associated with a further reduction of the excretion of the water and sodium. This combination of hemodynamic and hormonal mechanisms in the kidney, even in the face of such restriction, may still accomplish complete protection of the ECF volume, and one may still expect to see the tendency toward dilution.

Changes in electrolytes

Following trauma the various volume shifts of body water are accompanied by changes in the electrolyte concentrations in the ICF and ECF. One might expect osmotic gradients to develop; however, the rapid fluid shifts will minimize the osmotic gradients. The tonicity of the ICF is maintained by movement of potassium ions from the cell into the ECF where they are rapidly excreted by the kidney. During the initial period following trauma, 60 to 80 mEq of potassium will be released into the ECF by endogenous water transfer. Cell destruction in traumatized tissue and lysis of red cells in accumulated blood is another rich source of potassium to the ECF. One should remember that normal potassium concentration is 4 mEq per liter in the ECF, and the total potassium content of the ECF will normally be 60 to 80 mEq. Thus it is easy to see how the serum potassium concentration can rise rapidly when renal excretion of potassium is impaired. The renal reduction of free water results in a urine osmolality of about 750 mOsm per kg and the reduction of sodium excretion in the urine results in a urine concentration of less than 10 mEq per liter. Therefore the osmolality of extracellular fluid is maintained by conservation of sodium. If the glomerular filtration rate is lowered by severe reduction of circulating blood volume, excretion of urea will be impaired and the resulting azotemia can increase the osmolality to a degree greater than one would expect from the serum sodium concentration. As a general rule the ADH effect following trauma tends to be stronger than the aldosterone effect; thus the body tends to maintain volume at the expense of tonicity. Nevertheless, the osmolality through all compartments will be equal. Thus if one sees extracellular hypotonicity, one can be sure there is an accompanying intracellular hypotonicity.

Diuretic phase

Beginning 1 to 5 days following trauma, the positive water and sodium balance reverses. This reversal is characterized by a diuresis of dilute urine containing increasing amounts of sodium. The negative potassium balance that characterizes the immediate posttraumatic period is rapidly reversed during the diuretic phase. If the patient was depleted of potassium by medication or other disease processes prior to injury, serious problems with hypokalemia can occur in the diuretic phase or afterward. The time of onset of the diuretic phase is, in part, a function of the magnitude of the trauma. In general the onset is not delayed by sepsis or starvation, but a continued blood volume deficit can delay the onset. The volume of the diuresis depends on the magnitude of the expansion of the ECF resulting from internal fluid shifts and on the magnitude of the water and salt loading given in the posttraumatic period. Although some of the fluid from the ECF will replace the transferred ICF, much of the expansion of the ECF is caused by endogenous water resulting from proteolysis. Replacement of this water in the ICF occurs with the onset of anabolism late in the posttraumatic period when there is an established positive nitrogen balance. Exogenous fluid loading during the posttraumatic period should be avoided because of the great risk of overloading ECF compartments of the lung and brain.

During the diuretic phase not only is the volume expansion of the extracellular compartment returned to normal but also the sequestered fluid from the ECF becomes functional. If renal blood flow and glomerular filtration rate are impaired because of heart failure or previous renal disease, there is a high risk of translocation of the returning sequestered fluid to the ECF in the lungs and brain. Usually this fluid becomes evident as subcutaneous edema, most evident under the skin of the back in the recumbent patient. If significant overloading of the ECF occurs in the posttraumatic period to replace the sequestered fluid into the "third space," the reabsorption of the sequestered fluid into the functional ECF can pose serious problems. This is especially true if one gives additional exogenous fluids. As a result of increased use of extracellular volume replacement in the posttraumatic period, the incidence of renal failure secondary to inadequate renal perfusion from a contracted ECF volume has significantly decreased in recent years. Simultaneously, there appears to be an associated increase in incidence of pulmonary problems, the so-called posttraumatic pulmonary insufficiency syndrome. The latter problem appears to occur most frequently during the period in which one would expect the diuretic phase.

ALTERATIONS IN PROTEIN, CARBOHYDRATE, AND FAT

In injuries that cause alterations in the balance of water, sodium, and potassium, the metabolic response is directed toward maintaining the volume of the extracellular fluid space. Of no less importance than the volume homeostatic mechanisms is the metabolic alteration of protein, carbohydrate, and fat that follows trauma. This catabolism is the principal source of energy for maintaining metabolism following injury. In most situations involving acute trauma, the added complication of chronic nutritional depletion does not need to be considered but will be discussed following a discussion of alterations caused by trauma in healthy individuals.

Supplying caloric needs

Acute starvation is one of the initiating factors of the metabolic alterations following injury. Indeed, many of the initial metabolic changes in water, electrolytes, and metabolic nutritional stores can be detected following a 24-hour fast in an uninjured person. The average person will burn about 2,000 calories per day, and this will be balanced with a nutrient intake equivalent to 2,000 calories. Most trauma of any significance will be associated with a total cessation of oral caloric intake. After trauma the caloric need will increase the basal metabolic requirements; however, the total energy requirements may remain unchanged since muscular activity is reduced to a minimum. The increase in basal metabolic requirement is usually only a moderate 10% to 15% in uncomplicated trauma but may rise to levels as high as 200% following extensive full-thickness burns.

Certain complications of trauma can markedly alter the metabolic caloric requirement. Sepsis and associated fever are obvious causes of increased caloric expenditure. Pulmonary problems cause increased caloric expenditures not only through increased muscular activity associated with labored respirations but also through metabolic effects of anoxia and associated temperature elevations. Following extensive burns there is a marked increase in evaporative water loss from the body. Most of the energy utilized as latent heat of vaporization is derived from the metabolic heat of the body. This is the probable reason for greatly elevated energy expenditures in extensive burns.

Following trauma the initial energy requirements are obtained through oxidation of body glycogen stores. In the normal adult these stores are probably not greater than 200 gm, thus limiting this source of energy to a total of 800 calories. After glycogen stores are rapidly expended, further energy sources are in fat and protein, although there is little utilization of protein as compared to fat.

Proteolysis

Obligatory proteolysis for caloric needs is one of the characteristic metabolic responses to injury. As protein is broken down, between 10 and 20 gm of nitrogen per day is excreted in the urine following significant trauma. Each gram of nitrogen in the urine represents a utilization of 30 gm of muscle mass. Although there is no loss of muscle cell integrity, this negative nitrogen balance represents a loss of 300 to 600 gm of muscle weight per day, and only 250 calories are provided during excretion of 10 gm of nitrogen per day. Therefore protein is not a good source of body energy.

Although negative nitrogen balance is a somewhat unavoidable response to injury, any measure that can be taken to minimize nitrogen loss is of considerable value in supporting homeostatic defense mechanisms. Intravenous infusion of 100 gm of glucose per day will decrease the negative nitrogen balance approximately 50%. Unfortunately, infusion of an equal amount of additional glucose will not show an equal reduction in negative nitrogen balance. In fact the glucose infusion is more effective in reducing the negative nitrogen balance of starvation than that which follows trauma, in which much of the excreted nitrogen comes from the breakdown of protein content of translocated fluids and blood retained in body cavities and tissues. The breakdown of this protein is a necessary part of wound healing, and it will not be altered by exogenous or endogenous sources of calories.

Fat catabolism

The principal source of energy for the body after injury lies in the breakdown of fat. Despite extensive catabolism of protein for energy sources, much of the weight loss following injury can be attributed to loss of body fat. One gram of fat provides 9 calories of energy. During starvation, 75 to 150 gm of fat is burned per day; after injury three or four times this amount of fat may be utilized for energy requirements, which can account for production of 2,000 to 4,500 calories per day. For each kilogram of fat utilized the body gains 1,050 ml of endogenous water. As stated before, endogenous water obtained from the catabolism of fat is important source of water for expansion of the ECF. Because of the ADH effect and resultant water retention, the net weight loss by the body is minimized.

Exogenous caloric supply

As one can see from the previous discussion, endogenous energy sources in order of importance are fat, protein, and carbohydrate. In managing the acutely injured patient one might like to administer foodstuffs in the same order of importance and efficiency as utilized by the body from its endogenous sources, but for all practicable purposes the availability of exogenous energy sources is reversed. Glucose remains the most available and important material for intravenous support. Other carbohydrates such as fructose and sorbitol can be used. Blood, plasma, and serum albumin are the only practical forms of protein for intravenous use. The use of protein hydrolysates has limited value in the management of acutely injured patients.

Emulsified fats have been used in the past but they carry a risk to the patient, and if they are used, they can be used only in limited amounts. For this reason fat sources for intravenous use have no practical value in the acute situation.

In the past decade, the development of parenteral alimentation has become one of the most significant advances in the metabolic care of surgical patients. Fluids for parenteral alimentation contain high concentrations of glucose (20%), potassium (60 to 120 mEq per liter), protein hydrolysates, and maintenance concentrations of other electrolytes. Recently the protein hydrolysates have been replaced with free amino acids representing each of the essential amino acids. The usual formulation of fluids for parenteral alimentation provides approximately 1 calorie per ml. Thus nutritionally depleted patients can be given 2,400 to 3,600 calories a day. Fluids of such concentrations must be given through a catheter placed in the central venous system. The efficient utilization of concentrated glucose and fluids containing protein hydrolysate (or amino acids) fluids administered intravenously is based on the discovery that high concentrations of potassium and adequate phosphate ions are essential for metabolic incorporation of concentrated nutrients. Parenteral alimentation has principal roles in treatment of patients with chronic nutritional depletion or nonfunctioning gastrointestinal tracts. It has only limited application in the management of acute trauma—the subject of this book.

Hormonal relationships

The mechanism for mobilizing the body's sources of energy appears to be related principally to the hormones of the adrenal gland: both the adrenocortical hormones and the catecholamines of the adrenal medulla. Epinephrine and norepinephrine from the adrenal medulla (along with other sources of catecholamines) appear to be involved in the mechanism for the rapid glycogenolysis that follows trauma. There is evidence that beta function of the sympathetic system is important for the mobilization of fat. The initial part of the negative nitrogen balance following injury can be imitated in normal persons by injection of cortisone or other glucocorticoids. Following trauma, importance of adrenocortical hormones in the vital defense mechanisms is clearly evidenced by the response of the adrenalectomized organism to stress without hormone substitution. The adrenalectomized animal cannot respond with volume protection mechanisms or with energy mobilization mechanisms. Because the mobilization of adrenocortical hormones comes from the stimulus of ACTH, hypophysectomized animals respond to stress in an identical manner.

FACTORS INITIATING THE METABOLIC RESPONSE TO INJURY

Initiating factors in the metabolic response to trauma fall into two groups: endogenous and exogenous.

The most important and principal endogenous factor in inducing the neurohumoral mechanism that controls metabolic response is volume reduction. As noted before, volume reduction can occur either in its most obvious form during hemorrhage or in the more subtle sequestration of extracellular fluid. No matter what the mechanism for reducing the functional volume of the ECF, receptors (both peripheral and within the central nervous system) act through the neurohypophysis to trigger both the ADH and aldosterone effects.

Exogenous factors are pain, sepsis, and pharmacologic agents. Pain, as well as emotional stimuli, can act through the neurohypophysis to initiate the metabolic responses described previously. Pain is the universal accompaniment of trauma, and it is one of the important factors in activating the homeostatic mechanisms.

Wound infection and sepsis are included here as exogenous factors for initiating metabolic response. More importantly, these probably constitute a principal factor in the continuing homeostatic defense mechanisms as a complication of trauma. Infection acts not only through pain from the tissues involved but also through toxins from the organisms that cause the infection or sepsis. In general infection has to be controlled before catabolism associated with the metabolic alterations can be reversed. However, parenteral alimentation has been used effectively to minimize the catabolic states associated with infection and sepsis by providing support for the patient until control is obtained with surgical drainage, antibiotics, or other measures.

Drugs can be an important contributing factor not only to the induction of the metabolic response but also to the magnitude and duration of the response. Ether and cyclopropane are potent stimulators of the catecholamine sources in the body. A number of vasodepressors, such as reserpine and chlorpromazine, can induce volume reduction mechanisms by blocking the catecholamines and by direct vasodilation, causing hypotension. A number of diuretics are well known for depleting the body of sodium or potassium or both, thus limiting the normal volume regulatory mechanisms. Certain central nervous system drugs can inhibit the normal response to the neurohypophysis in controlling volume.

QUESTIONS

1. List four hormones that play an active role in the metabolic response to trauma. For each, briefly outline the effect of that hormone in restoring homeostasis.
2. What happens to endogenous fat and protein following acute major injury? Which is the principal energy source in starvation in the posttraumatic state?
3. Why are restoration of circulatory volume and support of cardiovascular function of prime importance in the resuscitation of the acutely injured patient?
4. What is meant by the phrase *the turning point* or the *diuretic phase* in the patient following trauma?
5. What effect do exogenous carbohydrates have on proteolysis following injury?
6. What is the principal stimulus inducing the metabolic response to trauma?
7. Which ion shifts from the intracellular to extracellular space following trauma? Under what circumstances is this potentially dangerous?
8. What is the effect of sepsis in the patient after trauma?

SUGGESTED READINGS

American College of Surgeons, Committee on Pre and Postoperative Care: Manual of preoperative and postoperative care, ed. 2, Philadelphia, 1971, W. B. Saunders Co.

American College of Surgeons, Committee on Pre and Postoperative Care: Manual of surgical nutrition, Philadelphia, 1975, W. B. Saunders Co.

Moore, F. D.: Metabolic care of the surgical patient, Philadelphia, 1959, W. B. Saunders Co.

CHAPTER 4

Shock

As is true with many major emergencies, the immediate treatment of the patient in shock may be multifaceted. If the causative factors still persist—such as continuing hemorrhage—efforts must be directed toward achieving hemostasis or control of hemorrhage. These efforts will not be discussed here but are detailed elsewhere. Because the shock victim may, of course, have received multiple injuries; the considerations mentioned in Chapter 9 are paramount. As with all emergencies, the patency of the airway and the adequacy of ventilation are of the first priority. Because of the reduced oxygen-carrying potential of the blood caused by reduced blood volume, oxygen should be administered if it is available. If one is satisfied that there has been no head injury, the patient should be kept in a supine or flat position or, better still, with his lower extremities moderately elevated (30 degrees). The patient should not be allowed to stand or sit. To reduce further soft tissue injury and to control pain, fractures should be splinted as soon as it is feasible and before transportation of the victim to the hospital.

DEFINITION

What is shock? Although shock, with its various aspects of circulatory derangement, may be considered a wastebasket term, there are certain features common to all forms. More than anything else, certainly, shock represents a defective or low perfusion rate of blood through the tissues. This inadequate oxygenation of tissues, regardless of its cause, sets up a cyclic reaction leading to generalized metabolic acidosis, decreased cardiac output, increasing hypotension, and further reduction of tissue perfusion; then another cycle begins. Effective immediate care dictates that this chain reaction be broken at the earliest possible time before irreversible changes have taken place.

A number of pathologic states may be defined as shock, such as electric shock, septicemic shock, cardiogenic shock, burn shock, or shock from the loss of blood.

DIAGNOSTIC DIFFICULTIES

What clinical features are common to most shock states? Early in the evolution of the shock state one will be impressed by the evidence of peripheral vasoconstriction: cool, moist, and clammy skin; a pale face; a subjective feeling of faintness and weakness; and an inability to remain in the upright or erect position. Usually the pulse is fast and less full than normal. If considerable blood loss is the etiologic factor, the patient will generally show signs of obvious apprehension and not infrequently be thirsty and request water. As a shock state increases in severity, mental sluggishness, increased restlessness, and further increase in the pulse rate will occur. Nausea may be present at an early stage. Respirations increase in rate and in depth as the shock state progresses, often to the state of gasping air hunger. Quite often the pupils are dilated.

As shock progresses, one can note increased pallor, increased repetitive heart rate, further agitation, dyspnea, and eventually an incoherent comatose state. Cyanosis is a particularly ominous sign because it portrays the fact that tissue perfusion is markedly deficient.

The blood pressure readings may be deceptively normal. Because of compensatory mechanisms, including increased peripheral vasoconstriction and increased cardiac output caused by sympathetic hyperactivity, a fall in blood pressure may not occur for some time. The amount of blood loss likely to produce a shock state may vary with the age of the patient, the preexisting health state of the patient, and associated pain factors. Generally speaking, most individuals show signs of peripheral vasoconstriction with cool, moist skin and an increased pulse rate if much more than 500 ml of blood is rapidly lost. Profound shock states may be present if more than one third of the blood has been lost. "Irreversible" shock is seen if profound blood loss is allowed to persist for more than a brief period of time.

Estimating the amount of blood loss at the scene of an accident is a difficult task even for the experienced physician. Even so, some approximation of the amount of blood visibly lost by the patient will be of help to those supplying definitive care in the hospital.

The amount of blood lost within the body cavity or in the soft tissue of the body is a factor more difficult to assess, but consideration of this possibility is not to be overlooked. For example, it is not uncommon for a patient with a fractured hip to lose more than 1,000 ml of blood into the soft tissues about the site of the fracture. Injuries of the thigh are notorious for harboring or sequestering huge quantities of blood in a hematoma.

Obviously large amounts of blood may also be sequestered in the abdominal cavity from a ruptured viscus. Not to be overlooked, however, is the possibility of considerable blood loss into the retroperitoneal space. It is important to be reminded that the previously mentioned features of hypovolemic shock are not often encountered in patients with head injuries. For this reason one should not assume that an obvious head injury is the cause of the shocklike state. Rather, one should assume that there is a source of bleeding in the sites mentioned.

As soon as possible the urinary output should be monitored, because the degree of oliguria is a particularly valuable means of monitoring defectiveness of the patient's blood volume. If the blood volume is less than 30 ml per hour, one can assume that the distal renal tubules are becoming ischemic.

This chapter does not delve to any great extent into the pathophysiology of shock but confines its discussion mainly to the immediate problem of hemorrhagic, or blood loss, shock. Other examples or etiologic factors are either elsewhere in this book or are beyond the scope of this presentation. These include shock of a neurogenic nature, psychogenic shock, septic shock resulting from infection, cardiogenic shock, metabolic shock, and anaphylactic shock as an allergic reaction.

RESTORATION OF BLOOD VOLUME

Several years ago a well-known professor of surgery in a Canadian school would talk to the medical students about hemorrhagic shock. Because of his conviction that whole blood is the preferable replacement for lost blood rather than a crystalloid or colloid solution, he would dramatically state that the treatment of hemorrhagic shock is with *blood* and with that he would throw a unit of blood against the blackboard, causing a considerable splash! No one in that class ever forgot the treatment for hemorrhagic shock!

Of paramount importance in the treatment of shock is the restoration of the circulating blood volume so that adequate tissue oxygenation may occur and so that irreversible damage to particularly susceptible organs such as the brain, kidney, and myocardium may be prevented. With evidence of a massive hemorrhage, emergency room physicians are alert to the need for establishing a rapid and secure intravenous route. If the veins are too much collapsed, a cutdown over one of the veins of an extremity will be required and either a needle or, preferably, a catheter may be inserted into the vein. The establishment of an intravenous route at the scene of the accident may be a lifesaving effort and should be done whenever possible. In such cases administration of lactated Ringer's solution or a solution of normal saline can be started. Ideally, a plasma expander should be immediately administered.

Most favor the use of Ringer's lactate solution to rapidly restore circulating blood volume and adequate perfusion of the capillary bed. Its immediate availability and freedom from pyrogens and substances that may cause allergic reaction make it a particularly attractive choice for rapid replacement of the blood volume. As much as 2 to 4 liters of Ringer's lactate may be required before adequately cross-matched blood is available.

Should one administer vasopressors in the immediate management of hypovolemic shock? Remember that the marked cutaneous vasoconstriction producing the pallor and decreased skin temperature is a result of the body's alpha adrenergic sympathetic response. The adrenal gland has been stimulated to release a large amount of epinephrine, and sympathetic postganglionic nerve endings have been triggered to release norepinephrine. These alpha and beta adrenergic responses of the body have been such that the addition of externally administered vasopressors may be detrimental. The use of vasopressors has been discussed in the chapter on cardiopulmonary resuscitation, to which the reader should refer.

As soon as the patient can be brought to the emergency room, after the management of the airway is adequately established, after obvious signs of external hemorrhage are identified, and after the hemorrhage is controlled, blood should also be drawn for blood gas determinations. As discussed in the chapter on the monitoring of the critically ill patient, a central venous pressure monitoring system should be established as an item of early priority. Knowledge of the central venous pressure allows one to know how much fluid the patient can tolerate and helps to prevent the induction of pulmonary edema or congestive heart failure.

Low molecular weight dextran (dextran 40) not only serves to enlarge the vascular space but also is extremely helpful in preventing the blood from clotting. In the shock state there is frequently a sludging of blood in the peripheral circulation that leads to intravascular thrombosis. If plasma is available, it is preferred to one of the artificial plasma expanders.

When an intravenous route is being established, blood should be drawn for immediate typing and cross-matching. In many instances the urgency of the situation is so great, however, that un-cross-matched blood from a universal donor (O, Rh negative) must be administered.

CONTROL OF PAIN DURING SHOCK

Much can be done to relieve the patient's pain without the use of drugs. Reassurance is vital. Tell the patient that you understand his situation and that he will receive the best possible care. Keep him informed of plans for his rescue, immediate comfort, and eventual professional aid. Proper positioning of and support for injured extremities can greatly decrease pain in these areas. *Ask* the patient: "Is this more comfortable or would that be better?" Let him know that you care. Slit or loosen tight clothing or shoes in any way that may increase comfort.

The difficulties with the indiscriminate use of pain medication are several. The patient's respirations are already depressed and use of narcotics may further aggravate the situation. Narcotics are particularly contraindicated when there is a possibility of intra-abdominal injury because these agents will, in many instances, almost completely block the symptoms of abdominal muscle guarding, peritoneal irritation, and other signs of an acute surgical abdomen. Furthermore, the administration of narcotics by either intramuscular or subcutaneous injection when there is marked peripheral vascular constriction will not be followed by an early uptake of the narcotic, and its desired effect will not only be delayed but perhaps compounded by a second narcotic injection given subsequently.

A more detailed discussion of the control of pain is presented in Chapter 6.

Should any fluids be given by mouth? Sometimes well-intentioned bystanders may offer the patient water and occasionally coffee, tea, or other fluids. Generally speaking, nothing should be given to the patient by mouth until it is clearly evident that no operative procedures will be indicated. This is a decision that should be made by the individual responsible for definitive care of the patient.

QUESTIONS

1. Explain the rationale in attempting to control pain as much as possible without drugs in the shock patient.
2. Describe emergency nondrug means of controlling pain.
3. Why is blood volume such a critical part of the total picture in shock?
4. Explain what is meant by shock as seen in the emergency patient.
5. Contrast the effects of actual blood loss and sequestered blood in the production of shock in the accident victim.
6. Discuss several of the various techniques available for restoring blood volume.
7. Explain the cyclic nature of shock.
8. Why is the cyclic nature of shock important in its treatment?
9. Describe the salient points in shock diagnosis.

CHAPTER 5

Monitoring of vital signs

From the time immediate care of the injured or acutely ill individual is begun, careful and meaningful observations must be made continuously until more definitive treatment is available. How does one adequately monitor the crucial physiologic functions of the patient? Under most emergency conditions sophisticated electronic and mechanical devices are not available. Instead one must rely on one's own clinical observations.

OBJECTIVES

What does one hope to achieve by effective monitoring? By periodic and almost constant attention to the patient's vital signs one hopes to receive early warning of impending catastrophe. For example, cardiac arrest or cardiovascular collapse may be preceded by changes in the pulse rate and rhythm. Internal hemorrhage may be suspected whenever the patient has a rising pulse rate, thirst, apprehension, and cool, moist skin, even though the blood pressure may remain at nearly normal levels. Respiratory obstruction, similarly, may be detected earlier by close observation of the respiratory rate, excursion pattern, color of mucous membranes, and sensorium.

As both ambulance care and equipment are being rapidly upgraded and as emergency rooms provide increasingly sophisticated immediate care, monitoring methods are changing. For example, at the University of Missouri Medical Center the emergency medical service provides ambulances equipped with electrocardiographic equipment, the readings of which can be transmitted via radio telephone to personnel in the emergency room and to the heart station where immediate interpretation and subsequent advice can be rendered. The value of attempting to stabilize the cardiac status prior to transportation of the patient is, of course, well documented. Continuous pulse and blood pressure monitoring can be initiated and continued throughout the patient's removal to the hospital.

In spite of mechanical devices, "eyeball observations" have no substitute, and one needs to continually improve one's knowledge of what to look for and one's ability to observe.

Basically, as mentioned, monitoring refers to qualitative and quantitative observations, over a period of time, of the physiologic functions in a clinical context. More specifically it refers to observation of the cardiovascular, respiratory, renal, and central nervous systems as well as observation of the electrolytic balance. Single observations of these systems, especially taken out of context, are of limited value in the evaluation of the therapeutic needs of the patient. Multiple observations naturally add a dimension of time and help to predict trends.

Urinary output, for example, needs to be monitored via the indwelling catheter. Not only does it provide proof of the adequacy of renal blood flow but also under some conditions, gives support to any decision regarding requirements for the use of intravenous fluids or osmotic diuretics.

The urinary output should be recorded at 15-minute intervals. If the output is less than 30 ml per hour, one may often assume that renal perfusion is deficient, and in the victim suffering from shock it is an indication of inadequate blood volume. On the other hand, however, if the patient is excreting more than 50 ml per hour one may assume a more optimistic view of general body perfusion.

Similarly, the monitoring of the patient's central venous pressure is a means of acquiring much-needed information that may mirror blood volume deficiency or excess. The greatest advantage of the central venous pressure reading is that it allows an estimate of whether the victim may tolerate additional quantities of whole blood or intravenous fluids without the likelihood of producing congestive heart failure or pulmonary edema. Although not always immediately available, its overall importance has prompted its inclusion in this chapter. A central venous catheter may be placed through a number of routes; each has certain advantages. Presently the subclavian or internal jugular vein approach is most commonly employed, although any vein approach may be used in an emergency, providing that it does in fact tap the central venous pool. In addition to providing readings of the central venous pressure, the catheter may be utilized for obtaining repeated venous pH and gas tensions as well as for fluid infusions. Although there are pitfalls in the interpretations of central venous pressures, one generally uses them as a guide to prevent overloading of patients with blood or certain intravenous fluids at a time when adequate estimation of blood loss is difficult. More accurately, central venous pressure is an index of the function of the right ventricle and the ability of the heart to handle returning blood volume at any given time. One may occasionally observe pulmonary edema in the presence of a low or normal central venous pressure.

The pulmonary artery pressure is becoming increasingly of interest to those concerned with techniques for adequate monitoring of resuscitative efforts in the injured patient, and there is some evidence that this may be the best single means for assessing adequacy of restoration of blood volume. False readings may reflect a mechanical obstruction of the returning venous blood that results from factors such as a pericardial collection of blood or fluid resulting in cardiac tamponade. Compression of the mediastinal structures can likewise give false elevations. Return flow may be slowed partially or obstructed by high intrathoracic pressures from a pneumothorax or from improperly employed artificial respirators.

Gas tension determinations are generally considered in definitive treatment because of their increasing availability in the emergency room. More and more reliance is placed on a monitoring of the gas tensions and blood pH level in the severely traumatized patient. These measurements provide a sensitive indication of respiratory and metabolic abnormalities. Repeatedly, these indicators have warned of serious problems before significant changes in pulse, blood pressure, electrocardiogram, venous pressure, or skin perfusion indicators. Blood pH and gas tension changes are particularly helpful when serial readings are performed. Prompt correction of abnormalities may prevent serious cardiovascular complications. Cardiac arrest, for example, is rare in the injured patient with a normal pH in the central venous blood.

Oxygen and carbon dioxide tension values are primary indices of ventilation and reflect pulmonary gas exchange. Venous oxygen tension values may serve to reflect the relationship between metabolic requirements for oxygen and oxygen transport by the circulating blood.

Monitoring requirements vary from patient to patient. The acutely ill person with sunstroke requires continuous temperature readings. Many acutely injured patients likewise need careful monitoring of their heat regulatory mechanism.

QUESTIONS

1. Discuss the adequacy of central venous pressure monitoring of fluid volume during resuscitative procedures.
2. Evaluate gas tension monitoring in the emergency medical situation.
3. Discuss the objective of monitoring the emergency patient's vital signs.
4. Which vital signs are most involved in monitoring the patient receiving emergency medical care?

SUGGESTED READINGS

Hartong, J. M., Dixon, R. S.: Monitoring resuscitation of the injured patient, J.A.M.A. 297:242-247, 1977.

CHAPTER 6

Control of pain

JOHN H. HENZEL

"Pain is always a sinister gift which diminishes man, and the strict duty of the doctor is to endeavor to suppress it, if he can. . . ." Had LeRiche included the trauma victim in his classic statement about the physician's duty toward pain relief, he would have admonished clinicians to suppress pain only when accurately indicated, at a stage when selective administration of a specific agent would not mask or confuse existing symptoms or further depress already obtunded vital functions.

Unfortunately, physicians inexperienced in the initial care of trauma victims still equate extensive injury with pain, despite the fact that experience has shown that most victims of major trauma do not complain of pain during the early period following injury.

VARIABLES AFFECTING PERCEPTION AND EXPRESSION OF PAIN

Individual awareness of and response to pain is tremendously variable and is not necessarily related to the severity of the trauma. Reaction to real pain and the degree to which an individual's mental and physical behavior and performance are affected are influenced by factors such as mental alertness, emotional stability, personal stoicism, and, in the case of the conscious trauma victim, anxiety about the extent and potential sequelae of his injury. In healthy, uninjured persons, painful experiences such as an abscessed tooth or migraine headache may either be ignored or be totally incapacitating, depending on coexisting psychologic-environmental variables. The abscessed tooth that throbs unbearably while the afflicted individual is at work may be almost ignored throughout an exciting football game.

Variables such as age, fatigue, and intelligence also influence perception and expression of pain. In addition, drugs and diseases affecting mental alertness and performance also modify response to injury and pain, a fact that is occasionally forgotten or overlooked in the tense atmosphere of the emergency room. A number of trauma victims, particularly older persons, are taking drugs that may have been primarily responsible for the accident and that may then have altered the patient's response to injury. Specific problems arise in the trauma victim who is receiving anticoagulants, digitalis preparations, and antihypertensive drugs. In evaluating any injured patient's clinical behavior relative to apparent pain, one should be alert to the possibility that the use of a tranquilizer or antihistamine has depressed the level of mental alertness prior to the accident, and such medication may be partially or totally responsible for obtunding both the level of consciousness and vital functions following injury. The well-known effects of alcohol are usually apparent. However, because it is often necessary to reexamine trauma victims repeatedly over a number of hours in deciding for or against surgical intervention, it is prudent to submit a specimen of blood for determination of baseline alcohol and barbiturate levels whenever one suspects that either of these agents may be contributing to the overall clinical picture. The effects of drug addiction can mimic pain, and the examining physician must also consider hard drug habituation or withdrawal in the inappropriately hyperactive or "wild" youthful victim. Finally, it is important to remain alert for the rare trauma victim whose abnormal conscious behavior is related to diabetic coma, adrenal insufficiency, or anticoagulant-related intracranial hematoma.

In the acutely injured patient, restlessness, groaning, or requests for relief (clinical behavior suggestive of pain) may be manifestations of something other than pain. The physician who evaluates or treats trauma victims must be familiar with those factors that can mimic or mask pain, and he must avoid administration of an analgesic until he knows the exact etiology of the pain.

ACCURATE INTERPRETATION OF CLINICAL BEHAVIOR

As the conscious trauma victim is being examined, an attempt should be made to alleviate anxiety by calmly informing him of the nature of his injury and describing insofar as possible the needed form of therapy. If the patient understands what has occurred and what to anticipate and is able to establish confidence in the examining physician, apparent need for analgesia will either decrease markedly or be eliminated. Although conversation may be difficult or impossible in an occasional situation in which seconds may make the difference between saving and losing a patient, in the long run the frequency with which trauma victims are afforded accurate diagnosis and efficient, safe management will be increased if one constantly remembers that *pain is a symptom complex that is occasionally controlled by little more than simple communication with the patient.* If the actual presence and intensity of pain are to be accurately evaluated, it is particularly essential that one pay attention to seemingly insignificant, often minimized, and frequently ignored parameters of patient comfort. Two case histories will illustrate this point.

Case 1. A 21-year-old injured man is lying on his left side and groaning loudly with his legs drawn up. Examination discloses a through-and-through gunshot wound of the right thorax about 2 inches directly lateral to the nipple. While intravenous fluids are being started, the junior surgical resident arrives on the scene and confirms the suspicion of alcohol on the patient's breath. He ascertains from the accompanying police officer that the youth was shot as he left a tavern after 2 hours of beer drinking with his friends. After examining the patient's thorax and abdomen, the surgical resident initiates nasal oxygen and inserts a chest tube and bladder catheter. After 1,050 ml of urine has filled the collection bag and while air from the pneumothorax is bubbling into the closed chest thoracostomy bottle, the injured youth stops moaning, relaxes, and appears surprisingly comfortable.

In this situation, clinical behavior suggestive of pain was, in actuality, the result of hypoxia related to pneumothorax and distended bladder in a semi-inebriated patient. Had morphine been administered hypoxia would have been aggravated, the level of consciousness further obtunded, and discovery of the full bladder delayed. As a result of accurate interpretation and precise nontoxic treatment, the patient was able to be discharged after 3 days.

Case 2. In the emergency room on a snowy November night, a disheveled middle-aged man is rolling from side to side and moaning in apparent delirium. Examination discloses shivering and pallor, a 2 cm superficial laceration through the right eyebrow, and a closed fracture deformity of the right lower extremity. It is ascertained that after the victim was struck by a slow-moving motorcycle while crossing the street against a green light, he had lain on the pavement in near-freezing rain for some 15 minutes while waiting for the ambulance to arrive. While wet clothing is being removed and the fracture immobilized, the patient's wife arrives. After learning that he is conscious, she produces a pair of glasses, concerned that her husband is "nearly blind without them." A half hour later, a calm, perfectly coherent, and surprisingly alert patient bemoans the pitfall of a shirtsleeve sprint across a busy street against a red light for a cup of coffee on a very cold night.

In this instance, environmental exposure, visual disadvantage, and fracture pain intensified by uncontrollable shivering combined to produce a clinical picture suggestive of severe pain. After wet clothing had been removed, warm covers supplied, and the patient's glasses made available, the relatively minor extent of injury became apparent. Appropriate x-rays ruled out additional trauma other than the closed tibial fracture, and the extent of total treatment amounted to suture of the supraorbital laceration, a long leg cast, and 24 hours of in-hospital observation.

Because restlessness, moaning, and excess motor activity may be erroneously interpreted as severe pain by the novice treating his first accident victim, such clinical behavior raises the *possibility of cerebral trauma or developing hypoxia*. While the novice requests a syringe of morphine, his experienced colleague is firmly reassuring the patient while simultaneously examining him for evidence of cerebral damage, occult hemorrhage, or pneumothorax, for example.

NARCOTIC OBTUNDATION OF SUBCLINICAL PATHOPHYSIOLOGY

Three principal reasons underlie the rationale for avoiding unnecessary analgesia in the acutely injured patient:

1. Drug idiosyncrasy may superimpose unnecessary and confusing symptoms on an already complex clinical situation. Undesirable drug side effects such as retching, excitement, fever, or allergic reaction will cloud those clinical parameters on which the physician must depend for early accurate diagnosis and precise therapy.
2. Not only may the pain threshold be increased but also the patient's ability to express concern about new or more intense symptoms may be blunted.
3. Perhaps most importantly, nonapparent and unsuspected subclinical depression of vital functions may unknowingly be further depressed at a time when compensatory factors are already straining maximally to maintain homeostasis.

It is in the third area that we have greatest concern, and only in recent years has clinical use of diagnostic methods previously confined to the experimental laboratory allowed us to detect and monitor subclinical, premorbid derangements in cardio-vascular-respiratory physiology.

During World War II, physicians noticed that certain clinical behavior suggestive of pain actually results from altering so-called vital functions. Restlessness, excitement, and hyperactivity were recognized as manifestations of acute head injury, and the term *traumatic wet lung* was affixed to characteristic x-ray changes that accompany the progressive asphyxia that results from certain types of thoracic trauma. However, accurate understanding of the exact changes, their prognostic significance, and the methods for reversing these changes had to await understanding and delineation of shock at the microcirculatory level and understanding of respiratory gas mechanics (relative to acid-base equilibrium) at the cellular and subcellular levels. During the past 10 years, however, trauma units have begun to use central venous pressure monitoring, sequential arterial blood gas analyses, pyruvate-lactate determinations, radioisotope-computer assessment of intra- and extravascular fluid dynamics, cardiac output determination, pulmonary-peripheral resistance determinations, and arteriovenous shunting during resuscitation and treatment of the severely injured patient. Ten years ago, the effect of 10 mg of intravenous morphine was barely evident to the experienced clinician, principally because the earliest changes of respiratory depression or oligemic acidosis are subclinical. Today sophisticated methodology readily documents the hypoxemia, hypercapnia, acidosis, and altered microcirculatory dynamics that occur in the face of narcotic overdosage.

Contraindicated or excessive narcotic administration does nullify or derange compensatory life-preserving processes. Knowing how narcotic administration can jeopardize already tenuous physiologic homeostasis in the trauma victim, physicians who treat these patients should be alert to three specific situations in which erroneous interpretation of clinical behavior may precipitate a vicious circle of diagnostic-therapeutic misadventure.

The first relates to trauma-precipitated changes in respiratory mechanics. Significant reduction in vital capacity is associated with such injuries as fractured ribs, pneumothorax, and peritoneal contamination by blood, bile, urine, or gastrointestinal content. Somewhat similarly, pulmonary contusion, massive fat embolization, and fluid overload atelectasis also result in varying combinations of hypoxia, hypercapnia, and acidosis. In each of these situations, irritability and restlessness related to and resulting from hypoxemia may erroneously be interpreted as pain. Administration of an analgesic further diminishes respiratory effort and hence compounds the overall situation.

A second, not uncommon pitfall is the interpretation of hyperventilation as pain in a hypotensive, poorly responsvie trauma victim when the increased respiratory rate is actually a necessary physiologic compensation for a developing metabolic acidosis. Administration of a narcotic may diminish or abolish this necessary compensation and thereby accentuate the acidosis.

The third pitfall constitutes an example of a situation in which partial knowledge precipitates well-meaning, partially correct, but dangerous therapy. When one interprets tachypnea and restlessness as being partially related to hypoxia in extensive thoracic cage trauma, both oxygen and a narcotic are administered. Hypoxia may be corrected, but coexisting hypercapnia is compounded as the respiratory rate is therapeutically diminished.

ADMINISTRATION OF INDICATED ANALGESIA

The actual indications for administration of an analgesic to victims of major trauma are rare and specific. Experienced trauma surgeons administer narcotics only when real and severe pain is present (usually after its cause has been determined), when there must be a delay before the completely evaluated and stable trauma victim can receive definitive treatment, and when a conscious trauma victim's clinical response to painful stimuli precludes definitive or accurate evaluation. There are no occasions when analgesia should be administered to a transportable trauma victim at the scene of an accident, and few if any instances in which the patient should receive a narcotic in the emergency ward prior to being evaluated by the physician who will be responsible for his care.

Because there is neither time nor place for indecision in managing the acutely injured person and because trauma respects neither age nor degree of health, it is best to adopt one drug for use in trauma, become familiar with its dosage and specific pharmacologic properties, and learn how to use it. Morphine sulfate has stood the test of time, and for one reason or another, most persons learn and retain the dosage and side effects of this narcotic. For these reasons and because of personal preference, discussion is limited to this drug.

Morphine relieves pain either by elevating the perception threshold of pain stimuli or by altering the patient's response to painful stimuli. In the latter action, this drug remains superior to other narcotics and as a result is uniquely applicable to the trauma victim, in whom profound responses (more profound than apparent stimuli warrant) may mask morbid injury or exaggerate minimal trauma. It is important that the route of administration be standardized and that the dosage be individualized. Undesirable side effects attributed to a specific drug are too frequently caused by lack of attention to the individual need of the patient.

Route of administration

Considering that all agents administered by either the intramuscular or the subcutaneous route require a relatively long period of time for absorption and that ideally the physician should be able to observe the effects of the analgesia, the intravenous route is the preferred method of administration. Direct injection into the bloodstream avoids the risks associated with inconstant absorption and minimizes considerations associated with using this route in the trauma victim. First, the drug should be given in markedly reduced dosages; second, the physician who administers the narcotic should remain in attendance to observe the immediate effects.

The frequent occurrence of cardiovascular shock is another reason for administering morphine intravenously to a trauma victim. Whether hypotension is present, impending, or a possible eventuality, the intravenous route assures controlled regulation of observable and effective therapy. Morphine should never be given via the subcutaneous or intramuscular route to patients in shock. During World War II it was observed that a number of the soldiers who received morphine on the battlefield experienced narcotic overload (respiratory depression in particular) once they reached the aid station and received definitive care. Morphine that sequestered in the periphery while the patient was in shock would suddenly be absorbed into the circulation all at once as administered blood or colloid returned blood pressure toward normal. Clinically, ineffectiveness secondary to lack of absorption (because of peripheral vascular collapse) may precipitate a second or third "shot for relief of pain." Toxic overdosage then results when the peripheral circulation suddenly becomes effective and several doses are absorbed at once. This potential danger, particularly in a cold environment, exists in any acutely injured patient and should constantly be borne in mind.

Individualized dosage

The ultimate determination of dosage depends on the patient's metabolic activity, which varies with age. Basal levels of metabolism are increased by pain and anxiety and decreased by debilitating diseases.

Although therapeutic levels of morphine affect cardiovascular dynamics minimally, excessive amounts will depress both respiration and vascular responses to oligemia. A safe dosage of morphine for the average adult is 0.05 to 0.1 mg per kg of body weight, diluted to a 10 to 20 ml volume. Injection through a 25-gauge needle will slow administration and thereby overcome a natural tendency for rapid injection. One should allow a minimum of 2 to 3 minutes for administering the total calculated amount and should then wait 10 to 15 minutes before giving additional drug. Experience with slow intravenous administration of diluted morphine sulfate, repeated if necessary, will produce the desired analgesia with minimal risk of diagnostic error, therapeutic complications, or iatrogenic catastrophe. Drugs are never given to relieve pain and restlessness when one is evaluating possible acute head injury. In those few instances in which convulsions or hyperactivity are too intense to allow accurate evaluation of suspected coexisting injury, 1 ml of paraldehyde may be diluted to a 10 ml total volume and administered intravenously.

QUESTIONS

1. Explain what is meant by the expression *narcotic obtundation of subclinical pathology.*
2. Certain factors of patient care in the emergency room may obviate the administration of analgesia to the acutely injured patient. Discuss these factors of patient care.
3. What particular aspects of patient behavior may easily be misinterpreted as severe pain in acutely injured patients?
4. Why is the discussion of analgesia in this chapter limited largely to administration of morphine sulfate?
5. What, if any, are the indications for administration of analgesia to the emergency care patient prior to evaluation by the physician who will be responsible for his care?
6. Drugs to relieve pain and restlessness are never given during evaluation of what specific injury—and for what rather obvious reasons?
7. Discuss the rationale involved in using the intravenous route for administration of morphine sulfate to a trauma victim.
8. Explain the relationship between the basic metabolic rate of the patient and individualization of analgesic dosage.
9. Briefly list three specific situations in which erroneous interpretation of clinical behavior may precipitate a vicious circle of diagnostic-therapeutic error.
10. For what reasons is response to pain not necessarily related to the severity of the trauma in a given situation?

PART THREE

Reaching the victim

CHAPTER 7

Rescue and extrication

FRANKLIN L. MITCHELL

EXTRICATION FROM AN AUTOMOBILE

An automobile crash resulting in serious injury does not always allow easy access to the injured person. Basic rescue and extrication equipment must be available in every ambulance, and the emergency medical technician must be well trained in the use of the equipment. The institution of lifesaving procedures is too critical to await the arrival of special rescue teams or equipment.

Minimal recommended ambulance extrication equipment*

1. Wrench, 12 inches, open end
2. Screwdriver, 12 inches, regular blade
3. Screwdriver, 12 inches, Phillips type
4. Hacksaw, 12-wire carbide blades
5. Pliers, 10 inches, visegrip
6. Hammer, 5 pounds, 15-inch handle
7. Fire-ax butt, 15-inch handle
8. Wrecking bar, 24 inches
9. Crowbar, 51 inches
10. Bolt cutter, 1, ¼-inch jaw
11. Portable power jack and spreader tool
12. Shovel, 49 inches, with pointed blade
13. Double action tin snips, 8 inches
14. Manila ropes, 2, 50 feet long, ¾-inch diameter
15. Rated chain with grab hook and running hook, 15 feet long
16. Fire extinguishers
17. Optional equipment:
    a. Power winch, front-mounted
    b. Power saw

In extricative maneuvers always bear in mind the following: *save the life, prevent further injury,* and *do not move the patient until he is stabilized.* Rescue and extrication procedures follow a logical sequence of events.

Achieve access to the patient. The emergency medical technician may need to

---

*List prepared by the American College of Surgeons.

enter the wrecked vehicle to maintain an airway or stop bleeding before extrication begins. If easy access is not apparent, entry through the rear window is frequently possible; otherwise forcing of doors or roof removal becomes necessary. *Never return a vehicle to the upright position* to gain access. Additional injury to the victim will undoubtedly result.

Initiate emergency medical care. Begin medical treatment as soon as access is achieved. Priorities of care are mentioned in Chapter 9. Stay with the victim while others proceed with extrication maneuvers. If extrication is prolonged, intravenous fluids may be initiated at this time.

Disengage automobile from patient. Peel the automobile from around the victim gently. With the listed equipment, steering wheels can be cut away, brake pedals divided, dashboards elevated, seats forced backward, doors popped open, and sheet metal skinned off. Never use the power saw unless firefighting equipment is present.

Stabilize the patient. Prevent additional injury. Before removing the patient from the vehicle, splint fractures, apply a short backboard, and dress wounds. Any *unconscious* patient is assumed to have a spine injury until proved otherwise.

Remove patient from vehicle. Make the portal of exit large enough to allow removal of the victim under your complete control. Apply long splints immediately after extrication if not previously possible. Do not remove the patient from the backboard.

GENERAL RESCUE AND EXTRICATION

Entrapments of a simple nature are handled in the same manner as automobile entrapments. As entrapments become higher above the ground, deeper below the ground, or under heavier material, specialists in rescue technique are essential. Usually fire departments are prepared for heavier rescue needs. Ambulance services, emergency rooms, and central dispatches should keep a ready list of the specialists who are capable of the various types of rescue work in their area.

Extrication techniques relating exclusively to automobile accidents include the important principles which are as follows:

1. Elimination of possible hazards to rescue personnel and on-lookers, such as live wires and gasoline spills
2. Penetration of the vehicle by rescue personnel to attend to life-threatening conditions such as airway obstruction and hemorrhage and to reassure the victim
3. Application of splints or a spine board if necessary
4. Removal of any part of the vehicle pinning in the victim and preventing safe extrication
5. Finally, removal of the properly splinted and bandaged patient for safe transport to a medical facility

These principles apply whether the victim is trapped in an automobile wreck, buried in a cave-in, or trapped in a collapsed building. Many jurisdictions have trained rescue personnel available, usually in the fire service. Where such service is not available, ambulance attendants must have some rescue capabilities and must carry certain minimum equipment for extrication. Frequently in rural and suburban localities the victims must await the arrival of the tow truck before being released from the wrecked vehicle; such a delay may well prove fatal. Adequate training in this phase of emergency care is very important since overturned vehicles are still being righted with victims in them, or victims are being improperly removed from a cave-in or collapsed building. Such improper handling is very likely to unnecessarily aggravate already serious injuries and can be prevented with proper training and supervision by the medical profession.

QUESTIONS

1. Name the three basic steps to bear in mind during extrication maneuvers.
2. What is assumed regarding any unconscious patient until proved otherwise?
3. Why should a vehicle never be returned to the upright position to gain access to the patient?

CHAPTER 8

Transportation

FRANKLIN L. MITCHELL

Medical care begins at the site of an accident or a sudden illness. The emergency medical care that the patient receives before he arrives in the emergency room may irreversibly influence his morbidity or mortality. Just as a physician has an obligation to monitor and improve the quality of the medical care given in his hospital, it seems no less important that he be knowledgeable of the ambulance and the personnel who transport his critically ill or injured patient. Ambulance service must be considered an integral part of the total medical care of the patient. Studies of emergency care reveal that 20% of persons killed in automobile crashes could have been saved if adequately trained ambulance service had been available. Recent work with trained mobile coronary care units has shown a significant reduction in deaths from myocardial infarctions. Increasing emphasis is being given to the prehospital medical care of the patients with excellent results.

The ambulance and its personnel should be thought of as an extension of the emergency room. The personnel need to be at least as well trained as the personnel who work in the emergency room. The equipment should complement the skills of the ambulance personnel. Medical students and physicians have an obligation to understand and improve the quality of their ambulance services.

GENERAL CONSIDERATIONS

Ambulance service guidelines include the following:
1. Two *trained* technicians on every ambulance call
2. Equipment to complement ability of technicians
3. Patient compartment space sufficient for resuscitation
4. Maximum of *two critically ill patients* in the ambulance
5. Two-way voice radio communication with hospital emergency room
6. Central dispatch for the area
7. No exceeding of posted speed limits
8. Written record of patient condition and treatment
9. No patient moved before emergency medical care given

The general priorities of emergency room medical care are followed in prehospital emergency treatment.
1. Save the life
2. Prevent additional injury
3. Transport the patient

Basic emergency medical care requires that any life-threatening condition be corrected at the site and be controlled during transportation. First consideration must be always given to conditions that threaten the patient's life (for example, airway obstruction, hemorrhage, shock).

Second priority is given to those conditions that may increase morbidity during movement or transportation. Injuries or illnesses that may be compounded by movement must be stabilized before transportation is begun (for example, spine injuries and fractures). Only the removal of the patient from a hostile environment, such as a burning car, takes precedence over these procedures.

AMBULANCE PERSONNEL

Ambulance personnel work independently of physician supervision most of the time. They make immediate decisions that may affect the ultimate outcome for the patient. They must be considered members of the medical team if effective medical care is to be achieved. An exchange of ideas must occur between emergency room physicians, medical students, nurses, and ambulance personnel if continued excellence is to be achieved.

National emphasis is being given to the paramedical profession of emergency medical technicians. A National Registry of Emergency Medical Technicians was established in 1971. The following is the topic outline of a suggested 81-hour basic training program for emergency medical technicians. This program was developed by the U.S. Department of Transportation, National Highway Traffic Safety Administration, American Academy of Orthopaedic Surgeons, American College of Surgeons, International Rescue and First Aid Association, and the National Research Council.

Curriculum	Hours
Responsibilities and equipment of emergency medical technicians	3
Airway obstruction and pulmonary arrest	3
Mechanical aids to breathing and pulmonary resuscitation	3
Cardiac arrest	3
Bleeding, shock—practice airway and cardiac resuscitation	3
Practice and test of above	3
Wounds and dressings	3
Fractures—upper extremity	3
Fractures—lower extremity	3
Injuries—head, face, neck, spine	3
Injuries—eye, chest, abdomen, pelvis	3
Practice and test of above	5
Medical emergencies—poisons, bites, heart attack, stroke, asthma	3
Medical emergencies—acute abdomen, infectious diseases, emotionally disturbed, alcoholic, epileptic, unconscious patient	3
Childbirth	3
Lifting and moving patients	3
Practice and test of above	3
Environmental emergencies—burns, heat, drowning, gas poisoning	3
Extrication from automobiles	3
Defensive driving—records—communications	3

Ambulance call procedures	3
Situational review	3
Final testing—practical and written	3
In-hospital experience—operating room, emergency room, delivery room, intensive care unit	10

This constitutes the minimum background training ambulance personnel should have. Do your ambulance personnel have this background?

Department of Transportation Advanced Emergency Medical Technician Training Program

The definition of a paramedic is open-ended as to how advanced the training of the individual must be, beyond the minimum. Paramedic courses show marked variation in minimum requirements. Of known courses, classroom hours vary from 68 to 720 hours and clinical experience varies from 16 to 800 hours. Most states have enabling legislation for paramedic activities. The individual state minimum training requirements also vary greatly.

In 1976 the U.S. Department of Transportation developed a detailed course for the emergency medical technician–paramedic. This course will be the nationally accepted norm. Because of the wide variation in state law requirements and present advanced emergency medical technician courses, and because of differing actual local needs, the course recommendations are flexible.

To provide flexibility in the course, the curriculum content is broken into medically related modules. The modules may be taken separately, in various combinations, or as a total course. As the levels of advanced emergency medical care may vary in local communities, so may the breadth of training vary. However, certification as an emergency medical technician–paramedic can be achieved only by completing all of the modules.

The curriculum content and objectives are outlined in detail. The actual lecture hours are presented as "average" hours required. The practical experience is not designated in hours but, more appropriately, as achievement of skill, proficiency, and competency. The advanced emergency medical technician continues clinical training until he has mastered the skills necessary to achieve the stated objectives.

The Department of Transportation Advanced Emergency Medical Technician Training Program provides many essential but frequently overlooked details that serve to ensure an organized course of good quality:

1. Course guide
2. Instructor lesson plan
3. Student study guide
4. Course planning considerations
5. Course implementation considerations
6. Detailed objectives and skills
   a. Emergency medical technician–paramedic
   b. Each module
7. Course outline to meet national standards of advanced emergency medical technicians
8. Optional skills of proved emergency medical care value

The emphasis of this training program has been on the development of student competencies irrespective of the number of hours required to develop those competencies. Further, the program allows for flexibility with respect to the level of knowledge required and the types of intermediate levels that can be identified.

To further explain the problem of the number of hours required for the training program, the following is presented. In a survey of some 30 training programs, each claiming to educate advanced-level emergency medical technicians, the number of classroom hours required ranged from 68 to 720 hours with a mean of 228 hours. The clinical experience had an equivalent variance with the range of 16 to 800 hours and a mean of 345 hours. As can be seen, in different states and different institutions varying amounts of time are required to complete the training.

Because of variances in training requirements, it is recommended that the medical director and course coordinator evaluate the program and determine the number of hours they think appropriate. The number of hours selected is, of course, only a reference to be used when planning the course and should not be used as a measure of successful completion.

Table 8-1 provides an *average* number of hours required to present each module. The hours presented should *not* be considered absolute, but should be used merely as a reference for planning. Table 8-2 gives prerequisites for these modules.

A well-documented and consistent training program is essential to obtain a uniform quality of advanced emergency medical technicians throughout the United States. I am hopeful that those persons contemplating advanced emergency medical technician training will review and consider the U.S. Department of Transportation Advanced Emergency Medical Technician Training Program. It is thoughtfully conceived, described in detail, and based on the experience of many advanced training programs.

Table 8-1. Average hours by module (for planning purposes only)*

Module	Average hours
I. The emergency medical technician	3.0
II. Human systems and patient assessment	10.0
III. Shock and fluid therapy	12.0
IV. General pharmacology	9.0
V. Respiratory system	27.0
VI. Cardiovascular system	48.0
VII. Central nervous system	12.0
VIII. Soft tissue injuries	10.0
IX. Musculoskeletal system	10.0
X. Medical emergencies	12.0
XI. Obstetric and gynecologic emergencies	12.0
XII. Pediatrics and neonatal transport	8.0
XIII. Emergency care of the emotionally disturbed	8.0
XIV. Rescue techniques	(Local option)
XV. Telemetry and communications	4.0
TOTAL	185.0 hours

* Excluding clinical experience.

Table 8-2. Prerequisites and clinical experience by module

Module	Prerequisite modules	Clinical experience*
I. The emergency medical technician	—	—
II. Human systems and patient assessment	I	Emergency department, ICU/CCU, morgue
III. Shock and fluid therapy	I, II	Emergency department, operating room, IV team
IV. General pharmacology	I, II, III	—
V. Respiratory system	I, II, III, IV	ICU/CCU, operating room, morgue
VI. Cardiovascular system	I, II, III, IV, V, XV	Emergency department, ICU/CCU
VII. Central nervous system	I, II, III, V	—
VIII. Soft tissue injuries	I, II, III, V, VII	Emergency department, operating room
IX. Musculoskeletal system	I, II, III, V, VII, VIII	Emergency department, operating room
X. Medical emergencies	I, II, III	—
XI. Obstetric and gynecologic emergencies	I, II, III	Obstetrics
XII. Pediatrics and neonatal transport	I, II, III	Pediatrics
XIII. Emergency care of the emotionally disturbed	I, II, III	Psychiatrics
XIV. Rescue techniques	I, II	—
XV. Telemetry and communications†	—	—

*Each program should include a vehicle internship with the trainee under the direct supervision of an experienced preceptor.
†The module dealing with communications should be included in any training program.

EQUIPMENT

The American College of Surgeons has established a guideline list of essential equipment for ambulances. This is a basic and minimum list.

1. Portable suction apparatus
2. Hand operated bag-mask ventilation unit
3. Oropharyngeal airways
4. Mouth-to-mouth artificial ventilation airways
5. Portable oxygen equipment with transparent masks
6. Mouth gags
7. Compartmentalized pneumatic trousers with inflation equipment
8. Universal dressings—10 × 36 inches
9. Sterile gauze pads—4 × 4 inches
10. Soft roller, self-adhering bandages—6 inches × 5 yards
11. Roll of aluminum foil—18 × 25 inches, sterile

12. Plain adhesive tape—3 inches
13. Two sterile burn sheets
14. Hinged half-ring lower extremity traction splint
15. Uncomplicated inflatable splints
16. Short and long spine boards
17. Triangular bandages
18. Large safety pins
19. Shears for bandages
20. Sterile obstetric kit
21. Poison kit
22. Blood pressure manometer, cuff, and stethoscope
23. Two-way radio to emergency department of a hospital
24. Light-duty extrication equipment

Emergency medical technicians-paramedics may well use additional equipment, especially if they are hospital based or linked by radio to the emergency room. This equipment would include the following:

1. Drug injection kit
2. Electrocardiograph—defibrillator
3. Cricothyrotome set
4. Pleural decompression set
5. Intravenous fluids with administration kits
6. Tracheal intubation set
7. Telemetry equipment

THE AMBULANCE

The ambulance should be envisioned as a four-wheel emergency room that could substitute for a treatment room in the emergency department. This room must have adequate space for the patient, emergency medical technician, emergency equipment, supply storage, and working area. There must be sufficient head room to enable attendants to effectively give cardiac resuscitation and administer intravenous fluids by gravity flow. (An unforgettable sight is the arrival of a hearse-type ambulance with the intravenous fluids being held out the window by the attendant.) The minimal workable internal dimensions of the patient compartment are as follows:

1. Minimum height—54 inches
2. Minimum width—72 inches
3. Minimum length—110 inches

Most modern ambulances are of the van type design or camper body–truck chassis configuration. Both meet these criteria for space.

Adequate power is needed to operate the medical equipment. Power for speed is unnecessary. Rarely will exceeding the speed limit favorably influence the patient's outcome. Much more commonly, the ambulance becomes involved in another accident, which can result in additional injury or death. Adequately trained technicians will have stabilized their patient and do not require excessive speed. A speeding ambulance indicates the presence of a sick patient with an untrained attendant.

COMMUNICATIONS

Too often an ambulance carrying a medical emergency victim arrives unannounced at the hospital. The staff is performing routine duties, and the physicians are not immediately available. Unnecessary loss of valuable time occurs.

Two-way radio communication between the ambulance and emergency room of each hospital is essential for effective and efficient medical care. The ambulance personnel will alert the emergency room regarding the condition of the patient being transported. If necessary the emergency room physician can give advice in the care of the patient to the emergency medical technicians.

Advanced ambulance services are sending electrocardiographs and other vital signs by radio telemetry to the hospital emergency room. Not only is the emergency room physician alerted as to the problem but also he can direct that additional appropriate medications or treatment be given by the ambulance personnel.

Ideally, each community should have a central dispatch for all emergency requests and responses. This provides coordination of fire, law enforcement, and health facilities.

QUESTIONS

1. State the minimum workable internal dimensions of the patient compartment of the ambulance.
2. Medical care begins at the site of an accident or a sudden illness. True or False? Explain.
3. What should be thought of as an extension of the emergency room?
4. Name the three general priorities of prehospital emergency treatment.

CHAPTER 9

Principles in management of multiple injuries

The emergency victim probably engenders more feelings of inadequacy in the examiner than any other regularly encountered medical problem. Confusion, frustration, and doubts of one's adequacy result from the simultaneous involvement of a large number of organ systems. By observing established principles of diagnosis and management, however, many pitfalls presented by the patient with multiple injuries can be avoided.

IS THE SITUATION LIFE THREATENING?

When faced with the responsibility of giving immediate care to an injured person, one can often assume that more than one organ system is involved. The first question to be answered is whether or not a life-threatening situation is present.

1. If the patient appears to be well oxygenated, is breathing without evidence of obstruction, and is conscious, the likelihood of any major respiratory problems is diminished.
2. If the patient's peripheral pulses are full and regular, if the skin is warm and dry, and if there are no outward signs of major blood loss, then the likelihood of an exsanguinating hemorrhage is diminished.
3. If the patient is able to communicate the lack of any neck or back distress, if there is no numbness or tingling in the hands or feet, and if the patient is able to move all extremities without difficulty, then there is a reduced likelihood of any injury to the spinal cord.
4. If the patient is conscious and relatively alert, he will generally be able to point to any obvious fracture site because of the pain and tenderness involved.

SPECIFIC PRIORITIES

Any effective management of the patient with multiple injuries is obviously predicated on an adequate system of priorities. Usually these priorities are centered on the necessity for establishing airway adequacy, recognition of and effective efforts to slow or stop exsanguinating hemorrhage with resultant hypovolemic shock, and, of course, the immediate institution of cardiopulmonary resuscitative techniques should circulatory arrest have occurred. Each of these priorities is a subject of detailed discussion in subsequent chapters.

Needless to say, the ability to maintain an adequate airway under even the most adverse situations and to thus allow for adequate respiratory exchange is a skill in which one should be well versed from the beginning. Similarly, an adequate ability to artificially maintain the circulation by closed-chest resuscitation should be a part of the armamentarium one takes to any emergency situation.

BLOOD LOSS

One should make an absolute effort to estimate blood loss not only at the scene of the accident but also during the trip to the hospital and in the emergency room. One should not hesitate to remove as much of the victim's clothing as may be required for immediate assessment of the necessary priorities.

PREVENTION OF ASPIRATION

One can take certain preventive measures at the scene of the accident or on the way to the emergency room that might be of a lifesaving nature. For example, many patients vomit shortly after an accident, regardless of the seriousness of the accident. To prevent aspiration of vomitus, the patient should be positioned so that his head is turned to the side. Any standard ambulance can provide an adequate suction apparatus to use in clearing the airway. Few situations permit giving the emergency patient liquids by mouth.

VITAL SIGNS

It will be helpful to establish baselines regarding all vital signs so that when the patient arrives in the emergency room any deviation from usually accepted norms can be evaluated. This is the subject of Chapter 5.

The suspicion of a rupture of the spleen or trauma to the intra-abdominal viscera should always be present if there has been any likelihood of a blow to or penetration of the abdomen. When the patient is seen in the emergency room, it is helpful to know what the abdominal findings were immediately after the accident.

Before moving the patient to the ambulance, one generally has time to inspect the head for any evidence of obvious injury to the skull or evidence of bleeding from the ears or nose, as well as observing any asymmetry of the pupils.

OBTAINING AN ADEQUATE HISTORY

Once the patient arrives at the emergency room of the hospital, there are a number of definitive examinations that can obviously be carried out immediately. At the scene of the accident evaluation is much more difficult. Because of the above-mentioned priorities, it is important to realize that evaluation and treatment may need to go hand in hand. In addition to careful attention to the all-important priorities, one should obtain as much of a reconstruction of the accident as possible. Were there witnesses? If so, they should be questioned closely to obtain valuable leads as to the nature of the impact, velocity on impact, and such further points as will help to evaluate anatomic areas that may have received the brunt of the force applied. For example, if one of the victims has been thrown against the steering wheel, the possibility of intrathoracic trauma including flail chest, hemothorax, pneumothorax, and cardiac tamponade should be considered. Was there a period of temporary unconsciousness? Did the victim walk about? Each of these observations deserves careful consideration.

TRIAGE OF THE INJURED

The initial management of simultaneous injury to a number of patients deserves some special consideration.

In cases of disaster such as tornadoes, fires, airplane crashes, or any accident that involves a number of persons, the concept of *triage* becomes important. Triage is simply another name for a sorting out of casualties so that the maximum effect can be achieved in the saving of lives and the prevention of crippling injuries by establishing proper treatment priorities based on the initial examination. Because of the need for hospitals to have a disaster plan, many persons have participated in a simulated hospital disaster program during which they have served as victims, stretcher bearers, aides, or various types of assistants.

During these disaster drills one is exposed to the various aspects of a disaster preparedness plan. These include an adequate notification system for all personnel and a continuous communication line using telephones, walkie-talkies, and other means of communication. Traffic control, equipment distribution, and the various logistics of transportation all play a part in the exercise.

At each sorting location it is essential that an adequate written record be maintained of any pertinent observations and any subsequent treatment rendered. Because the clinical picture may vary considerably within a short period of time, it is most important for the physician treating the patient to have a complete account of all findings.

Sorting of casualties occurs at several places along the line. Basically, *triage is an establishment of proper priorities* regarding each patient and the needs for his effective care. Effective triage allows for immediate attention to patients with airway insufficiency problems, hemorrhage, and cardiorespiratory collapse. Every effort is made to avoid diversion to less urgent problems and to center on the life-threatening ones.

SUMMARY

If broad general principles are recognized in the management of the injured person, a sizable percentage of stabilized patients will reach the hospital where definitive care can be administered. It is estimated that approximately 20% of the traffic fatalities in the United States could be averted if proper attention were given at the scene of the accident to maintenance of the airway, control of hemorrhage, and recognition of the potential presence of severe neurologic injury. Much of this book is devoted to these key considerations.

QUESTIONS

1. Explain the importance of adequate triage in emergency situations.
2. How much time should be spent in assessing which aspects of an emergency are life threatening?
3. Briefly list specific priorities in the administration of emergency care.
4. Explain the statement that evaluation and treatment need to go hand in hand.
5. What special challenge lies in the treatment of the patient with multiple injuries?

PART FOUR

Cardiorespiratory emergencies

CHAPTER 10

Airway obstruction

Few emergencies create such panic in the victim or in the observer as sudden airway obstruction. There are few considerations of an emergency nature that require a more thorough understanding of the anatomy and physiology involved than those associated with the respiratory emergency. Cardiopulmonary resuscitation has been considered in some detail in Chapter 12. A number of the principles considered in that chapter are also applicable here. Furthermore, Chapter 11, Near Drowning, includes special aspects of artificial ventilation.

Airway emergencies include a wide range of etiologic factors. According to the National Safety Council, there were 3,100 deaths from foreign body obstruction of the airway in 1975. Aspirated foreign bodies are responsible for an inordinately large percentage of accidental deaths of young children, and in adults there is the condition termed the cafe coronary. Airway obstruction can also be caused by such factors as the tongue of an unconscious person.

Complete obstruction of the airway for any period lasting between 5 and 10 minutes will cause death. The resulting accumulation of carbon dioxide obviously represents an emergency of almost exactly the same proportions as does sudden cessation of cardiac output. The heart may continue to beat, in fact, for several minutes under conditions of asphyxia, but all available oxygen stores are rapidly depleted, cardiac output becomes ineffective, and ventricular fibrillation may begin.

Airway obstruction should be easily recognized, but this is not always the case. Merely positioning the unconscious patient, neck in a partially flexed position with neck muscles and head relaxed, may be sufficient to obstruct the airway even if the tongue does not become so relaxed as to press against the posterior pharyngeal wall. Not all victims become cyanotic. Vasodilatation may be initiated by hypoxemia; therefore even the color of the nail beds, mucous membranes, or conjunctiva may be misleading, particularly if the patient is a dark-skinned person. The presence or absence of noticeable respiratory movements of the chest or abdomen cannot be relied on. Patients who are somnolent from hypercarbia or those suffering from massive drug overdoses may present such a profound state of hypoventilation that one may need to hold a wisp of cotton in front of the mouth or nose to detect any air current. There are various degrees of partial airway obstruction. Depending on the degree of obstruction, intrathoracic pressure fluctuations are increased along with the efforts of breathing. Gradually the respiratory center becomes less sensitive to the usual stimulation from a buildup of carbon dioxide.

Marked activity of the accessory muscles of respiration in the neck and supraclavicular and intercostal areas should alert one to the presence of severe or even complete airway obstruction. If the airway obstruction is complete, no air flow can be heard; if it is incomplete, various degrees of noise intensity may be provoked, depending on the degree of obstruction. Snoring is probably the best known example of partial airway obstruction and is produced simply by hypopharyngeal obstruction by the tongue. The wheezing effect of the asthmatic patient caused by partial bronchial obstruction is well known. Laryngospasm produces a characteristic crowing sound. Foreign matter obstructing the airway may occasionally produce a gurgling noise.

CAFE CORONARY

The phrase *cafe coronary* was coined by Haugen to describe a condition that appears to be a sudden heart attack but that is actually a result of sudden airway obstruction by food while the victim is eating. The victim whose airway is suddenly obstructed by a large bolus of food is unable to cough, speak, or breathe if the obstruction is complete. After clutching at his throat the victim becomes cyanotic and collapses. Gordon recommends that if the victim can cough, speak, or breathe, no action is necessary except the victim's own spontaneous coughs. One must act immediately, however, if the victim cannot cough, speak, or breathe.

BASIC PROCEDURES FOR OPENING THE AIRWAY
"Artificial cough" maneuvers

There are three basic maneuvers designed to produce an "artificial cough" to clear the airway. These are abdominal compression (the Heimlich maneuver), low chest compression, and back blows.

Abdominal compression. Few emergency care measures have received such widespread interest among laymen as the so-called Heimlich maneuver for removing the foreign body obstruction of the airway by manual upper abdominal compression.

In doing the abdominal thrust, one should never place one's hands on the xiphoid process of the sternum or on the lower margin of the rib cage. One stands behind the victim and wraps one's arms around the victim's waist and grasps one's fist with one's other hand. The thumb side of the fist should be placed against the victim's abdomen between the xiphoid and the umbilicus. The fist can be pressed into the victim's abdomen with a quick, upward thrust.

If the victim is lying down, one should position him with the face up (supine) and place one's knees close to his hips. The heel of one's hand should be placed against the victim's abdomen between the xiphoid and umbilicus. The other hand should be placed on top of the first and pressed into the victim's abdomen with a *quick upward thrust.*

If one is alone and has choked on food, one can perform this maneuver on oneself by pressing the fist into the upper abdomen with a quick upward thrust or by leaning forward and pressing one's abdomen abruptly against a firm object. Gordon believes that chest compression should probably be used in preference to abdominal compression, which may initiate regurgitation and aspiration when the patient is in a supine position.

Abdominal compression also has, on occasion, produced laceration of the liver or rupture of the stomach.

Chest compression. While there are no significant differences in the airflow, pressure, and volume between abdominal and chest compression, the latter is best used in advanced pregnancy and in markedly obese individuals.

Guildnar recommends that if one witnesses a so-called cafe coronary and the victim is unable to talk, cough, groan, or breathe, total obstruction is probably present. One should quickly position oneself behind the patient (often still standing or sitting), lean the patient forward, and promptly and vigorously apply the low chest squeeze. The technique can be utilized with children by placing only one arm around the chest. The rescuer should pick up the child and invert him over the rescuer's arm while administering a quick compression between the shoulder blades.

Chest compression may produce fractures of the ribs, pneumothorax, or both.

Back blows. The National Research Council for Emergency Medical Services recommends a rapid series of sharp blows delivered with the heel of the hand over the spine between the shoulder blades. These back blows may be given with the patient in a sitting, standing, or lying position. They should be applied rapidly with force.

If the victim is standing or sitting, one should deliver the forceful blows with the heel of one's hand over the patient's spine between the shoulder blades from a position slightly behind him, or he can be supported by placing one's other hand on the chest. Ideally the head should be lower than the chest in order that gravity may aid in the release of the foreign body from the patient's throat. Therefore if the victim is lying down, one should kneel and roll him onto his side so that he faces the rescuer with his knees against his chest. In this manner one can deliver sharp blows to the back in the same area as when the patient is standing or sitting.

In small children and infants with complete airway obstruction, the patient should be placed face down on one's forearm with the head down. Sharp blows are then delivered to the back.

Eliminating obstruction by tongue

The hypopharynx can be opened in 70% to 80% of unconscious victims simply by tilting the head backward. By simply tilting the victim's head backward as far as possible, one can open the airway in most instances. However, if this is not the case, one can perform the head-tilt maneuver by placing one hand beneath the victim's neck and the other on his forehead. The tongue is lifted away from the back of the throat when the neck is in this extended position by lifting the neck with one hand and tilting the head backwards by pressure with the other hand on the forehead.

Neck lift. The National Research Council's Emergency Medical Services Committee recently identified several difficulties with the neck-lift technique. Cervical spine injuries, to the extent of fracture with cord transection, may result from the use of excessive force in the neck-lift procedure. The main application of the technique is in the unconscious patient with absent respiratory movements. In such instances, the neck should be lifted gently, with extension of the head occurring at the occipitoatlantal articulation. The neck should be lifted by placing the hand close to the occiput so that cervical spine hyperextension can be prevented.

Jaw thrust. If airway patency in the apneic, unconscious patient is not effectively achieved by the neck-lift method, the jaw-thrust maneuver should be instituted. By placing one's fingers behind the angles of the patient's jaw and forcefully displacing the mandible forward at the same time, one can tilt the head backward. In addition, one's thumbs are used to retract the lower lip to allow breathing through the mouth as well as the nose. The jaw-thrust maneuver is aided if the rescuer's elbows rest on the same surface as the patient.

Chin lift. If the unconscious patient is breathing spontaneously, the chin-lift maneuver is recommended. In so doing, one lifts the lower jaw and moves it forward with the fingers of one hand. This maneuver brings the tongue forward and away from the back of the throat. The rescuer's other hand tilts the head back by pressing on the victim's forehead. Although the lips remain separated, the chin should be brought forward so that the teeth are nearly together. Dentures are allowed to remain in place to help provide a mouth-to-mouth seal.

Guildnar compared the three techniques for opening the airway obstructed by the tongue and found that the chin-lift technique provides the most consistent adequate airway. Surprisingly in a large number of unconscious patients the neck-lift method does not relieve the airway obstruction produced by the backward movement of the tongue when the jaw is relaxed. To provide an open airway the lower jaw often needs support to adequately lift the tongue away from the throat. When the chin is lifted, the lower jaw moves forward, followed by the tongue. The chin-lift maneuver has the added advantage of facilitating holding the patient's dentures, if present, securely in position.

Emergency procedure

External cardiac compression is naturally of little value in foreign body obstruction unless both cardiac arrest and foreign body obstruction have occurred. However, if one encounters an unconscious person and there are no witnesses to provide information about the cause of unconsciousness, one obviously is not aware of whether a foreign body obstruction is present. Therefore one should proceed as in a case of unwitnessed cardiac arrest. The following procedure is recommended by Gordon.

1. Kneel at the victim's side.
2. Determine whether he is unconscious.
3. If the patient is unconscious, tilt the head and check for breathing.
4. If the victim is not breathing, give four quick breaths.
5. If you are unable to ventilate him, use the jaw-lift maneuver and attempt one-finger extrication of a foreign body.
6. If this is unsuccessful, roll the victim toward you onto his side and deliver a series of two to four back blows.
7. Roll the victim onto his back and deliver a series of four to six compressions on the side of the chest.
8. Repeat the jaw-lift and one-finger extrication maneuvers, as the foreign body may have been forced into a position where you may then be able to retrieve it.
9. If this is unsuccessful, attempt mouth-to-nose ventilation.
10. If this is unsuccessful, repeat the series of back blows, chest compression, jaw-lift, and finger extrication maneuvers with attempts to ventilate because,

as Gordon emphasizes, the muscles of the victim's throat become increasingly relaxed as the victim becomes more hypoxic; thus the efforts may become increasingly effective.

ARTIFICIAL VENTILATION

Once the airway is patent, artificial ventilation may be satisfactorily accomplished by intermittent inflation of the lungs with positive pressure applied to the airway. Mouth-to-mouth, mouth-to-nose, mouth-to-tube, or a bag-mask ventilation apparatus may be used. In many immediate care situations the most available technique is either mouth-to-mouth or mouth-to-nose ventilation.

During mouth-to-mouth respiration, the nose should be compressed with one hand; the other hand should be used to apply pressure over the patient's upper abdomen and epigastrium to prevent distension of the stomach by air. The mouth of the patient may be covered by several thin layers of gauze, a handkerchief, or even a thin paper towel. Prior to expiration, the operator should take a deep inspiration and then immediately apply his widely opened mouth over the mouth of the patient and made a forcible exhalation. The uninitiated will be surprised at the degree of inflation produced by this method. The patient's chest can be observed to expand as the air is blown into his mouth, and when the operator raises his mouth from that of the patient, a rush of air can be heard coming from the patient's lungs. This latter aspect can be improved by forcible pressure on the patient's chest. As in all other methods of artificial respiration, the tongue must be brought forward, because it may occlude the oral pharynx. Again it should be emphasized that one may have confidence in one's ability to perform mouth-to-mouth respiration when it is recalled that 16 mm Hg pressure is the level of oxygen pressure developed by most of the positive-negative pulmonary resuscitators. Men can exhale with a force of 50 mm Hg, and this pressure may even reach 100 mm Hg. A rate of at least 12 times per minute is suggested. One should exhale twice one's normal resting tidal volume (about 1,000 ml). Inadequate oxygenation is often the result of exhalations that are too slow.

Caution should be observed in the use of mouth-to-mouth respiration with infants, because a pressure may be exerted by the operator that is sufficient to rupture some of the alveoli. As in all types of artificial respiration, there is the problem of keeping the airway patent. This can be aided by pulling the tongue forward or, most ideally, by insertion of the endotracheal tube or catheter. If one uses excessively high inflation pressures during artificial ventilation, some of the air is forced into the stomach by way of an open esophagus. The esophageal obturator airway was developed because of concern about the inflation of the stomach that occurs in the course of routine mouth-to-mouth respiration.

Artificial respiration may be best applied by the mouth-to-nose technique in several instances. For example, the individual applying artificial respiration may be unable to completely seal his mouth around the patient's mouth. If transient rigidity, trismus, or convulsions are present, mouth-to-nose respiration should be used. A patient with a broken jaw may have his teeth wired. Even so, blowing between the teeth may be successful.

The mouth-to-tube device ensures that adequate volume of sufficient gas composition is delivered to the patient. Unlike other forms of artificial respiration, the mouth-to-tube method does not depend on the operator's observation and judgment to determine whether ventilation of the patient is adequate. The mouth-mask or mouth-to-tube methods have advantages over the simple mouth-to-mouth procedure in that both hands of the operator are available to maintain patency of the upper airway. The operator is able to sense any increase in pulmonary resistance by the amount of exertion it takes to deflate his own lungs.

The mouth-to-tube method of respiration has several points in its favor besides that of prevention of hypocapnia in the operator. These include the prevention of cross-contamination between the operator and the patient if a disposable filter is placed in the breathing tube. The method can be continued for long periods of time, and no special position of the patient is required by the operator. The equipment is of minimal expense, and adequate ventilation is ensured despite abnormalities in airway resistance and in lung compliance.

Generally, automatic resuscitators have little place in emergency artificial respiration, particularly in conjunction with cardiac resuscitation. External cardiac compression triggers the termination of the inflation phase prematurely, and flow rates and pressures are usually inadequate.

Mouth-to-mouth or mouth-to-nose ventilation may produce gastric distension and subsequent vomiting; therefore the danger of aspiration is ever present. Gastric distension is common in the infant or child after mouth-to-mouth or mouth-to-nose ventilation because the amount of pressure that allows air to enter the stomach is less. To relieve the gastric distension one should place the infant in the prone position or onto one side while exerting pressure with one hand over the epigastrium between the xyphoid and the umbilicus. By maintaining pressure in the epigastric area, one may help prevent recurrence of gastric distension.

Face masks

Certainly deserving of attention in discussing artificial ventilation is the use of face masks. Valuable time should not be expended in passing an endotracheal tube during the early stages of resuscitation when simple mouth-to-mouth or face-mask-and-bag techniques can more quickly ventilate the patient. The face masks that are available include the simple oronasal mask, the oronasal mask with mouthpiece, and the oronasal mask with bag or bellows. Such masks are successfully used by most physicians, but in the hands of the inexperienced there may be a problem with leakage. Inspiration may occur through the nose, and expiration may be blocked by a valving action of the soft palate.

Respirator bags

Since the AMBU (Air-Mask-Bag Unit) bag was developed by Rubin and reported in the literature in 1955, various types of AMBU systems have evolved that now deliver 100% oxygen. The AMBU bag provides satisfactory artificial respiration by manual compression of the bag, or it may be attached to an endotracheal tube. Self-inflating respirator bags achieve adequate ventilation when they are used with well-fitted face masks or when they are connected to either an endotracheal tube or a tracheostomy tube. There are at least nine commonly used resuscitative bags that all give an increased concentration of oxygen with an increase in oxygen flow, but none gives 100% oxygen when the oxygen flow is twice the minute ventilation. Although it is beyond the scope of this presentation to go into detailed features of each bag, the AMBU, the AMBU compact bag with E-2 valves, and the AIR-VIVA bag seem to be the most suitable ones. The AMBU appears to give a slightly higher percentage of oxygen and the AIR-VIVA is usually easiest to clean and to sterilize. The Lierdal bag has the advantage of extreme portability. Any regurgitation is immediately visible because the bag and mask are transparent.

ARTIFICIAL AIRWAYS

Mouth-to-mouth resuscitation is usually, of necessity, instituted without the advantage of an airway; however, various types are available.

Labiodental airways simply provide a channel through the victim's lips and teeth incorporating a mouth guard to provide a seal and a short blow tube. Unfortunately these airways do not overcome any obstruction in the front of the mouth that may result from opposition of the tongue against the palate. Oral airways are of sufficient length to ensure the passage of air through the victim's lips, teeth, and front of the mouth. Hyperextension of the head prevents obstruction by the tongue and the throat, and in the Brook airway a nylon bite block maintains a channel between the teeth while a mouth guard provides a seal. A flexible extension facilitates resuscitation when the victim must be less than ideally positioned. A nonreturn valve diverts the victim's expired air from the rescuer's mouthpiece.

Pharyngeal airways transverse the victim's mouth and reach the back of the throat. Safar's Resuscitube contains a large mouthpiece to provide a seal. Because of their length, these airways may cause retching or vomiting with subsequent aspiration of stomach contents unless the victim is deeply unconscious. Occasionally the epiglottis may be impacted and the larynx may be obstructed by use of an oversized pharyngeal airway.

The various S-shaped airway adjuncts range from simple pipes with mouthpieces and bite blocks to more elaborate devices that incorporate valves in their construction. The limitations of the S-tubes include the following features:
1. They may induce vomiting if they are improperly used.
2. They do not reduce potential transmission of infection.
3. They require particular attention to safe and effective use.
4. The seal provided is not generally considered to be as effective as that provided by either direct mouth-to-mouth or mouth-to-mask ventilation.
5. They require that the person administering aid move the victim's head and reposition the S-tube to inflate the lungs between chest compressions in the event that cardiac assistance is required. They do, however, offer the useful feature of overcoming aesthetic problems involved in direct mouth-to-mouth contact. They assist in maintaining a patent airway, and they do obviously keep the mouth open.

Esophageal obturator airway

The esophageal obturator airway is a relatively new device that has the advantage of requiring rather minimal training while providing excellent ventilation and preventing aspiration of gastric contents. It consists of an endotracheal tube modified so that it may be inserted into the esophagus instead of into the trachea. An inflatable cuff just proximal to a soft rubber obturator blocks the distal end of the tube. Air injected into this Silastic cuff distends it symmetrically when the attached plastic syringe and check valve are put into operation allowing the syringe to be removed without escape of air. Sixteen serial openings in the upper one third of the tube provide a total opening that exceeds the diameter of the tube itself.

Insertion requires little or no visualization of the anatomic structures. The rescuer merely lifts the mandible between the thumb and index finger of one hand while he inserts the tube into the mouth and pharnyx and advances it into the esophagus with the other hand. With the mask then seated onto the face the rescuer performs mouth-to-airway resuscitation.

The obturator blocks the distal end of the esophageal airway while the air escapes from the openings in the upper portion of the tube and inflates the lungs. Because the openings are located in the back of the mouth and the upper pharynx, fluids do not interfere with ventilation. These reusable tubes provide at least as much ventilation as mouth-to-mask ventilation (since air does not pass into the stomach) and are far easier to introduce than standard endotracheal tubes. Personnel should be trained in their use, first on an anatomically suitable mannequin and then on actual anesthetized patients whenever possible. The airway should never be used with a conscious patient.

Inadvertent tracheal introduction of the tube may occasionally occur, but this has not proved to be a problem in more than 1,000 insertions made in actual cases by highly trained personnel. If the chest rises, the tube is in the esophagus; if the chest does not rise, the tube is in the trachea. If it is in the trachea, it is immediately removed, of course, and some other from of artificial ventilation is used until it can be placed properly.

It should not be removed until appropriate steps have been taken: Adequate suction should be available to clear the airway in case of vomiting, which frequently occurs on removal of the tube. Obviously the cuff of the esophageal airway should always be deflated prior to its removal. The mask may be removed when the patient resumes spontaneous respiration; the tube, however, should be left in place until the patient is reacting or is sufficiently conscious to permit extubation under the previously mentioned conditions.

The stomach should be decompressed prior to the removal of the esophageal airway by passing a nasogastric tube to the area of the cuff in the esophagus, temporarily deflating it while the nasogastric tube is passed into the stomach, and then reinflating it as the stomach is being decompressed. Alternatively, the unconscious patient may have an endotracheal tube introduced while the esophageal obturator airway remains in place. The esophageal airway can be removed without hazard of aspiration after the cuff on the endotracheal tube has been deflated.

The size of the tube (which comes in one adult size only) does not overdistend any normal adult, flaccid esophagus, and it is so designed that the inflatable cuff always lies central to the carina of the trachea in tall individuals and may lie deeper in the esophagus in small or short individuals but will not extend into the stomach. Only about 30 ml of air should be used in inflating the cuff to prevent over distending the esophagus. Rapid and careless introduction, as in any similar procedure, could naturally cause damage to the mucosa and wall of the esophagus, but proper training and care should eliminate this problem.

The esophageal airway's appeal rests largely on the ease with which both physicians and paramedical personnel can be trained in its use in contrast to the training of individuals in tracheal intubation.

Critics of the esophageal airway point out that the inflated cuff is too small to uniformly prevent gastric distension and regurgitation except in small individuals. In addition, blind insertion of the esophageal device into the trachea may produce total airway obstruction and massive gastric distension. If the inflated cuff is inadvertently withdrawn prior to deflating, esophageal lacerations may occur.

Elam's esophageal pharyngeal airway with an inflatable cuff effectively seals the esophagus against regurgitation and gastric inflation. Provision is made for monitoring cardiac sound and cardiac pacing with low wattage, as well as the use of ventricular countershock and defibrillation.

CRICOTHYROID MEMBRANE PUNCTURE

Acute obstructive laryngeal edema from an allergic reaction to penicillin, from hemorrhage into neck tissue planes, or from an engorgement of particulate matter such as food in the larynx provides indications for immediately establishing an airway via the cricothyroid membrane puncture. If an inability to inflate or deflate the lungs is noted during mouth-to-mouth respiration, obstructions of this nature can be suspected. Therefore, if the emergency measures previously listed fail, cricothyroid puncture and insertion of a 6 mm tube have been recommended for adults.

There are several advantages to this approach through a relatively avascular membrane. It is easily reached because of its superficial position and adjacent landmarks of cartilage. The cricothyroid space is large and can accept fairly large tubes. Posterior perforation is unlikely because of the heavy posterior projection of the cricoid cartilage. Elective tracheotomy can be done later if necessary. This approach should not be utilized for much longer than 24 hours.

The larynx is stablized between the left thumb and the middle finger, the skin is incised over the cricothyroid space, and the scapel or scissors is guided down the index finger to puncture the membrane. As soon as the knife blade enters the trachea, the resistance gives way and the incision can be enlarged to at least 1.5 cm. A tracheostomy tube can be put in place if one is available.

If one notices that the suprasternal notch is drawn upward when the patient takes a breath, one may suspect that the foreign body has lodged above the level of the cricothyroid membrane puncture site and that the emergency procedure may be lifesaving.

A "mini-tracheostomy" may be performed wherein a standard intravenous transfusion needle is inserted into the trachea through the cricothyroid membrane. This technique is often used when anesthetic apparatus is unavailable. At negative pressures reached during obstructed inspiration, the volume of air that can be drawn into the needle is believed to be sufficient both to prevent asphyxia and to enable the patient to make forced expiratory efforts. Use of a No. 13 needle may temporarily provide an adequate airway in an infant but it will probably not do so in a child or adult who has an acute obstruction of the upper airway; indeed the percutaneous insertion of a No. 13 needle into the trachea of an infant is not always easy to accomplish. It must be emphasized that, to be effective, cricothyroid membrane puncture should generally be done with a large bore cannula of at least 6 mm to allow for breathing, suctioning, or ventilation.

TRACHEOSTOMY

Tracheostomy is often described and is frequently used as an emergency procedure. Actually it is poorly suited as an emergency technique and for all practical purposes should not be strongly considered at this point. Tracheostomy should be performed under ideal situations, most frequently in the operating room with the patient well oxygenated via an endotracheal tube, if possible. The tracheostomy is best reserved for individuals who will need to have assisted ventilation for a prolonged period of time. Theoretically the tracheostomy might be reserved for upper airway obstruction if the cricothyroid membrane puncture is not effective. Usually the tracheostomy is indicated for patients who, for one reason or another, cannot bring up their secretions. These are usually patients with neurologic trauma or injuries, severe inanition, or chronic lung disease and bronchitis. Patients who have had severe trauma, particularly those with a flail chest, may commonly require a tracheostomy. Patients with conditions such as a fractured larynx or an acutely obstructing carcinoma of the larynx may require an emergency tracheostomy, but in each instance a cricothyroid membrane puncture can be more rapidly accomplished.

Tracheostomy is not a procedure to be lightly considered. Occasionally death results from massive tracheal hemorrhage. The patient with a tracheostomy requires continuous observation by experienced personnel. Complications of the procedure include severe endotracheitis, pneumothorax, improper positioning of the cannula, aspiration, delayed arterial bleeding, atelectasis, diminution of the tracheal lumen, mediastinitis, and wound infections.

Because of the belief that an emergency tracheostomy is generally outside the scope of this book, a detailed description of the technique is not included.

Occasionally a bronchoscopy may be necessary as an emergency procedure for lower airway obstruction, aspiration, and atelectasis. However, this should be reserved for the individual skilled in its use and for an environment in which such a procedure is feasible.

QUESTIONS

1. Define "cafe coronary" and discuss treatment of this emergency.
2. Describe the various artificial airways and delineate their use in airway obstruction.
3. How urgent is the problem of the obstructed airway?
4. Discuss the relative importance of head tilt in treating the obstructed airway.
5. What is the place of tracheal intubation in treatment of the obstructed airway?
6. What is the accepted rationale in the use of the face mask?
7. Discuss the advantages and disadvantages in use of the esophageal airway.
8. What are the indications for use of both cricothyroid membrane puncture and tracheostomy in the management of the obstructed airway? What are the hazards?
9. Describe the technique and precautions of cricothyroid membrane puncture.
10. What is the Heimlich hug and how is it best applied in airway emergencies?

CHAPTER 11

Near drowning

Resuscitation of the nearly drowned patient is basically an extension of the general principles of cardiopulmonary resuscitation. Because of the wide variety of circumstances in which the patient can be involved, there is a need to be familiar with the pathophysiology of the near-drowning patient. New considerations and numerous adjuncts in the management of the near-drowning victim have evolved from some of the conventional approaches used in the past. For example, it is important for the rescuer to realize that precious time should not be spent in an effort to remove water from the patient's lungs, but that the first priority is to establish an airway that allows for assisted ventilation, if needed.

Drowning is the fourth most common cause of accidental death. As a cause of accidental death in young males under 25 years of age it ranks first or second. Because of greatly accelerated interest in water sports, the importance of adequate rescue teams becomes obvious. For example, statistics compiled by the National Surf Lifesaving Association of America from the major lifeguard agencies on the California coast in 1972 indicate that 297 resuscitation attempts were made that year for more than 200 million beach visitations. There were more than 37,000 near-drowning rescues, but the only fatalities were recorded in the unguarded areas.

The complexities of resuscitation of the near-drowning victim may be accentuated by the prior occurrence of a heart attack, or the drowning may have been precipitated by a drug overdose or frequently by the injudicious use of alcohol. Serious injuries may accompany the near-drowning episode, and the victim may have been hit by the propeller or the bow of a boat. The water skier may have been tangled in the guide ropes. More important, a serious spinal cord injury may have precipitated the near-drowning incident. Increasingly larger numbers of apparent drowning victims are divers who had been using self-contained underwater breathing apparatus (SCUBA).

Drowning may, of course, occur in any fluid, but the vast majority of drownings are associated with either fresh or salt water. Drowning in chlorinated pools is common.

Unfortunately each year a number of drownings involve underwater competition or accompany voluntary hyperventilation. Young swimmers should be cautioned against hyperventilation prior to breath holding under water. Normally the partial pressure of carbon dioxide increases after breath holding to the point that an individual cannot resist the urge to breathe. However when hyperventilation occurs, the individual exhales an excessive amount of carbon dioxide, and the increase of the carbon dioxide during the breath hold is slower and the breath holding ability is increased. Partial pressures of oxygen may be decreased to such a dangerously low value that unconsciousness occurs before the urge to breathe becomes excessive. In such instances the swimmer may be unaware that loss of consciousness is eminent and may continue to swim up to the point of collapse. Observers of the swimmers can seldom detect trouble until the collapse occurs.

It is obvious that death by drowning is a costly killer when one considers that the victim is usually young and in a vigorous state of health. Unfortunately drowning is not a reportable accident in most states, and precise figures regarding the frequency of drownings are not available.

IMMEDIATE EFFORTS

Immediate efforts to combat hypoxia should receive top priority. As soon as the victim is removed from the water, one should check for breathing movements. If breathing movements and coughing are present, one should direct efforts to maintain adequate ventilation. The oral airway should be checked quickly, and by sweeping the back of the pharynx, any foreign material should be removed, including dentures. By using the conventional means of establishing an open airway already described in this book, mouth-to-mouth exhaled ventilation should be started promptly. As emphasized repeatedly, efforts to drain water from the lungs usually simply detract from the main effort and do not represent a primary concern. The amount of water aspirated by the victim is seldom sufficient to produce life-threatening changes in serum electrolyte concentration, whereas even small quantities of fluid can produce persistent arterial hypoglycemia. Mouth-to-mouth ventilation enables one to use somewhat greater exhalation pressure than ordinarily employed because of the beneficial effects of positive pressure breathing on any interpulmonary shunts and any pulmonary edema that may be present.

Obviously ventilatory support is of no benefit unless adequate circulatory efforts are taking place. If carotid or femoral pulses cannot be detected, closed-chest cardiac massage should be employed as outlined elsewhere in the book.

An important note of caution should be interjected: The victim may have been submerged in water for periods of a minute or more to even 20 or 25 minutes with eventual recovery. He may have fixed, dilated pupils even after prolonged resuscitative efforts and may remain unconscious for some hours with eventual and complete recovery.

Although transportation of the victim to the nearest medical facility is urgent, it is even more important that adequate attention be given to the ABC's of cardiopulmonary resuscitation at the scene of the accident.

During transportation to the hospital, 100% oxygen administration via positive pressure breathing is desirable. Closed-chest cardiac compression should be continued if there is an ineffective or absent cardiac output. On an empiric basis, an adult may be given an ampule of sodium bicarbonate, intravenously (44.6 mEq), and small children may be given sodium bicarbonate in a dosage of 1 mEq per kilogram of body weight. Maximum ventilatory support is of major importance. Although electrocardiographic monitoring is important, ventricular fibrillation is not commonly encountered in the near-drowning patient, contrary to previous theories that were based on experimentally controlled tests on animals. Marked hypoxia in addition to a profound metabolic acidosis (and in many instances marked hypothermia) may, however, induce ventricular fibrillation. Frequent oronasal suctioning should be instituted as soon as facilities are available. A cuffed endotracheal tube may facilitate ventilation and may prevent aspiration of vomitus during resuscitative procedures. Gastric decompression with nasogastric suction should be instituted.

EMERGENCY ROOM CARE

As soon as the victim arrives at the hospital emergency room, every effort should be directed toward an improvement in pulmonary function and adequate gas exchange. If spontaneous heartbeat has not resumed, then continued efforts should be employed, including intravenously administered 1mg doses of epinephrine. If an endotracheal tube is in place, a mechanical ventilator should be connected for ventilatory support. The use of a positive end expiratory pressure respirator (PEEP) provides an ideal mechanism to adequately remove carbon dioxide and minimize mismatched ventilation perfusion ratios. In any event, intermittent positive pressure breathing (IPPB) with 100% oxygen should be started if positive end expiratory pressure ventilation is not available. In addition to assisting ventilatory control, passage of the endotracheal tube aids in the clearing of pulmonary edema and allows suctioning of vomitus and other particulate matter.

Since further intensive pulmonary care depends on laboratory data, arterial oxygen and carbon dioxide tensions should be determined as well as the acid-base status as provided by the pH and base excess studies. Blood pH levels of less than 6.96 and base deficits of −26 mEq per liter have been reported in near-drowning victims who subsequently recovered.

FURTHER OBSERVATION

As noted, the near-drowning victim may be in any stage of distress. Although the victim may quickly regain consciousness and appear to be reasonably alert, hospitalization is indicated. Serious degrees of pulmonary insufficiency may not become apparent for some hours. Monitoring of the patient in the pulmonary intensive care unit should include careful attention to cardiovascular performance. Whenever possible, a Swan-Ganz catheter should be placed in the pulmonary artery to determine pulmonary capillary wedge pressures and cardiac output. Such a procedure removes much of the guesswork in determining adequate intravascular fluid replacement and the need for cardiotonic drugs.

Whether large doses of corticosteroids should be administered to the near-drowning victim has not been clearly resolved. There are conflicting reports as to the beneficial effect. Proponents urge the intravenous administration of 1 gm of methylprednisolone sodium succinate to assist in maintaining alveolar membrane integrity and to decrease pulmonary inflammation and diminish cerebral edema. As with the use of steroids, no available data indicate that antibiotics should be administered routinely to the near-drowning victim. Ampicillin has often been the antibiotic of choice on an empiric basis to prevent secondary pulmonary complications.

Any rush to obtain a chest film should be resisted so that previously sought priorities can be accomplished. Typically the pneumonitis of the near-drowning victim shows patchy, perihilar infiltration of the lungs that may persist for several days. Antifoaming agents such as 20% to 30% ethyl alcohol (as an aerosol) may be helpful in treating pulmonary edema, and when combined with isoproterenol hydrochloride, they may aid in the treatment of bronchospasm and pulmonary edema. Isoproterenol may be given as a dose of 0.25 ml in 40% alcohol (3 ml) by nebulized IPPB for 5 minutes.

Initially Ringer's lactate may be given intravenously at the rate of 10 ml per kilogram of body weight for the first hour. Plasma is the fluid of choice for both freshwater and saltwater drowning and can be given after adequate oxygenation is established. Because aspirated fresh water finds its way almost immediately into the vascular tree, hemolysis and hemodilution in addition to hypovolemia may be encountered. Therefore the use of packed red blood cells is preferable, although whole blood may be given if the central venous pressure is carefully monitored.

A urinary catheter should be placed and urinary output should be monitored.

QUESTIONS

1. Discuss preexisting medical conditions that may cause complications in the near-drowning victim.
2. What is the significance of hyperventilation in the near-drowning victim?
3. Explain the importance of ECG monitoring in the near-drowning victim.
4. Describe the use of respirators for the near-drowning victim.

CHAPTER 12

Cardiopulmonary resuscitation

This chapter is intended to provide essential information for basic life support of the patient until transportation to an advanced life support station can be accomplished.

Within recent years the training of firemen, policemen, lifeguards, and other rescue workers in the application of cardiopulmonary resuscitative techniques has accelerated. Likewise, training in the basics of resuscitative techniques has been extended into the high schools of the nation and among the lay public. Certainly it seems logical that medical personnel should be exposed as early as possible to a period of sophisticated training in all of the ramifications of effective cardiopulmonary resuscitation. Unfortunately some are completely lacking in the knowledge of even basic resuscitative techniques.

Sudden, unexpected death, in terms of absolute loss of life, does pose the greatest single medical problem today. It is the most common mode of death in the adult population. The actual incidence of sudden death represents almost 30% of all natural deaths. It is estimated that ventricular fibrillation in structurally good hearts occurs more than 900 times a day in the United States in victims outside a hospital. Approximately 70% of deaths from arteriosclerotic heart disease occur in persons who die outside a hospital or who are dead on arrival. Advancements and refinements in cardiopulmonary resuscitation should significantly reduce these deaths. Few, if any, advances have so dramatically altered the area of emergency medical care as the advent and widespread application of mouth-to-mouth ventilation and closed-chest augmentation of circulation.

It should be repeatedly emphasized that the crux of successful resuscitation centers on a realization that time is of the essence in successful resuscitation because irreversible cerebral damage may occur as early as 3½ to 4 minutes after sudden cessation of cerebral circulation. Establishment of an open airway and immediate application of mouth-to-mouth artificial ventilation and closed-chest compression for circulatory augmentation, if applied properly, may maintain life for a lengthy period of time, allowing for further definitive measures to be applied, leading to eventual successful resuscitation of the patient.

Medical personnel are likely to encounter patients requiring resuscitative efforts in a variety of circumstances and always at unexpected moments. Because these personnel are in the proximity of high-risk patients, it behooves them to develop confidence and ability in the application of resuscitative techniques.

RECOGNITION OF CARDIAC ARREST

Cardiac arrest seldom occurs without some warning signs. Yet these signs may be subtle and varied. Frequently the blood pressure and pulse may suddenly disappear and on inspection the heart is found to be in complete standstill or more often fibrillation. Even in a hospital setting, cardiac arrest may well represent a "sudden and unexplained" occurrence. On very sophisticated intensive care wards, a life-threatening arrhythmia may occur without warning. Six instances of ventricular fibrillation and two cases of sudden ventricular tachycardia occurred among 50 patients being monitored by extremely sophisticated equipment in one intensive care study. Previous to the events, no important physiologic changes could be identified in three of these eight patients, but in five cases, there were serious pulmonary malfunctions or ventilatory disturbances prior to the arrhythmia. Hypoventilation and hypercapnia may not be as easy to identify as one might assume because patients often fail to show classic signs of these conditions.

There is a period of time in which reversibility (and resuscitation) is possible in *almost every case* of cardiac arrest. More patients lose the chance for total recovery during the critical period between arrest and diagnosis than at any other time in the resuscitative period.

Although the absence of heart sounds on auscultation usually indicates inadequate cardiac output, complete cardiac standstill is not necessarily implied. Prolonged stethoscopic auscultation should be avoided. Once the blood pressure and pulse have ceased, the time factor obviously precludes spending much time in reviewing what may be unreliable evidence of heart action. As a general rule, however, heart sounds resume about the same time that circulation does.

Abrupt cardiopulmonary failure may not always begin with cardiac arrest. It may simply involve a respiratory failure with subsequent cardiac collapse. Hyperventilation and convulsive action may characterize sudden, complete anoxia, and there may eventually be agonal, gasping respiratory activity. The blood pressure usually rises temporarily, only to fall precipitously. These abrupt failures may occur as a result of airway obstruction, near-drowning, drug overdose, electric shock, and a variety of other causes.

Unfortunately the first thing noted is sometimes cessation of respirations, even though actual circulatory arrest may have been initially present. Sudden cessation of heart action may frequently be followed by a few agonal respiratory efforts. In any case, if effectiveness of respiration cannot be quickly ascertained, it is wise to conclude that ventilation is inadequate, regardless of the cause.

Ophthalmologic evidence of cardiac arrest has received attention, but as with most of the so-called classic signs, there is considerable dispute. Pupillary diameter does increase to a marked degree when circulatory arrest occurs; yet because of the appreciable lag (30 to 40 seconds) between cessation of cardiac output and full dilatation, it is desirable that resuscitation be started before such dilatation occurs. The pupils may, indeed, be small even after death in certain cases. This is specifically true if the patient has been administered morphine sulfate or other opiates. Patients who are receiving atropine, quinidine, or epinephrine—as well as those with hypothermia—may continually exhibit varying degrees of pupillary dilatation. Funduscopic examination may show segmentation of retinal venous columns and disappearance of the retinal arterial pattern within a minute or more after cardiac output ceases. Although these ophthalmologic findings are of considerable diagnostic value, they are academic because other physical findings are more easily available at an earlier stage.

The term *cardiac arrest* has continued to be somewhat a "wastebasket diagnosis," but in discussing problems related to the acutely arrested circulation no better term seems to be available. Although many different terms have been substituted to denote more precisely the actual situation, none have been used successfully. The term *cardiac arrest* may perhaps be compared to the term *cystosarcoma phylloides*, a breast tumor that has been given at least 60 new and different names over the last hundred years; yet physicians fully realize what is meant by the diagnosis of cystosarcoma phylloides. Similarly, the term *cardiac arrest* serves an equally useful purpose despite some obvious disadvantages implied by the title. Most patients who require cardiopulmonary resuscitation present no initial clear-cut delineation of the etiology involved, thus obviating the use of a more appropriate term for the state of an acutely arrested heart, whether it be in ventricular fibrillation or in asystole.

Definitions of the term *cardiac arrest* vary. They range from a description of the clinical picture of cessation of circulation (sudden, unexpected unconsciousness, pulselessness of large arteries, cyanosis, and apnea) to failure of the heart action to maintain an adequate cerebral circulation in the absence of a causative and irreversible disease.

CAUSES OF CARDIAC ARREST

When we refer to the term *cardiac arrest* we are speaking of the sudden, superficially unexplained, and unexpected cessation of an effective cardiac output. Sudden cessation of an adequate cardiac output to maintain consciousness or adequate cerebral oxygenation may be caused by the absence of all cardiac activity, which is cardiac asystole. The same inadequate cardiac output may result from the sudden onset of ventricular fibrillation, which represents a wild, uncoordinated, and disorganized myocardial contraction resulting in the complete absence of any cardiac output. A third condition may occasionally prevail: The heart may be beating feebly, but at such a depressed rate or with such an ineffective stroke volume that the net result is much the same as with cardiac asystole or ventricular fibrillation. In any event, all three conditions require immediate efforts to artificially reestablish circulation so that irreversible brain damage may be avoided.

It is now generally recognized that the majority of deaths from acute myocardial infarction occur within 24 hours of the onset of symptoms. At least 50% of these deaths occur within the first hour after the onset of difficulty. As mentioned, ventricular fibrillation is commonly associated with the early stages of an acute myocardial infarction. Following an acute myocardial infarction, it is reassuring to know that the probability of ventricular fibrillation is not necessarily related to the size of the infarct. The electric stability of the heart can be a fragile affair. Areas of anoxic change in the myocardium may trigger electric discharges sufficient to throw the heart into fibrillation.

Vagal reflex patterns may play an important role. When the cardioinhibitory nerve is stimulated, one will commonly notice an effect on the cardiac conduction mechanism involving a depression of the sinus node, depression of the atrioventricular node, and impairment of atrioventricular conduction, resulting in auricular or ventricular slowing or, as a matter of fact, standstill in all degrees of atrioventricular heart block. Clinical evidence supports the view that the sensitivity of the heart is more affected by vagal stimulation under hypercapnic states or in patients with an increased serum potassium level or hyperpotassemia. Hypercapnia simply refers to an increase in carbon dioxide often associated with respiratory acidosis. These factors are particularly reflected in the increased frequency with which sudden cardiac arrest, most frequently ventricular asystole, is seen in the burned patient. Severely burned patients have an increased serum potassium level as a result of tissue breakdown. Patients with obstructive jaundice (caused by a stone in the common duct or a cancer of the ampulla of Vater or head of the pancreas) may be very sensitive to vagal influences.

Those persons who have studied neuroanatomy will understand why pressure on the eyeball often results in a slowing of the patient's radial pulse. In many instances the bradycardia associated with operations about the eye, particularly involving the rectus muscles, may involve a certain risk of cardiac arrest. The efferent limb of the reflex arc consists of the vagus nerve, whereas the trigeminal nerve constitutes the afferent limb. This reflex, which we call the oculocardiac reflex, results from stimulation of the first division of the trigeminal nerve (ophthalmic). While there is pressure on the globe or when the extraocular muscles are stretched, electrocardiographic tracings often reflect abnormalities supporting the role of the vagus nerve in the production of various cardiac arrhythmias.

Mention should again be made of sudden cardiac arrest following severe anaphylactic reactions in such instances as the injection of penicillin, local anesthetic agents, vaccines, and various types of sera. Systemic reactions following stings by bees, hornets, wasps, and yellowjackets may, as is generally known, cause severe anaphylactic reactions in certain individuals.

Another explanation for sudden cardiac arrest in a sizable percentage of patients involves a block in the conductive system of the heart. *Stokes-Adams disease* is a term applied to many of the conditions characterized by sudden failure of the ventricles to contract. It may be associated with markedly slowed idioventricular beats, ventricular tachycardia, or ventricular fibrillation. Patients with Stokes-Adams disease may suddenly have an attack without any warning. Within the last decade a large percentage of diagnosed Stokes-Adams cases have been managed successfully with long-term implantation of electric cardiac pacemakers.

There are many other diseases and conditions associated with a high instance of cardiac arrest. For example, cardiac arrest following carotid sinus pressure may occur.

Factors that mechanically block an effective cardiac output may produce the same ultimate damage as that which results from a sudden cardiac arrest. A pericardial tamponade is such an example. The pericardial sac becomes quickly distended and may interfere with the cardiac input and, to a degree, with the output of the heart. This condition may be caused by penetrating wounds of the heart or contusions in such accidents as a steering wheel injury. The relief of the cardiac tamponade is urgent. Air emboli forming a large bolus in the outflow tract of the right ventricle or between the right atrium and right ventricle may effectively block cardiac output, as will a large pulmonary artery embolus.

IMMEDIATE RESUSCITATIVE MEASURES

Once it has been determined that the patient's respiratory activity and circulation are absent or even markedly depressed, immediate application of resuscitative techniques is indicated.

The first step of emergency resuscitation usually requires assurance that the airway is open and prompt artificial ventilation by mouth-to-mouth or mouth-to-nose techniques. Which should one start first: closed-chest resuscitative efforts or artificial ventilation? Physicians may debate the merits of each as a priority. The truth of the matter generally involves an almost simultaneous beginning of both aspects of resuscitation. The most crucial point in question is that of cerebral circulation. The first priority involves artificial augmentation of the circulation with oxygenated blood. Obviously the circulating blood, if unoxygenated, has limited value. Likewise a well-ventilated lung is of no value to the patient unless the circulation is moving. Again, it should be emphasized that one effort without the other is virtually worthless. Unfortunately in the excitement of an emergency this obvious fact is frequently overlooked. When rare situations of marked cardiopulmonary collapse occur while the heart is still beating, the patient may be revived by artificial ventilation alone.

Airway management and ventilation

The basic life-support measures relating to artificial ventilation (as adopted by the National Conference on Standards for Cardiopulmonary Resuscitation and Emergency Cardiac Care at the Washington Conference in May, 1973) need to be continually stressed in teaching airway management to hospital personnel. Except in certain circumstances of a cardiac arrest that is witnessed or an individual who is being monitored, first attention should be directed toward establishment of an adequate airway, followed by ventilation. The patient's head is first tilted backward as far as possible to ensure an open airway by placing one hand beneath the patient's neck, lifting the neck with one hand, and then tilting the head backward by pressure with the other hand on the forehead. The neck is extended and the tongue is thus lifted away from the back of the throat. In teaching airway management to others one should continually emphasize the frequency with which the tongue can occlude the airway by dropping against the back of the throat.

Occasionally, the simple head-tilt maneuver may not be adequate to establish an airway and a so-called triple airway maneuver is employed to promote forward displacement of the lower jaw. Another maneuver is to place one's fingers behind the angles of the patient's jaw, forcibly displacing the mandible forward while at the same time tilting the head backward and using one's thumb to retract the lower lip to allow breathing through the mouth as well as the nose.

Frequently spontaneous respiration can be observed immediately after an adequate airway is established, but, of course, cardiopulmonary arrest requires both artificial ventilation and circulation. Rescue breathing must be started promptly—by either mouth-to-nose or mouth-to-mouth breathing.

Again, it must be emphasized that one of the most common errors in resuscitation of the unconscious patient is the failure to maintain an open airway. In the excitement involved in meeting the crisis of cardopulmonary arrest, one may temporarily overlook the simple physiologic fact that there must be a clear and open pathway for the oxygen to reach the lungs of the patient before any other resuscitative activities can help him, no matter how sophisticated they may be.

In our experience, one of the most difficult aspects of training personnel for cardiopulmonary resuscitation has been the establishment of a patent airway and adequate ventilation. We have been impressed with the difficulty many physicians have shown in establishing ventilation, even using the Resusci-Anne mannequin. In this context, the words of Coryllos are appropriate: "Life is continued as long as exchanges of oxygen and carbon dioxide in the tissues are carried on in a normal way. Gas exchanges depend upon and are regulated by their respective positive pressures."* These pressure must, whatever the metabolic needs of the different tissues, always be maintained at constant levels. Circulation of the blood is but a part of the total respiratory picture, since the supply of oxygen and the removal of carbon dioxide are accomplished by the circulating blood. Too little training is given in practical demonstrations of pulmonary resuscitation and consequently grossly ineffective maneuvers are being used on anoxic patients.

Mouth-to-mouth artificial respiration

When the method of mouth-to-mouth artificial respiration was first mentioned by Karpius as long ago as the late 1700's, interestingly it was recommended that the larynx be pressed against the spine to prevent entry of air into the stomach. Then the method was not widely used, however, because expired air was not considered to be of any great value and was even thought by some to be of possible harm. Bellows were sometimes used to provide fresh air for artificial respiration.

In starting mouth-to-mouth ventilation, place one hand behind the patient's neck to maintain the head in the position of maximum backward tilt. Pinch the nostrils together with the thumb and index finger of the other hand while continuing to exert pressure on the forehead to maintain the backward tilt of the patient's head. Opening the mouth widely, take a deep breath, make a tight seal with the lips around the patients' mouth and blow into his mouth. Break contact and allow the patient to exhale passively, watching the chest fall. The initial respiratory maneuver should be four quick, full breaths without allowing time for full lung deflation between breaths.

To prevent distension of the stomach by air, the patient's nose should be compressed with one hand while the other hand is used to make pressure over the upper abdomen and epigastrium. The operator should take a deep inspiration, immediately apply his widely open mouth to the mouth of the patient, and make a forcible exhalation. The patient's chest expands quite noticeably as the air is blown into his mouth, and when the operator raises his mouth from that of the patient, a rush of air can be distinctly heard coming from the patient's lungs. Forcible pressure on the

---

*From Coryllos, P. N.: Mechanical resuscitation in advanced forms of asphyxia: a clinical and experimental study in different methods of resuscitation, Surg. Gynecol. Obstet. **66:**698-722, 1938.

chest augments expiration. As in starting all methods of artificial respiration, one must remember to bring the patient's tongue forward because it may occlude the oropharynx. One should exhale twice his normal resting tidal volume (about 1,000 ml).

In most cases of mouth-to-mouth breathing, the head tilt method is effective. If it is not, one of several jaw-thrust methods may be required. The fingers may be placed behind the angles of the patient's jaw to forcibly displace the mandible forward while the head is tilted backward; the thumb is used to retract the lower lip to allow breathing through the mouth as well as through the nose. This maneuver is best performed from a position near the top of the patient's head while his mouth is kept open with the thumbs. The nose may be sealed by placing the cheek against it. This maneuver is difficult to teach on practice mannequins and is more tiring to perform than the head-tilt method. In mouth-to-nose ventilation, the jaw-thrust technique involves using the cheek to seal the patient's mouth and does not involve retracting the lower lip with the thumb. The problems that are associated with practice on the mannequin, in addition to the special details just described, usually limit use of the jaw-thrust technique to specially trained personnel. In any event if the patient does not resume spontaneous breathing, the rescuer must soon move to his side to perform mouth-to-mouth or mouth-to-nose ventilation.

Several precautions and possible pitfalls are inherent in performing mouth-to-mouth resuscitation. Because of the limited endurance of the individual performing the resuscitation, the question of physical fatigue must be considered. The operator may experience a degree of hypocapnia and subsequent vertigo as a result of his prolonged efforts. Although the decrease in the carbon dioxide concentration of the blood is not sufficient to cause any real discomfort, additional personnel should be available to take over the procedure at the appropriate time.

Either the mouth-to-mask or mouth-to-tube method is advantageous over the simple mouth-to-mouth procedure in that both hands of the operator are available to maintain patency of the upper airway. Any increase in pulmonary resistance can be judged by the amount of exertion it takes to deflate the rescuer's lungs. Several other advantages of the mouth-to-tube method of respiration should be noted in addition to that of preventing hypocapnia in the operator: cross-contamination between the operator and the patient is prevented if a disposable filter is placed in the breathing tube. Efforts can be continued for long periods of time, and no special positioning of the patient is required. The equipment is minimal in expense, and adequate ventilation is ensured despite any abnormalities in either airway resistance or lung compliance.

A drawback in the mouth-to-mouth procedure is the danger in some instances that the operator may be exposed to infectious diseases, such as pulmonary tuberculosis. Anaerobic suppuration of the lungs and its associated foul odor present an added difficulty, and the rescuer may be reluctant to contact the lips of a dying patient. Prevention of cross-contamination can be implemented by the use of a handkerchief, and of course the mouth-to-tube method also obviates this objection.

To alleviate the problem of gastric dilatation, the operator may press his hand on the epigastrium of the patient periodically to prevent the accumulation of air. There is the possibility of lung rupture, particularly if too much expiratory effort is applied by the rescuer—especially in the case of infants. With the very young infant, a mere puffing motion with the cheeks may suffice and will eliminate any danger of too much pressure.

If one uses excessively high inflation pressures during artificial ventilation, some of the air will be forced into the esophagus. Additionally, pressure on the sternum may provoke regurgitation of stomach contents into the upper airway. Both active and passive regurgitation and air venting into the esophagus can be prevented if the esophagus is compressed against the cricoid cartilage. Apply posterior pressure to the skin over the anterior surface of the cricoid and compress the esophagus between the cricoid and the anterior surface of the cervical vertebrae. Moderate pressure will prevent air from entering the esophagus and prevent gastric contents from regurgitating through it. Two fingers of the hand supporting the chin and tongue are free to displace the cricoid backward with sufficient strength to occlude the esophagus. Care must be used to apply pressure to the cricoid cartilage and not to the thyroid cartilage.

An opening at the front of the base of the neck will identify the patient who has had a laryngectomy. Direct mouth-to-stoma artificial ventilation will be required in these individuals, who have a permanent stoma connecting the trachea directly to the skin, and neither head-tilt nor jaw-thrust maneuvers will be needed. If the patient has a temporary tracheostomy tube in place, the rescuer must seal the mouth and nose with his hand or with a tightly fitting face mask to prevent leakage of air while blowing into the tracheostomy tube. This problem is, of course, avoided if the tube is provided with an inflatable cuff.

Mouth-to-nose respiration

As an alternative to mouth-to-mouth respiration, mouth-to-nose respiration may be useful if the individual applying artificial respiration is unable to completely seal his mouth around the patient's mouth. Transient rigidity, trismus, or convulsions may make mouth-to-nose respiration a viable alternative. The patient with a broken jaw may have his teeth wired together, but blowing between the teeth has been successful in these cases. It may become necessary to open the patient's mouth or to separate his lips to allow the air to escape during exhalation because the soft palate may cause obstruction of the nasopharynx.

In infants and small children, the rescuer may cover both the mouth and the nose of the child with his mouth and, of course, use less volume to inflate the lung *once every 3 seconds.* Forceful backward tilting of the neck of the infant may obstruct breathing passages because of the marked pliability of the neck; therefore the tilted position should not be exaggerated.

The advantages of the nasal insufflation route include less likelihood of gastric regurgitation and subsequent aspiration. It is generally accepted that gastric inflation is uniformly produced when pressure in the upper airways is more than 25 cm water but almost never occurs if pressures are lower than 15 cm water. With increased resistance to airflow via the nasal route as opposed to the oral one, there is a reduction of the air pressure in the pharynx and at the gastric cardia. Ruben has demonstrated that regurgitation is less likely to occur in instances of expired air resuscitation when the nasal insufflation route is used. The use of the mouth-to-nose technique, of course, eliminates maneuvers such as pinching the nostrils or resting the cheek against the nostrils to prevent an air leak. Not only is the incidence of nasal blockage extremely low (probably less than 2%) but also the tilt angle is less critical when the mouth-to-nose technique is used.

Suction devices

Both portable and installed equipment adequate for pharyngeal suction should be available for resuscitative emergencies. The installed unit should be sufficiently powerful to provide an airflow of more than 30 liters per minute and a vacuum of at least 300 mm Hg. The amount of suction should, of course, be controllable for use with children and intubated patients. Either a Y or T connection or a lateral opening between the suction tube and the suction source should be provided as an off-on control. The tube should reach the airway of any patient regardless of his position, and the apparatus must be designed for easy cleaning and decontamination.

If a nasogastric tube is to be used for gastric decompression, it should be inserted after the airway has been isolated by endotracheal intubation. If gastric distension interferes with adequate ventilation, however, then a nasogastric tube may be inserted before the endotracheal intubation by well-trained personnel.

USE OF 100% OXYGEN

The patient naturally receives only expired air at the initial phase of cardiopulmonary resuscitation. If the AMBU bag is used, he receives room air; therefore one should strive to administer 100% oxygen if possible. There is no excuse for using less than 100% oxygen at the start of resuscitative measures despite the vasodilatative effect of a 7% to 10% carbon dioxide mixture or a mixture of helium and oxygen. A complete saturation with oxygen is the desired first goal. Under conditions of total anoxia, no additional stimulus to the respiratory center from either carbon dioxide or helium is needed. Lower oxygen concentration should, however, be used in prolonged resuscitative efforts because of the possible complications of prolonged high oxygen concentrations (such as intra-alveolar hemorrhage, fibrosis, and inhibition of the mucociliary apparatus).

TECHNIQUE OF CLOSED-CHEST COMPRESSION

The patient should be placed in the supine or flat position, preferably on a hard, nonyielding surface, while efforts are made to compress the heart between the sternum and the thoracic vertebrae. When this maneuver is properly instituted, cardiac output is sufficient to maintain adequate cerebral circulation as well as adequate blood flow to the myocardium and to other vital tissues (as much as 35% of the normal blood flow). Intermittent pressure is applied to the lower one third of the sternum with minimum pressure to the adjacent rib cage, by using the base of the palm. One should, ideally, be positioned directly above the patient, with the elbows rigidly extended to exert pressure from the shoulders downward. If the pressure is directed at an angle to the chest wall, it is more likely to produce complications such as rib fractures and soft tissue injuries. The uninitiated tend to apply the initial compression too vigorously. One usually begins with an intermittent depression of the sternum that gradually increases in depth as the sternum and the rib cage become slightly more mobile and elastic.

One should stand or kneel at either side of the patient and place the heel of one hand over the lower half of the sternum and the heel of the other hand on top of the first. (The lower hand should not be placed over the lower tip of the sternum.) The sternum is then downwardly displaced approximately 1½ to 2 inches toward the spine. It should be held down for a fraction of a second and then should be released rapidly. Contact with the chest is maintained during relaxation, and a rate of 60 to 80 compressions per minute is probably best in most cases. In children, however, the rate should probably be raised to between 100 and 120 compressions per minute. Undue fatigue will be avoided if the operator utilizes the entire weight of the body rather than just the strength of the arms in applying the compressions. The fingers should be carefully maintained in a raised position to avoid undue pressure on the rib cage.

In children the principles are the same, but much less pressure is used. In small children the force of the heel of one hand is ordinarily sufficient, and with infants moderate pressure should be applied to the center of the sternum with the tips of the fingers only. Care must be used because the infant's myocardium is easily bruised. The infant's sternum should be depressed ½ to ¾ inch and that of the young child should be depressed ¾ to 1½ inches. The rescuer should encircle the chest of a small infant with his hands while the midsternum is compressed with both thumbs.

Evaluating the effectiveness of closed-chest compression is naturally desirable. If a blood pressure cuff is available and if a person is available to use it, maintenance of a blood pressure above 60 to 70 mm Hg indicates that the cardiac output is adequate to sustain life. Otherwise a palpable pulse and maintenance of the pupils in the constricted state are generally indicative of satisfactory augmentation of the circulation. Merely observing the patient for a well-oxygenated appearance can be helpful and reassuring in the absence of other measures.

Two immediately applicable measures may be helpful at the *very start* of closed-chest resuscitative efforts: Placing of the patient in a supine position with the head slightly downward provides a restorative action and produces an actual, significant, rapid, and demonstrable increase in the blood pressure to the brain. The head-down position appears to extend that delicate time period between reversibility and irreversibility of cerebral cortical inactivity. Additionally, the Trendelenburg position has a tendency to prevent aspiration of vomitus and gastric contents following pressure on the sternum and epigastrium.

Rhythmic sternal compression may have some value in artificial respiration. It is generally believed, however, to be minimal in value. Safar and associates attempted to evaluate this feature under several different conditions. In 30 curarized patients with natural airways, no respiratory tidal exchange was produced by using closed-chest compression when the head was unsupported and there was probable upper airway obstruction. If the airway was improved with elevation of the shoulder and backward tilting of the head, some improvement in the respiratory tidal exchange occurred, but this was still minimal. If an artificial airway was introduced, tidal volumes as high as 390 ml were recorded, with tidal volume being inversely proportional to rate of chest compression. Tidal exchange was also studied in 12 patients on whom closed-chest massage had been started while an endotracheal tube was in place. No basic tidal exchange was detectable, and it was therefore assumed that closed-chest compression should not be relied on to produce much tidal exchange. Occasionally, this procedure does seem to benefit patients; however, adult patients with a more rigid chest probably receive less benefit than do the younger persons.

As previously mentioned, if the cardiac arrest occurs in a hospital bed, a firm support should be provided beneath the patient's back when cardiopulmonary resuscitation is performed. A simple serving tray or support of comparable size is useful but not the best support. Optimally a bed board should extend from the shoulders to the waist and across the full width of the bed. A special cardiac arrest board is available that is shaped to position the patient's neck in the properly extended position. Spineboards should be used for ambulance services and mobile support units. They are also useful for extricating and immobilizing patients. They may be used directly on the floor of the emergency vehicle or on a wheeled litter.

Simultaneous closed-chest and mouth-to-mouth resuscitation

If one is alone with the patient, how does one combine external cardiac compression with intermittent positive pressure artificial ventilation? The best combination makes use of alternating two mouth-to-mouth lung inflations with 15 chest compressions at about 1-second intervals. With only one operator, chest compression should be given at a more rapid rate: approximately 80 compressions per minute. Two full lung inflations are delivered in rapid succession, within a period of 5 or 6 seconds, without allowing full exhalation between breaths. In the event that a second person is available to apply artificial respiration, he should *interpose* one deep lung inflation after every fifth sternal compression. It has been emphasized that interposed breathing must occur without any pause in compressions because cerebral perfusion drops to zero whenever there is a cessation of compression.

The person administering closed-chest resuscitation counts aloud as follows: "One one-thousand, two one-thousand, three one-thousand . . . ." At each count of five, the individual responsible for the mouth-to-mouth effort should administer one good exhalation to the patient's mouth. In effect, one can imagine blowing the compressing hands off the chest wall as one exhales just at the end point of the fifth compression. The reversal of roles between the two rescuers should be so coordinated that *no* interruption of perfusion occurs. Even with the most effective technique of closed-chest resuscitation the perfusion rates remain only one-third that of normal. *Obviously any detraction from the proper technique will drop perfusion to an ineffective level.*

If the person administering the chest compression tires after prolonged efforts, it may be desirable to change operators. In this case the count by the person compressing the chest may be as follows (adhering to the previously counted rhythm): "Next-time-change-on-*three*." After administering a breath to the patient on the word "three," the person administering the mouth-to-mouth technique should immediately move to the chest area. Placing his hands beside those of the compressor of the chest so that he is almost literally ready to shove these hands aside, the operator should continue with the count "four one-thousand" at the proper time in the next cycle. Then the other person should immediately move to the head of the patient and be ready to administer the next breath to the patient on the following count of five.

Even experienced personnel who are effective at either of these techniques alone may prove to be quite awkward at the time of coordination and change over. Practice with mannequins is essential.

Mention should be made in this context of the urgent necessity for practice on mannequins by all health care personnel who are likely to be in a situation requiring cardiopulmonary resuscitation. If the recording Resusci-Anne mannequin can be used for a demonstration and various hospital personnel can be allowed to demonstrate their techniques, amazing procedural inadequacies are almost invariably demonstrated—even by those considered to be experienced in the area of resuscitation.

The recording mannequin has two distinct aids to teaching closed-chest massage and mouth-to-mouth breathing: First, a series of lights on a panel beside the mannequin indicates the effectiveness of the efforts applied. A single green light glows at the instant of sufficient pulmonary ventilation, and independently a red light and an amber light demonstrate the effectiveness of the chest compression (the red light indicating either misapplied chest compression or an effort of too great a magnitude and the amber light indicating correctly applied compression of the proper magnitude). A first effort by even the supposedly experienced resuscitator will frequently fail to illuminate either of these lights.

The second feature of this mannequin involves an internal recorder that delivers, through a slit in the side of the mannequin, an ECG-type printout on a paper strip that shows the effectiveness of the efforts applied.

A training session with this mannequin quickly separates the bone crushers, the too-gentle chest caressers, and the ineffectual puffers from the truly lifesaving administrators of correctly applied cardiopulmonary resuscitative measures.

Precordial precussion or thump

Precordial thumping of the chest is a simple but sometimes effective technique that can be immediately employed—even during the brief time spent in making a diagnosis. The technique involves simply striking the left chest in the precordial area with a clenched fist. A sharp blow delivered high on the chest with the clenched fist or with the ulnar border of the hand may activate the heart and produce several ventricular complexes, and in some instances reestablish the heart beat.

The precordial thump is *reserved* for those situations in which the victim can be given the precordial blow within a few seconds after onset of the cardiac arrest has been observed. The effectiveness in other situations appears limited. In fact, indiscriminate use of the precordial thump has been the subject of some criticism, because the technique lacks objective data to support its value in resuscitating the arrested heart. After a controlled evaluation of precordial thump, it has been concluded that many aspects are more dangerous than beneficial, particularly when applied in the management of ventricular tachyarrhythmias. In experimental animals, no beneficial effect was produced during either cardiac standstill or ventricular fibrillation.

VENTRICULAR FIBRILLATION

Ventricular fibrillation refers to an irregular, uncoordinated activity of the ventricles of the heart or to a quivering motion with almost complete absence of any cardiac output. Death will result from ventricular fibrillation in the untreated patient as quickly as it will result from cardiac asystole.

Because ventricular fibrillation can seldom be diagnosed without either the aid of an electrocardiogram or direct visualization of the heart action, it is probable that ventricular fibrillation can only be a suspected diagnosis in cardiac arrests occurring outside the hospital. It should again be emphasized that the need to defibrillate the heart does not in itself constitute a first priority in the scheme of one's efforts, although defibrillation is highly desirable at the earliest possible moment. Providing that adequate cardiac output is being maintained by closed-chest resuscitation and that adequate oxygenation is being provided by mouth-to-mouth or mouth-to-nose respiration, the patient can be maintained in a reasonably satisfactory state for some time. Most patients can be transported to a defibrillator, or vice versa, in the necessary time period.

I recall such a situation in the early 1950's when I was a resident at Bellevue Hospital in New York City. At that time we had one of the few cardiac defibrillators in the city. One morning we received a call from a hospital more than 100 blocks away on the opposite side of Manhattan. Ventricular fibrillation had occurred in a patient while he was on the operating table. Adequate resuscitative efforts were carried out by the hospital personnel during the time that it took us to arrive by ambulance through heavy traffic to the hospital. The patient was promptly defibrillated and the surgeon proceeded with the operation.

Defibrillation can be accomplished by electric countershock with either direct or alternating current. Generally speaking, the direct current countershock defibrillator is preferable. Using a direct external countershock, a setting of 400 watt-seconds is frequently used to defibrillate the adult heart and 100 watt-seconds is used for a child's heart. This recommended energy level may have to be raised in large, diseased hearts or under certain other conditions that make defibrillation difficult.

It is important to remember that electrode paste must be applied generously to the skin or to the electrodes, which should be free of old, dried paste from previous defibrillatory attempts. Saline-soaked gauze sponges are good conductors. One electrode is placed just below the right clavicle medially and a second electrode over the apex of the heart beneath the left breast. We prefer to apply our own countershock either by a foot or hand switch rather than to delegate this to an assistant because of the danger of inadvertently shocking the resuscitation personnel. The objective of defibrillation is to produce a synchronized depolarization of all heart muscle, to eliminate all uncoordinated ectopic foci of activity, and to converge all electric activity into one single contractile effort.

If the patient appears to be resistant to defibrillatory attempts, the intravenous or intracardiac injection of epinephrine may change the fibrillatory action of the heart to a coarser nature and increase the likelihood of defibrillation. Sodium bicarbonate injections may need to be repeated just prior to a defibrillatory attempt. Between countershocks, of course, the patient should be well oxygenated and closed-chest compression should be continued. It is important to remember that almost all hearts can be defibrillated.

Occasionally the heart can be successfully defibrillated prior to either ventilatory assistance or external cardiac massage. This situation probably arises only in an area such as the coronary care unit where the electric activity of the heart is constantly being monitored. During former President Eisenhower's last illness he required 14 separate attempts at defibrillation. These were successful in several instances even without a loss of consciousness by the patient. "Blind defibrillation" in the unconscious, pulseless patient is becoming increasingly employed even though ventricular fibrillation has not been confirmed electrocardiographically, provided that artificial ventilation and chest compressive efforts are not delayed.

One can seldom rely on the possibility of spontaneous defibrillation. It does occur, however. For example, ventricular fibrillation suddenly developed in a young woman during a cardiac catheterization procedure. Full monitoring observations were available and within a few seconds of adequate closed-chest compression the heart was seen to spontaneously defibrillate.

We soon shall see no doubt the widespread introduction of portable external cardiac defibrillators as more satisfactory models become available.

All medical personnel should be knowledgeable in the use of the external cardiac defibrillator.

PHARMACOLOGIC AIDS IN CARDIAC RESUSCITATION

Although there are more than 30 drugs that may play a part in helping to successfully resuscitate a heart, in the majority of cases one only need be concerned with a relatively few agents.

The proper use of drugs, including timing, proper dosage, and intended pharmacologic effect, has provided the necessary measure for success in many instances of cardiopulmonary resuscitation. In this consideration, we enter a rapidly changing field, and one is always confronted with the question of exactly how far to go in presenting highly specialized material in a fairly general discussion. A chapter much longer than this one would indeed be required to adequately present all the details of the sophisticated pharmacologic routines available to the modern resuscitator. In fact, in the fourth edition of the text *Cardiac Arrest and Resuscitation*, complete chapters are devoted to presentation of the material on each of four of the more specialized areas in this field. Therefore the present discussion of drugs is restricted to the guidelines set up in the *Standards for Cardiopulmonary Resuscitation and Emergency Cardiac Care* by the National Conference on Standards of the National Academy of Sciences.

Any discussion of the pharmacology of resuscitation inevitably turns our attention to the four basic properties inherent in a normal beating heart: excitability, contractility, rhythmicity, and conductivity. These properties of the beating heart are the ones we seek to control, inhibit, or enhance. The pharmacologic agents that are presented can be divided into two categories, although this categorization—as is true with any—can probably never be absolute. The categories are essential drugs and useful drugs.

Essential drugs

Essential drugs listed by the National Conference on Standards of the National Academy of Sciences include sodium bicarbonate, epinephrine, atropine sulfate, lidocaine, morphine sulfate, and calcium chloride. Oxygen is also considered because it is obviously essential.

Sodium bicarbonate. Sodium bicarbonate is necessary to combat metabolic acidosis. It is administered intravenously in an initial dose of 1 mEq per kilogram by either bolus injection or continuous infusion for a 10-minute period. Once effective spontaneous circulation is restored, further administration of sodium bicarbonate is usually not indicated and may even be harmful. The average dosage forms available for sodium bicarbonate are prefilled syringes of 50 ml of 8.4% solution (50 mEq) or 7.5% solution (44.6 mEq); 50 ml of ampules of 7.5% solution; and 500 ml bottles of 5% solution (297.5 mEq). Bolus administration is much preferred to continued infusion.

If ventricular fibrillation is present, defibrillation should be attempted immediately, before sodium bicarbonate is administered. If effective circulation is not restored after defibrillation and the initial dose of bicarbonate, a repeat dose of 1 mEq per kilogram should be given. In hospitalized patients, further administration of sodium bicarbonate should be governed by arterial blood gas and pH measurements.

Sodium bicarbonate administration must always be accompanied by effective ventilation to remove carbon dioxide from the arterial blood. When blood gas pH determinations are not available, one half of the initial dose may be administered at 10-minute intervals. Excessive therapy may lead to metabolic alkalosis and hyperosmolality. Catecholamines may be given either simultaneously or in rapid succession with sodium bicarbonate, but they generally should not be added to continuous infusions of the bicarbonate, which may inactivate them.

Patients with cardiac standstill or persistent ventricular fibrillation should not receive sodium bicarbonate alone. Repeated doses of epinephrine and sodium bicarbonate should be administered while external cardiac massage and artificial ventilation are continued. This combination may convert cardiac standstill into ventricular fibrillation, which can then be defibrillated. During ventricular fibrillation, the use of both drugs improves the status of the myocardium and enhances the effectiveness of defibrillation.

Epinephrine. Epinephrine may initiate ventricular fibrillation, but its action in restoring electrical activity in asystole and in enhancing defibrillation is well known. It increases myocardial contractility, elevates perfusion pressures, lowers the defibrillatory threshold, and occasionally restores myocardial contractility in electromechanical dissociation.

It is unlikely that pharmacologic assistance in cardiopulmonary resuscitation will be readily available for the case occurring outside the hospital, at least not until the ambulance arrives. As previously emphasized, immediate efforts should be geared to doing as much for the patient as possible prior to transporting him to the hospital. In other words, much can be done to stabilize the patient's condition. For example, an intravenous route can be established through which drugs can be administered. Although epinephrine can be given directly into the heart, such an injection usually takes time away from the external cardiac compression that is being given. In addition, some difficulty may be experienced in getting the drug into the heart chamber because of the size of the needle, site of the injection, or intrathoracic pathology.

In any event epinephrine probably should be given as soon as possible, particularly if there is no evidence of an immediate return of a spontaneous heartbeat. If the intravenous route is available, a dose of 0.5 mg (5 ml of 1:10,000 solution) may be given. If the heart is in asystole, the epinephrine may help initiate the heart action once it is circulated through the myocardium. If weak ventricular fibrillatory actions are present, epinephrine encourages the strength of the contractions and helps to promote successful defibrillation.

Some physicians recommend an initial dose of epinephrine within the first 2 minutes of cardiopulmonary resuscitation. I am somewhat more inclined to wait a few extra minutes before the use of epinephrine because a considerable number of cardiac resuscitations can be achieved without the use of drugs. A cardiotonic drug may, however, provide the additional needed contractile force to help maintain myocardial oxygenation. If epinephrine is not available, then either calcium chloride or calcium gluconate can be used. Epinephrine acts by improving coronary perfusion pressure, by improving myocardial conduction through direct effect on the myocardium and on the conduction tissue, thereby producing more forceful contractions of the myocardium, and by lowering the defibrillation threshold. It increases the speed of atrioventricular conduction.

There is a sizable group of pressor drugs available to the clinician. All of the pressor drugs are derivatives of epinephrine, but they differ from it in their potency and predominant mode of action. In addition, their stability varies in the presence of aminoacidosis. Because of differences in their molecular structure, some act primarily as vasoconstrictors and others act principally on the heart and may cause vasodilation. Of the two kinds of receptors at sympathetic nerve endings, the alpha receptors are concerned with excitatory efforts such as pupillary dilation, peripheral vasoconstriction, and mobilization of glucose from liver glycogen. The beta receptors at the nerve endings are chiefly concerned with inhibitory effects and thereby produce vasocilation of blood vessels that supply skeletal muscles, reduction of tone of the smooth muscle supplying the bronchial tree, and an increase in the rate of the heartbeat and cardiac output.

Because epinephrine stimulates some nerve endings while inhibiting others, it is regarded as both an alpha and a beta receptor. Levarterenol (norepinephrine) produces its effect chiefly by action on the alpha receptors. It increases the rate of contraction of the heart in the presence of heart block. In addition to causing vasoconstriction, pupillary dilation, and a rise in blood glucose level by liberation of glycogen from the liver, levarterenol also increases coronary flow and may produce slowing of the heart through reflex vagal inhibition as the blood pressure rises. Marked constriction of the vessels of the gut and reduction of bowel motility may occur with levarterenol infusion. Adrenergic blocking agents are able to block the alpha receptors but are not effective in blocking the beta receptors.

Among the pressor amines, other drugs are phenylephrine, methoxamine, and metaraminol. By acting mainly on the alpha receptors, this group of drugs raises the systemic arterial blood pressure during vasoconstriction of peripheral vessels. The force of contraction of the heart is not appreciably altered, but coronary blood flow and cerebral blood flow are increased when hypotension is present.

Other pressor amines that act mainly on the heart and in the production of vasodilation, in addition to epinephrine, are ephedrine, methamphetamine, and mephentermine.

In administering vasopressors during cardiac resuscitation and in the immediate postresuscitative period, care should be taken to avoid local tissue necrosis by using large catheters in large veins and by using dilute solutions. Obviously one should use the smallest dose that will provide the desired effect. The action of pressor amines is less effective in the presence of uncorrected metabolic acidosis. Vasoconstrictors increase diastolic pressure during cardiac resuscitation and materially improve the chances for return of spontaneous circulation. The vasopressors, which act mainly on the alpha receptors, do raise diastolic pressure; their value seems to lie primarily in the improvement of the peripheral vascular tone.

There is complete absence of body perfusion during either cardiac asystole or ventricular fibrillation. This state is often followed by the marginal perfusional status of cardiopulmonary perfusion efforts; therefore both situations add up to a severe metabolic acidosis. The acidosis contributes to atony of the myocardium, to decreased peripheral vascular tone, and to interference with catecholamine (endogenous epinephrine and norepinephrine) production and action. Whenever severe metabolic acidosis is present in association with attempts to resuscitate the fibrillating heart, success is unlikely because the arrhythmia rapidly recurs, even after defibrillation.

As previously mentioned, cardiac arrest represents a *zero* perfusion state. During resuscitative efforts, this situation may improve only to the point that a low perfusion state exists. In any event, metabolic acidosis enters the picture along with its own inherent adverse features such as decreased arterial pressure, reduction in cardiac output, and a gradual rise in both central venous pressure and peripheral resistance. Cardiac slowing, sinus arrhythmias, sinus pauses, and sinus arrest (all suggestive of increased vagal activity) may be seen. Certainly the threshold for ventricular fibrillation is lowered.

Lidocaine. Lidocaine raises the fibrillation threshold and increases the electrical stimulation threshold of the ventricle during diastole, therefore exerting an antidysrhythmic effect. There is no significant change in myocardial contractility, systemic arterial pressure, or absolute refractory period when lidocaine is given in the usual therapeutic doses. It is particularly effective in depressing irritability when successive defibrillatory attempts revert to fibrillation. This drug is also particularly effective in the control of multifocal premature ventricular beats and in episodes of ventricular tachycardia.

Fifty to 100 mg (approximately 1 mg per kilogram) should be administered slowly as a bolus intravenously and may be repeated as often as every 3 to 5 minutes if necessary. A continuous infusion of 1 to 3 mg per minute should follow, usually not exceeding 4 mg per minute. Lidocaine is of no value in asystole.

Morphine sulfate. Morphine is not directly indicated in cardiopulmonary resuscitative emergencies, but it is important in cases of myocardial infarction to relieve pain and in the treatment of pulmonary edema. For pain relief in acute myocardial infarction, 1 ml of morphine sulfate (15 mg) should be diluted to 5 ml (3 mg per milliliter). Of this solution, 1 ml (3 mg) to 1.5 ml (4.5 mg) should be given intravenously every 5 to 30 minutes as required. Small doses frequently provide the desired effect while avoiding significant respiratory depression.

Atropine sulfate. Atropine sulfate accelerates heartbeat in cases of sinus bradycardia, reduces vagal tone, and enhances atrial ventricular conduction. In cases of hypotension it is particularly useful to prevent arrest in profound sinus bradycardia secondary to toxic myocardial infarction. Atropine sulfate is indicated for the treatment of sinus bradycardia with a pulse of less than 60 beats per minute accompanied by premature ventricular contractions or a systolic blood pressure of less than 90 mm Hg. Its usage is indicated for high-degree atrioventricular block that is accompanied by bradycardia, but it is of no value in ventricular ectopic bradycardia in the absence of atrial activity. The recommended dosage is 0.5 mg administered intravenously as a bolus and repeated every 5 minutes until a pulse rate greater than 60 is achieved. The total dose should not exceed 2 mg except in cases of third degree atrioventricular block, which may require larger doses.

Calcium chloride. Calcium chloride increases myocardial contractility, prolongs systole, and enhances ventricular excitability. Following rapid intravenous injection, it suppresses sinus impulse formation and sudden death, especially in fully digitalized patients. Calcium chloride is useful in treating profound cardiovascular collapse (electromechanical dissociation), it may restore an electrical rhythm in instances of asystole, and it may enhance electrical defibrillation.

The dosage is difficult to define adequately and varies widely. The usual recommended dosage of calcium chloride is 2.5 to 5 ml of a 10% solution (3.4 to 6.8 mEq CA^{++} ions) injected intravenously as a bolus at 10-minute intervals. Calcium gluconate provides fewer calcium ions per unit volume and if it is used, the dose should be 10 ml of a 10% solution (4.8 mEq). Alternatively, calcium gluceptate may be administered in a dose of 5 ml. Hypercalcemia is a definite hazard of large doses. No form of calcium should be administered at the same time as sodium bicarbonate, because the mixture results in formation of a precipitate.

Alternate drug routes. In the event of failure to establish an intravenous lifeline, epinephrine can be effectively instilled directly into the tracheobronchial tree via an endotracheal tube, using 1 to 2 mg per 10 ml of sterile distilled water. Lidocaine may be similarly used in the amount of 50 to 100 mg per 10 ml of sterile, distilled water. Endotracheal use of other drugs for cardiopulmonary resuscitation has not yet been established.

Atropine sulfate (2 mg) or lidocaine (300 mg) can be given intramuscularly to establish therapeutic and prophylactic blood levels for control of dysrhythmia; this route, however, requires the presence of adequate spontaneous circulation.

Useful drugs

In addition to the vasoactive drugs (levarterenol and metaraminol), isoproterenol, propranolol, and corticosteroids are included in the category of useful drugs.

Some physicians challenge the use of potent peripheral vasoconstrictors because of the possibility of reducing cerebral, cardiac, and renal blood flow. The choice of a vasoconstrictor or a positive inotropic agent remains controversial in the treatment of cardiac arrest and in the immediate postresuscitative period. Blood pressure must, however, be supported when it (and inadequate cerebral and renal perfusion) gives evidence of shock—both during cardiac compression and in the postresuscitative period.

In cases of peripheral vascular collapse identified clinically by hypotension and the absence of significant peripheral vasoconstriction, levarterenol (Levophed) bitartrate in high concentrations of 16 μg per ml or metaraminol bitartrate (Aramine) in concentrations of 0.4 mg per milliliter of dextrose in water should be given intravenously. Metaraminol can be given intravenously as a bolus of 2 to 5 mg every 5 to 10 seconds. Continuous administration is required to maintain a satisfactory blood pressure and adequate urinary output. Both of these drugs are potent vasoconstrictors that have a positive inotropic effect on the myocardium. They are especially useful when systemic peripheral resistance is low.

Isoproterenol. If a bradycardia is demonstrated to be the result of complete heart block, isoproterenol (Isuprel) hydrochloride should be infused in amounts of 2 to 20 μg per minute (1 to 10 ml of a solution consisting of 1 mg in 500 ml of 5% glucose in water). The flow should be adjusted to increase heart rate to approximately 60 beats per minute. This regimen is useful in cases of profound sinus bradycardia that have proved refractory to atropine.

Propranolol. Propranolol is a beta adrenergic blocking agent that possesses useful antiarrhythmic properties. It is useful in instances of repetitive ventricular tachycardia or repetitive ventricular fibrillation in which maintenance of a restored beat cannot be achieved by use of lidocaine. The usual dose of propranolol is 1 mg given intravenously and repeated to a total of 3 mg under careful monitoring. Caution is required in patients with chronic obstructive pulmonary disease or cardiac failure.

Corticosteroids. Cardiogenic shock or shock lung that occurs as a complication of cardiac arrest may be treated with pharmacologic doses of synthetic corticosteroids (5 mg per kilogram of methylprednisolone sodium succinate or 1 mg per kilogram of dexamethasone phosphate). When cerebral edema is suspected in cases of cardiac arrest, methylprednisolone sodium succinate in a dosage of 60 to 100 mg every 6 hours may be beneficial. Postaspiration pneumonitis or other pulmonary complications may indicate the use of dexamethasone phosphate in a dosage of 4 to 8 mg every 6 hours.

Drug treatment after cardiac arrest

Cerebral edema, which may follow successful resuscitation, may require potent diuretic agents, hypothermia, and controlled hyperventilation in addition to corticosteroids. Furosemide and ethacrynic acid in doses of 40 to 200 mg may provide the desired diuresis, but hyperosmolality may be aggravated by these drugs.

Drug dosage for infants and children

The drugs previously discussed are recommended in these dosages for infants and small children:

Epinephrine: intracardiac, 0.3 to 2 ml diluted 1:10,000 (0.1 ml per kilogram).

Calcium chloride (10%): intravenously, a maximum dose of 1 ml per 5 kg (30 mg per kilogram); intracardiac, 1 ml per 5 kg diluted 1:1 with saline. Caution should be used in giving calcium chloride to digitalized children.

Sodium bicarbonate: intravenously, 1 ml (0.9 mEq) per kilogram diluted 1:1 with sterile water. Dose should be repeated after pH is obtained and a base deficit has been calculated.

Levarterenol (Levophed) bitartrate: intravenously, infants should be given 1 mg in 500 ml of 5% dextrose in water; children, 2 mg per 500 ml of 5% dextrose in water. Should be titrated to give the desired effect and should not be used in cases of endotoxic shock or renal shutdown.

Metaraminol (aramine) bitartrate: intravenously, 25 mg per 100 ml of 5% dextrose in water. Should be titrated to give the desired effect.

Mephentermine (Wyamine) sulfate: intravenously, 0.05 mg.

Lidocaine (Xylocaine): intravenously, infants should be given 0.5 mg per kilogram, not to exceed 100 mg per hour; children, 5 mg. Should be repeated until the desired effect is obtained. May also be administered as an intravenous drip, 6 mg per kg per 4 hours (100 mg in 500 ml of 5% dextrose in water).

Isoproterenol (Isuprel) hydrochloride: intravenous drip, 1 to 5 mg per 500 ml of 5% dextrose in water. Should be titrated to achieve the desired effect.

PRECAUTIONS IN CARDIOPULMONARY RESUSCITATION

Although complications of cardiopulmonary resuscitative efforts inevitably occur, these complications can be minimized by an effective training program that also embodies periodic retraining efforts. One should be aware of the potential pitfalls and precautions necessary to prevent complications. Some of these complications are discussed in the following paragraphs.

Multiple rib fractures are likely to occur during closed-chest ventilation, especially in the elderly patient whose rib cage is relatively inflexible. The broken ends of the rib present sharp edges that may lacerate the lung. Various studies report a 24% to 40% incidence of fractured ribs in large series of patients. It appears that the incidence of rib fracture as a result of external cardiac massage probably depends on the skill and experience of the individual who performs the resuscitation. Additionally, 2% of these studies have reported fracture of the sternum during closed-chest massage, as well as at least one case of a fracture of the scapula.

The incidence of fat embolization following closed-chest massage is probably at least as high as 30% to 50%. The actual embolizing mechanism has been a source of some speculation. There is now some consensus that the concussion of bones or the act of bending and compressing bones such as the rib cage may lead to microfractures within the medulla of ribs and sternum with an increase in marrow pressure. Thus fat is permitted to enter the venous circulation from the marrow. Significantly, pulmonary marrow embolization may occur in the absence of demonstrable fractures. In fact, because of the semiliquid nature of the sternal marrow and the communication of the marrow cavities with the venous system, such embolism may occur even more often than is realized by the reported incidence of successful closed-chest cardiac massage. Diffuse pulmonary fat and marrow emboli were found in random microscopic sections of the lungs of 10 of 16 patients treated by external cardiac massage by Lane and Merkel.* Pure fat emboli were five times more common than bone marrow emboli in this series, and four of the patients showed embolization without demonstrable fractures of either ribs or sternum. These authors raise the question of whether emboli may cause the acute cor pulmonale that is responsible for some of the failures of resuscitation. Although it has been generally assumed that mental deterioration following cardiac resuscitation results from the effect of prolonged anoxia on cortical cells, the question now is whether to consider cerebral fat emboli as another etiologic factor.

---

*Quoted by Neely, W. A., and Youngmans, J. R.: Anoxia of canine brain without damage, J.A.M.A. **183:**1085, 1963.

Pneumoperitoneum is a recognized hazard of closed-chest cardiac massage because free abdominal air under sufficient pressures severely compromises ventilation. The mechanism of air entry into the peritoneal cavity may involve a rupture of the wall of a viscus; hence closed-chest resuscitation could, of course, be the precipitating factor. Air extravasated from the pulmonary parenchyma to the mediastinum following external massage may dissect within the esophageal wall to the stomach or intestine (or enter the peritoneal cavity through the serosal surface of the intestine or stomach). Obviously it is important that this complication be recognized. Its immediate effects can be managed simply by aspiration of the air from the abdomen or, in the case of pneumothorax, from the chest.

Gastroesophageal laceration is a not infrequent complication of closed-chest cardiac massage. The laceration is commonly a linear one along the lesser curvature of the stomach that extends upward through the fundus and the cardia into the esophagus. The combination of mouth-to-mouth artificial respiration with closed-chest massage is particularly prone to produce such tearing. Pressures as low as 120 to 150 mm Hg produce mucosal slits in the adult stomach. Varying degrees of hemorrhage have been associated with this complication; therefore any bleeding from the nose or mouth following resuscitative efforts should alert one to this condition, which is similar to the Mallory-Weiss syndrome. Delayed perforation of the transverse colon has appeared as a sequel to mouth-to-mouth resuscitation and external cardiac massage. Edema and interstitial hemorrhage of the bowel wall, as well as hematoma of the mesentery and transverse colon, doubtless follow the trauma sustained during resuscitation. Ultimately this progresses to necrosis and perforation of the bowel wall.

Numerous reports of hepatic lacerations following closed-chest cardiac compression have appeared in the literature. This may well be the most common serious complication of external cardiac compression in infants and children; it apparently results from simultaneous compression of the chest and abdomen, thus limiting free movement of the liver. The patient with pectus excavatum or funnel chest is particularly susceptible to this hazard of sternal depression. In these patients, the funnel chest serves literally as a battering ram that compresses the liver forcibly against the vertebral bodies.

Gastric dilatation is a fairly common complication of closed-chest cardiac massage. It can easily occur with pharyngeal pressures of 20 to 25 cm water, such as may commonly be used during mouth-to-mouth or bag-and-mask resuscitation. In addition to regurgitation and aspiration pneumonia, several ill effects result from overdistension of the stomach. Gastric dilatation may further impair function in patients who already have difficulty with hypoventilation and hypotension. Further, increased vagal tone and decreased venous return to the heart may occur—even to the point of being the actual cause of bradycardia, sinus arrest, or cardiac standstill. Gastric pressure can easily force air out of the stomach, allowing gastric secretions to enter and even block the upper airway. One must be cautioned that the patient should be in a head-down position if epigastric pressure is being employed, and one should be reasonably certain that the stomach is empty (preferably by passing a gastric tube). Ideally the gastric tube with suction is the safest means of preventing or handling the problem of gastric dilatation.

One should be aware of the fact that vomiting may occur with a high degree of frequency in situations requiring oral resuscitation, particularly in asphyxiated patients. Although vomiting is not present in all cardiac arrest situations, it does represent a potential complicating hazard. Use of suction equipment is possible in many situations, but when it is not available the patient should be placed in a position that prevents the aspiration of vomitus. Mechanically tilting the patient and turning his head to the side often prevent aspiration.

Many of the postresuscitative complications of cardiac arrest depend on how quickly resuscitative efforts are employed and how effectively they are used. For example, the renal problems that ensue after cardiac arrest are much the same as those after any shock-producing cardiovascular collapse. Any impairment of renal function caused by hypoxia with associated metabolic acidosis and hyperkalemia is a serious threat. The definitive care of the postresuscitative victim is outside the scope of this book, but certainly the problems can be minimized if the patient receives properly applied resuscitative efforts.

Doubtless there are instances in which direct trauma to the lungs is a hazard of closed-chest resuscitation. Increased right atrial and vena caval pressures during application of the closed-chest technique have been confirmed by numerous studies, and it seems likely that pulmonary edema may be more common than has been clinically recognized.

Sudden or jerking motions should be avoided when one is compressing the chest. The compression should be smooth, regular, and uninterrupted. One half of the cycle should be compression, and half of it should be relaxation. Quick jabs increase the possibility of injury and produce quick jets of flow; however they do not enhance stroke volume or mean flow and pressure.

While closed-chest compression is being performed continuous pressures should not be maintained on the abdomen to decompress the stomach. Such action may trap the liver and could cause it to rupture.

If the patient with cardiac arrest is lying on a mattress or other soft surface, it is probably best to start closed-chest compression immediately; however the resilience of the mattress may dampen the effort applied in compressing the chest. If a bed board is available and can be inserted by the personnel, it should be quite helpful. Actually the floor may be the best place for application of closed-chest massage. When the patient is lying on a bed or a high-wheeled litter, the rescuer must stand on a step or chair or kneel on the bed or litter. With a low-wheeled litter, the rescuer can stand at the victim's side.

The rescuer's fingers should not rest on the patient's ribs during compression. Interlocking the fingers of the two hands may help to avoid this. Pressure with fingers on the ribs, or lateral pressure, increases the possibility of rib fracture and costochondral separation.

The most serious and dreaded complication of cardiac resuscitation results when cerebral anoxia produces serious neurologic sequelae. Depriving the brain of adequate oxygenation for even 3 to 4 minutes may have an adverse effect on the central nervous system. Any time longer than this may result in irreversible damage. The amount of time that the brain will withstand complete ischemia without permanent damage has never been altogether established. Even if this were known, other factors such as age, oxygenation of the patient at the time of the arrest, and temperature of the patient and the environment all play a part. The brain apparently is somewhat more sensitive to metabolic derangements at some ages than at others. The first sign of brain damage is, of course, unconsciousness. The respiratory center is knocked out, the pupils are dilated, the body is without reflexes, and electroencephalographic activity may be extremely slow or absent. Hopefully, however, most of these features can be reversed if oxygenated blood is quickly rushed to the most critical portion of the body, the brain.

What can be done on an immediate basis to reduce the likelihood of cerebral damage? Although the technique is somewhat controversial, I believe that a patient should be immediately tilted in a 10- to 15-degree Trendelenburg position (head down). Not only does this position improve venous return to the heart but also there is some evidence that it can delay irreversible brain damage.

The crucial period of time can be compromised by several factors. Of first importance is the effectiveness of the individual rescuer's ability to compress the heart manually. Ordinarily if one is not able to maintain a systolic blood pressure of at least 60 to 70 mm Hg, produce an easily palpable pulse in the peripheral vessels, maintain normal skin color of the patient, and keep the pupils constricted, the likelihood of neurologic damage is great.

If there is a possibility that severe brain damage may have occurred, the sooner one can apply effective measures the better. Therefore even on the way to the hospital, large doses of steroids may be started and the patient's body temperature may be lowered with whatever means are available. Because of the adverse effect of metabolic acidosis produced by anaerobic metabolism in the absence of oxygen, sodium bicarbonate should be given as soon as possible. Lactic and carbonic acids, products of the anaerobic metabolisms, rapidly lower the pH of body tissues. This action is thought by some to cause coagulation of the blood in the small vascular channels, such as those within the brain.

Certain psychiatric complications of closed-chest cardiac resuscitation that may be of considerable concern have been demonstrated. Severe personality decomposition is occasionally seen in patients subjected to highly mechanized and anxiety-provoking emotional distress during treatment in areas such as the coronary care unit, intensive care unit, recovery room, or burn and trauma units. Likewise the post–cardiac resuscitation victim is no exception as he may require some type of prolonged artificial assistance. An endotracheal tube may prevent him from communicating easily, and he may be totally unfamiliar with the purpose of the monitoring apparatus and the strange sounds, tubes, and equipment. The impersonal nature of his confinement, often in a windowless room, may compound the difficulties. In addition, his psychologic problems may prolong an acute brain syndrome that was provoked by an excessive period of anoxia or hypercapnia. We can aid in the situation considerably by giving as much personal attention and direct communication as possible. It is usually impossible for a patient to clearly remember the events surrounding cardiac arrest followed by successful resuscitation. The emotional adaptation of patients following cardiac resuscitation has been, in my experience, quite varied.

The psychiatric study by Druss and Korneld of a group of 10 survivors of cardiac arrest is significant. These physicians wondered how patients might react to the unique and remarkable experience of having been "dead." Their group of 10 patients was taken from 16 patients successfully resuscitated and discharged from Columbia Presbyterian Hospital. They represented a group of 85 patients who had experienced cardiac arrest outside the operating room. Prolonged psychiatric interviews were carried out with both the patient and the relatives. The control group consisted of 10 additional men who had been in the intensive care unit although they had not had cardiac arrest. Nine of the 10 patients with cardiac arrest had a mild to severe organic brain syndrome that included symptoms of confusion, delusional thinking, and uncontrollable agitation. At least four defense mechanisms were elicited, including denial and isolation, displacement, rejection, and hallucinatory or delusional behavior. Eight of the patients reacted by an isolation of affect and by denying that they had been afraid. Eight of the 10 patients experienced dreams of violence and violent death. When questioned about their attitude toward death, patients replied that they had been in no pain; therefore death was believed to be painless. No overt alterations in patients' religious attitudes were uncovered. Persistent long-term symptoms were often present, the most common being insomnia. Tenseness, anxiety, restlessness, and irritability were common. A majority of these patients experienced difficulty in concentration and a lack of memory for recent events.

Several suggestions have been made by psychiatrists. A great deal might be done to make the intensive care unit or the coronary monitoring unit a less frightening place. Increasing the degree of privacy would be helpful so that patients would be less aware of the life and death struggle of other patients. Monitoring equipment might be placed outside the unit to reduce the frightening aspects to the patient. Each patient experiencing a cardiac arrest should be talked to in detail and given as much reassurance as possible.

The psychic trauma to the physician himself might well be mentioned. I know of one physician who was so severely depressed by an occurrence of cardiac arrest during a tonsillectomy that he ceased performing any type of surgery.

Any interruption in the continuity of cardiopulmonary resuscitation, of course, presents a great and obvious hazard to the patient. Cardiopulmonary resuscitation should not be interrupted for more than 5 seconds for any reason except under the following circumstances. Endotracheal intubation, if absolutely necessary, may require up to 15 seconds for accomplishment by those well practiced in the technique when the patient has been properly positioned and all preparations have been made well in advance. When moving a patient up or down a stairway, it is difficult to continue effective cardiopulmonary resuscitation. It is best to perform cardiopulmonary resuscitation at the head or the foot of the stairs and then interrupt it at a given signal and move quickly to the next level where the resuscitation can be resumed. Such interruptions should not exceed 15 seconds. The patient should not be moved to a more convenient site until he has been stabilized and is ready for transportation or until arrangements have been made for uninterrupted resuscitation during movement.

In this section we have given a rather formidable list of possible pitfalls in, and complications of, closed-chest cardiac massage. Each of these complications can be minimized by careful attention to details of performance. It must be remembered that during cardiac arrest effective cardiopulmonary resuscitation is required even if it results in complications because the alternative to effective cardiopulmonary resuscitation is death.

CONTINUATION OF RESUSCITATIVE EFFORTS

If one compresses the heart for a prolonged period of time without success and if artificial ventilation is adequate, one should systematically review all the potential sources of error before deciding that further resuscitative efforts are of no avail. Prolonged heart massage for more than 3 hours with complete recovery has been reported in several instances.

As a general rule cardiac resuscitative efforts should be maintained at least until the patient can be brought to the hospital where electrocardiographic and even electroencephalographic tracings can be made.

In spite of precordial concussion, artificial ventilatory efforts, and closed-chest cardiac compression, very frequently a regular heart rhythm will not resume. Ventricular fibrillation is often directly related in a high percentage of arrests occurring outside the hospital. Fibrillation is particularly likely in cases of arrests associated with accidental electrocution, coronary occlusion, and occasionally near drowning. Ordinarily a heart that is fibrillating in such circumstances does not spontaneously defibrillate; electric defibrillation is indicated. The main point to remember is that life can be maintained and cerebral damage can be prevented simply by *augmentation* of the cardiorespiratory system. This can be accomplished for an indefinite period if performed in optimal fashion. Generally it can be maintained for a long enough period to allow the patient to be brought to a hospital or to allow more definitive care to be brought to the patient.

OPEN-CHEST COMPRESSION

Although opening the chest for direct cardiac massage is certainly not a part of immediate care, in the sense in which the term is used in this book, it is pertinent that we be aware of situations that are not likely to yield successfully to closed-chest compressive efforts. Pathophysiologic considerations that contribute to ineffective closed-chest compressive techniques can be managed more effectively via the direct or open-chest route.

Open-chest cardiac compression and defibrillation should definitely be a part of every physician's armamentarium, whether he is a surgeon or not. There are times when closed-chest cardiac compression is less likely to be successful. Some situations that might be best managed by the open-chest approach include the following:
1. Pectus excavatum or marked pectus carinatum
2. Massive air embolism
3. Cardiac tamponade
4. Bilateral pneumothorax or tension pneumothorax
5. Lack of availability of an external defibrillator in the presence of ventricular fibrillation
6. Failure to respond adequately to closed-chest compression (should the patient be in the operating room under a well-controlled situation, one should open the chest in 2 to 3 minutes)
7. Some instances of severe mitral stenosis (commissurotomy may be the emergency procedure of choice)
8. Pregnancy (third trimester)
9. Flail chest

10. Massive pulmonary embolism
11. Evidence of intrathoracic hemorrhage or severe trauma to the chest
12. Penetrating thoracic injuries
13. Ventricular herniation after cardiac surgery
14. When the heart's anatomic position is not in the midline
15. When one desires visual monitoring of the heart
16. With other causes of intracardiac obstructions, such as a left atrial myxoma
17. When the chest is already opened

PROGNOSIS

How often are cardiopulmonary resuscitative efforts likely to be needed outside the hospital? The full scope of the picture is yet to emerge, but it is known that more than 800,000 individuals in this country die each year of heart attacks. More than 50% of those patients dying of heart attacks die before reaching the hospital. In fact, more than 50% of those dying of severe injuries die before reaching the hospital. There is evidence that a substantial percentage of these patients could be saved if adequate resuscitative efforts were immediately available.

What can one expect of his resuscitative efforts? At the time of this writing, even resuscitative efforts under the most ideal conditions in the hospital seldom produce successful results in more than 20% of the instances. There has been a permanent success rate in more than 16% of over 5,000 reported cases. Since resuscitative efforts outside the hospital are fraught with many additional problems, it seems unlikely that the success rate will soon approximate that within the hospital. It is likely, however, that these efforts should ultimately yield considerable dividends with improved ability to reach the victim quickly through more effective communications and through the proper training of large numbers of individuals capable of providing resuscitation.

The crux of successful resuscitative efforts revolves around the vital importance of the *time factor*. Certainly this principle is most important and needs to be reemphasized. Beyond the need for active resuscitative measures, the need for consciousness of the urgency of this situation must play a part in any thoughts relative to cardiac arrest. If the percentage of permanent survivals is to be increased, and if neurologic complications are to be reduced, then every possible source of delay in beginning immediate manual systole must be eliminated. In an early study of the first 1,200 recorded cases of cardiac arrest, it became apparent that 94% of the successfully and permanently resuscitated patients had cardiac massage within the first 4 minutes. In other words, cerebral circulation must be artificially augmented within this time or permanent irreversible changes will occur.

It is still too early to know what can be accomplished with cardiopulmonary resuscitation for the patient experiencing a sudden arrest from a myocardial infarction. Adequate numbers of cases are still not available. Permanent success with 15% to 20% of such cases has been reported in relatively small series. A group of the Royal Victoria Hospital in Belfast, Northern Ireland, has had remarkably high success rates with their mobile coronary care unit.

There may be a number of factors that contribute to the failure to successfully resuscitate the heart. Although much of the success rate may be dictated by the nature of the pathology, some degree of blame can probably be placed on the fact that there may have been an inexcusable delay in instituting proper resuscitation, the resuscitative measures were not adequate, or the individual applying resuscitation had inadequate knowledge. Obviously proper means of compressing the heart will be completely negated if there has been a failure to establish adequate ventilation. Premature discontinuance of resuscitative efforts may be involved. Of 300 fatal cases of cardiac arrest in one series, for example, almost one third were associated with totally inadequate attempts at resuscitation.

It seems reasonable to assume that in the near future all medical personnel will be well versed in the techniques of cardiopulmonary resuscitation at an early stage. Practice sessions on resuscitation of the dog heart are essential. There are few better ways to acquaint one with the technique of cardiac resuscitation than by following actual experience in the animal laboratory with observation of resuscitative efforts on the ward. Formal periods of instruction in cardiac arrest and resuscitation should be repeated each year. There is no reason to neglect training physicians in cardiopulmonary resuscitation, especially at a time when every effort is being made to provide lifesaving technique training to members of the nursing and allied health professions and members of rescue squads.

QUESTIONS

1. Distinguish between useful drugs and necessary drugs in the treatment of cardiac arrest.
2. Discuss the importance of using mannequins in teaching cardiopulmonary resuscitation.
3. What are the two obvious phases of cardiopulmonary resuscitation, *and* how should they be coordinated?
4. List the main hazards of closed-chest massage.
5. Discuss the extreme importance of the time factor in cardiopulmonary resuscitation.
6. List and explain each of several common pitfalls in applying cardiopulmonary resuscitation.
7. When is mouth-to-nose artificial respiration likely to be more useful than the mouth-to-mouth technique?
8. What is the Trendelenburg maneuver and what is its place in cardiopulmonary resuscitation?
9. How long should cardiopulmonary resuscitative effort be continued in the absence of obvious success?
10. Discuss the psychologic aspects of cardiopulmonary resuscitation to the patient and the physician.

CHAPTER 13

Cardiac arrhythmias and the myocardial infarction victim

RICHARD H. MARTIN

It is customary to organize a discussion of the treatment of cardiac arrhythmias by specific diagnostic categories. When considering the definitive therapy of each arrhythmia such an organization is appropriate because a correct diagnosis should generally be established before treatment is begun. Unfortunately in emergency circumstances the equipment necessary to make a definitive diagnosis may not be available. Occasionally it may be necessary to begin therapy without electrocardiographic confirmation of the specific type of arrhythmia based on careful consideration of the probable diagnoses that might be present, the risk of delaying therapy, and the potential hazard of immediate therapy.

The organization of this chapter therefore is based on the clinical presentation of the patient before an electrocardiogram is available. The discussion stresses emergency measures that can be carried out with reasonable safety before reaching the hospital and deals only with those steps of diagnosis and treatment that are appropriate in the home, the field, or the emergency room. The treatment of rhythm disorders requiring hospital or coronary care unit admission is beyond the scope of this discussion; however it is well covered in numerous other sources. Similarly there is no attempt here to cover details of electrocardiographic diagnosis of arrhythmias, which can be reviewed in standard textbooks of electrocardiography.

REGULAR TACHYARRHYTHMIAS

In the adult 100 beats per minute is the arbitrary upper limit for the resting heart rate. An infant may have a normal sinus rhythm as fast as 200 per minute at 1 month of age, but the resting sinus rate should not exceed 140 per minute after 1 year of age. It is not unusual to find a heart rate of 200 per minute in a young adult during extremely strenuous exertion. Other causes of physiologic sinus tachycardia are fever, emotional stress, and severe pain. In general the sinus tachycardia accompanying these conditions in the adult does not exceed 150 per minute. A potentially more serious cause of sinus tachycardia is thyroid storm complicating thyrotoxicosis.

In a patient with a rapid, regular pulse the diagnostic considerations are sinus tachycardia and three types of ectopic tachycardia: (1) supraventricular tachycardia (a categorical term that includes atrial tachycardia and atrioventricular junctional tachycardia), (2) atrial flutter, and (3) ventricular tachycardia. *Sinus tachycardia* requires no treatment except that which may be required for the underlying cause. In the presence of serious underlying heart disease, any rapid ectopic tachycardia can potentially lead to the serious complications of pulmonary edema or cardiovascular collapse.

Certain features are useful in attempting to establish a preliminary diagnosis. Ectopic supraventricular tachycardias usually produce a heart rate in excess of 150 per minute, in contrast to sinus tachycardia, which is rarely faster than 140. It is important to listen to the heart tones to establish the heart rate, because a peripheral pulse deficit at very fast rates may be a result of pulsus alternans in the patient with serious myocardial disease. The rate of sinus tachycardia generally varies by 5 to 15 beats per minute over a period of several minutes, in contrast to ectopic tachycardias, which are likely to be quite constant.

Carotid massage characteristically slows sinus tachycardia slightly, but this may not be detectable without an electrocardiographic recording during the massage. In contrast, there occurs either no change in rate or an abrupt return to normal sinus rhythm during carotid massage in the patient with supraventricular tachycardia. Atrial flutter may show a stepwise decrease in pulse rate because of increased atrioventricular block resulting from the augmented vagal tone induced by carotid massage. Ventricular tachycardia does not change during carotid massage. A hallmark (but not a sine qua non) of ventricular tachycardia is the presence of atrioventricular dissociation. This may be detected by the presence of jugular venous A waves dissociated from the first and second heart sounds and intermittent jugular cannon waves caused by right atrial contractions during ventricular systole against a closed tricuspid valve. The jugular veins on occasion may also establish a diagnosis of atrial flutter by revealing flutter waves (at a rate of 250 to 350 per minute).

The most important determinant of the potential need for treatment before an electrocardiogram can be obtained is the clinical setting in which tachycardia is observed. A healthy young woman with the sudden appearance of tachycardia of 170 per minute, moderate dyspnea, and lightheadedness is likely to have *paroxysmal atrial tachycardia*. There is often a history of previous episodes or possibly a diagnosis of mitral valve prolapse or Wolff-Parkinson-White syndrome. She generally does not require immediate treatment. Indeed, carotid massage should be deferred until an electrocardiogram is recorded to establish a diagnosis. After the diagnosis has been documented on one or more occasions, it is acceptable to treat recurrences in the home. Often the patient can be taught to terminate paroxysms by a Valsalva maneuver or gagging, both of which augment vagal tone. Carotid massage, although generally somewhat more effective, is not without hazard, particularly in the elderly patient. It should not be maintained for more than 5 seconds and should never be applied bilaterally. If drug therapy is required, the patient should be electrocardiographically monitored in an emergency room or the physician's office. Normotensive young patients may convert when mild hypertension is induced by giving methoxamine, 10 to 20 mg intramuscularly or 5 to 15 mg intravenously. Edrophonium (Tensilon), 5 to 10 mg administered intravenously after a test dose of 1 mg is usually well tolerated and has effectively terminated supraventricular tachycardia in many patients since this use of the drug was introduced in 1969. If the tachycardia is well tolerated, a hypnotic drug may allow the paroxysm to terminate during sleep. If more urgent conversion is warranted, digitalis glycosides are generally the most effective drugs, particularly if manifestations of congestive failure are present. After administration of 0.5 mg of digoxin, carotid massage should be repeated because the vagal effect of both measures is additive. Propranolol, 1 to 2 mg given intravenously, may also be effective. If the situation is critical or if rapid certain conversion to sinus rhythm is desirable for other reasons, synchronized precordial shock (cardioversion) under light sedation with diazepam or sodium pentothal usually terminates supraventricular tachycardia immediately.

Atrial flutter is relatively uncommon and usually accompanies underlying mitral valve or congenital heart disease. It occasionally complicates acute pulmonary embolism, which should be suspected in a previously healthy individual who suddenly develops atrial flutter or atrial fibrillation associated with acute dyspnea, with or without chest pain or hypotension. In contrast to atrial fibrillation, which is differentiated at the bedside by its irregular ventricular rate, the ventricular rate in atrial flutter often fails to slow after administration of digitalis. Misguided efforts to slow the pulse rate in atrial flutter with large doses of digitalis commonly result in digitalis intoxication. Because of this problem, it is often best to promptly terminate acute atrial flutter with synchronized percordial shock before administering digitalis, which can make cardioversion somewhat hazardous. Quinidine may also terminate atrial flutter. It should never be administered in an attempt to convert atrial flutter until after adequate digitalization has been accomplished because of the risk of reducing atrioventricular block, leading to a 1:1 ventricular response to each flutter wave at a rate in excess of 200. Quinidine should not be given in doses exceeding 0.4 gm every 6 hours because of the risk of cardiac or respiratory arrest with high doses of this drug. High-dose quinidine therapy has been replaced by cardioversion, which is much safer and much more likely to terminate the arrhythmia.

Tachycardia detected in a patient with crushing substernal pain, diaphoresis, and a sensation of impending doom (the classic symptoms of acute myocardial infarction) may represent sinus tachycardia, supraventricular tachycardia, atrial flutter, or ventricular tachycardia. *Ventricular tachycardia* is a particularly life-threatening problem in this setting. It usually produces a heart rate between 100 and 180 per minute. It is more likely to cause hypotension or loss of consciousness than are the supraventricular arrhythmias. If ventricular tachycardia is a significant consideration in a patient with severe cardiovascular distress, an attempt should be made to terminate the rhythm without delay.

Occasionally a sharp blow delivered with the fist to the precordium terminates a paroxysm of ventricular tachycardia; this is particularly true if the blow is delivered within a few seconds of the onset of ventricular tachycardia induced by a premature ventricular beat occurring in the vulnerable period of the cardiac cycle. If such a blow does not promptly break the arrhythmia, lidocaine should be administered in a dose of 100 mg intravenously. If the rhythm is actually sinus or supraventricular tachycardia, lidocaine is ineffective but the dose does no appreciable harm. If a precordial blow or lidocaine administration terminates the arrhythmia, a continuous drip of lidocaine, 1 to 4 mg per minute, should be maintained while the patient is transported to a hospital or coronary care unit. After electrocardiographic confirmation of the diagnosis, if lidocaine has not been effective, precordial shock should be administered as soon as possible because ventricular fibrillation may supervene as a result of several factors that include further reduction in coronary blood flow to already ischemic areas of the myocardium.

IRREGULAR TACHYARRHYTHMIAS

A rapid, irregular rhythm may result from premature atrial (or junctional) contractions, premature ventricular contractions, atrial fibrillation, or multifocal atrial tachycardia. Multiple premature beats generally produce a patterned irregularity, whereas atrial fibrillation and multifocal atrial tachycardia cause the rhythm to be totally irregular. Premature beats commonly occur in normal individuals and usually require no treatment. Acute *atrial fibrillation*, likewise, is usually fairly well tolerated, allowing time for transport to a hospital for definitive diagnosis and treatment. When atrial fibrillation results in a very rapid ventricular response in a patient with a serious underlying heart disease, emergency treatment may be indicated prior to admission to the hospital. In the presence of mitral stenosis, the sudden onset of atrial fibrillation with a fast ventricular response may quickly lead to pulmonary edema.

Efforts should be directed toward slowing the ventricular rate rather than immediate conversion. This can usually be accomplished with digitalis glycosides. Because such patients have often already been receiving digitalis, care should be taken to avoid overdosage. Digoxin given intravenously in 0.25- or 0.125-mg increments every 2 to 4 hours is usually effective. Rarely propranolol may be necessary, in combination with digitalis, to secure adequate slowing. Caution is required with use of propranolol, however, for its myocardial depressant effects may aggravate congestive heart failure. It is containdicated if there is a history of bronchial asthma. Conversion of acute atrial fibrillation is most safely and surely accomplished by cardioversion, which should be carried out unless the prognosis for prolonged sinus rhythm is very poor or unless conversion occurs spontaneously, after digitalization, or after administration of quinidine, 0.2 to 0.4 gm every 6 hours (given primarily to minimize the likelihood of reversion to atrial fibrillation after cardioversion).

Multifocal atrial tachycardia is impossible to differentiate from atrial fibrillation without an electrocardiogram. It is usually encountered in severe, life-threatening illnesses such as septic (or less commonly hemorrhagic) shock or acute respiratory failure. There is no effective means of controlling this arrhythmia or slowing the heart rate in this condition; giving large doses of digitalis in attempting to do so is a certain way to produce digitalis intoxication. The arrhythmia generally resolves when the primary problem is successfully treated.

Premature beats in the setting of a suspected acute myocardial infarction frequently warn of impending, more serious arrhythmias. The peripheral pulse may feel as though there are dropped beats and thus may suggest intermittent second degree heart block. Auscultation of the heart while palpating the carotid pulse should resolve this problem. It is impossible to differentiate between atrial and ventricular premature beats without an electrocardiogram (even with one this is often difficult). There are so many exceptions to the "rule" that premature ventricular contractions have a fully compensatory pause that this feature is useless in making decisions regarding therapy. It is reasonable to act on the assumption that all premature beats early in the course of an acute myocardial infarction are premature ventricular contractions. Thus premature beats in this setting should be treated promptly with administration of intravenous lidocaine (1 to 1.5 mg per kilogram bolus followed by a drip of 1 to 4 mg per minute during transport to the hospital and coronary care unit), particularly if the frequency of premature beats exceeds 6 per minute. As in the case of sustained tachycardia during an acute myocardial infarction, it would appear to be far safer to administer lidocaine unnecessarily (and ineffectively) for atrial arrhythmias than to allow a ventricular arrhythmia to progress to ventricular fibrillation because a relatively innocuous drug has been withheld.

BRADYARRHYTHMIAS

Although the accepted lower limit of normal sinus rhythm in adults is 60 beats per minute, it is not unusual to see physiologic *sinus bradycardia* with a rate of 40 or 50 per minute in healthy adults of all age groups. Sinus bradycardia may be seen in patients under treatment with propranolol for prevention of tachyarrhythmias, reserpine for hypertension, and occasionally a variety of other drugs. Any condition that is associated with increased vagal tone—for example, nausea and vomiting—may produce sinus bradycardia, as may myxedema, hypothermia resulting from prolonged cold exposure, obstructive jaundice, and cerebrovascular accidents associated with increased intracranial pressure.

A particularly common syndrome in which profound sinus bradycardia is a frequent finding is *vasodepressor (vasovagal) syncope*, the common fainting spell. Such fainting may occur at any age but is most characteristically seen in young healthy individuals subjected to a sudden emotional stress, such as threatened or imagined bodily injury. The patient has generally been noted to have collapsed to the floor, usually without warning. He may appear to be near death, with profound hypotension, marked pallor, and diaphoresis. The pupils may be dilated. Respiration may be either shallow or deep and sighing. There may be alarming bradycardia (rates of 20 to 30 beats are not uncommon). Heart tones may be distant, suggesting severe cardiac disease. Clonic movements may occur, localized to the face and upper body or occasionally generalized.

The ultimate mechanisms underlying vasodepressor syncope have fascinated investigators for many years and remain the subject of some uncertainty. It is evident that there is profound autonomic activity during the faint; this factor is responsible for the bradycardia (vagal effect). The hypotension results from pooling of blood in capacitance vessels of the body so that venous return cannot keep up with the demand for increased cardiac output that would ordinarily accompany the drop in peripheral resistance characteristic of this syndrome. These physiologic mechanisms provide the rationale for therapy, which consists of placing the victim supine with the head and trunk lower than the legs (to augment venous return), giving reassurance verbally, and maintaining a calm environment about the patient. The syndrome usually clears quickly without further therapy; occasionally administration of intravenous atropine, 0.5 to 1.0 mg, may be necessary to reverse the marked bradycardia, and rarely vasopressor agents may be needed if hypotension is prolonged.

Some patients may develop a syndrome similar to vasodepressor syncope during acute myocardial infarction. The age of the patient and the presence of severe chest pain (usually but not invariably present) help to differentiate this life-threatening problem from the benign simple vasodepressor faint. Diaphragmatic wall myocardial infarction is particularly likely to produce this *bradycardia-hypotension syndrome,* which, like vasodepressor syncope, is usually associated with diaphoresis and other signs of autonomic hyperactivity. Bradycardia in this setting may be particularly dangerous because it may predispose to the development of ectopic beats that may lead to ventricular tachycardia or fibrillation. In addition, the bradycardia, coupled with the limited stroke volume of an acutely damaged left ventricle, impairs cardiac output and intensifies the hypotension that initially results from inadequate peripheral resistance and venous pooling. Hypotension may then beget further reduction in myocardial perfusion and further myocardial ischemia or necrosis or both and may lead to a vicious circle and death. Morphine, given appropriately to relieve chest pain and to allay anxiety in the patient before transport to the hospital, causes dilation of arterioles and veins that can intensify this process. Therapy consists of elevating the lower extremities to increase venous return to the heart, administration of vasopressors, if necessary, to maintain a systolic blood pressure of 90 to 100 (in a previously normotensive subject, higher in the hypertensive patient), and the immediate intravenous injection of atropine, 0.5 to 1.0 mg. Atropine should be injected slowly (over 1 to 2 minutes) in this circumstance because on rare occasions rapid injection of the drug may cause a sudden release of acetylcholine from cardiac vagal nerve endings and produce a paradoxic vagal effect with complete asystole or heart block.

Marked bradycardia or asystole may also result from *heart block* or less commonly from *sinoatrial arrest*. These two conditions generally occur in patients older than 50 years of age as a result of degeneration of the specialized fibers of the cardiac conduction system and sinus node or as a result of coronary heart disease. Such patients most commonly seek help because of an episode of syncope or near-syncope. There is usually no associated chest pain. The pulse pressure is usually wide because of the large stroke volume accompanying the slow idioventricular rhythm that generally becomes established after several seconds of asystole. Once an escape rhythm appears, hypotension is unusual. Ausculation may reveal atrial sounds dissociated from first and second heart sounds, and occasional cannon waves may be seen in the jugular veins. Asystole may recur at any time in such patients, who should be observed continuously until such time as effective therapy with a transvenous pacemaker has been established.

In this electronic age, physicians often feel helpless without an oscilloscopic electrocardiographic monitor in such circumstances. They forget that each patient has been endowed with a very effective built-in heartbeat detector: the peripheral pulse. A finger continuously on the pulse will detect recurrent asystole before sufficient time has elapsed for the patient to lose consciousness. A sharp blow to the precordium during this interval may do little to further a budding doctor-patient relationship but usually mechanically stimulates the myocardium sufficiently to trigger ventricular depolarization and obviate the need for cardiac massage, a difficult procedure during transport to a hospital. In the absence of a specific electrocardiographic diagnosis in such a patient, it is reasonable to administer atropine, which may increase the heart rate and reduce the risk of recurrent asystole if the mechanism has been marked sinus bradycardia, sinus arrest, or heart block in the atrioventricular junctional region. Atropine has no effect in the statistically more likely event that the block in such a patient occurs below the atrioventricular node, in the bundle of His, or its more distal ramifications. Isoproterenol increases the irritability of myocardial cells with pacemaker potential in the sinus node, atrium, atrioventricular junction, and ventricle; in addition, its effect on the atrioventricular node may reduce block at that level. Thus this drug may be effective regardless of the cause of the asystole. If atropine has not resulted in a heart rate of at least 60 per minute within 5 minutes, an intravenous drip of isoproterenol should be begun (1 to 2 mg in 500 ml at an infusion rate of 0.01 to 0.03 μg per kg per minute). Even if this treatment does not increase the heart rate, it may reduce the chances of prolonged asystole or it may make the myocardium more responsive to the occasional precordial blow required for episodic asystole. The patient should be transported to a hospital with facilities for artificial pacemaker implantation without delay. Therapy for heart block with sodium lactate infusion, corticosteroids, or potassium solutions has no place in the emergency treatment of the patient with asystole.

An increasingly common cause of asystole and bradycardia is sudden failure of an implanted cardiac pacemaker. Pacemaker failure generally results from cessation of effective pacing, and the patient should be dealt with in the manner previously outlined. Less commonly an implanted pacemaker may accelerate to a dangerously high rate also leading to near-syncope. In this circumstance antiarrhythmic drugs are not effective; therefore the pacemaker must be inactivated and replaced by another unit as soon as possible.

PROPHYLACTIC ANTIARRHYTHMIC DRUGS IN ACUTE MYOCARDIAL INFARCTION

The major impact of the coronary care unit in reducing the mortality of acute myocardial infarction has resulted not from the original goal of prompt resuscitation of cardiac arrest but instead from *prevention* of cardiac arrest. This has been accomplished by identifying warning arrhythmias and initiating antiarrhythmic therapy before the appearance of ventricular tachycardia, ventricular fibrillation, or asystole. It has been established that the risk of serious arrhythmias resembles a logarithmic function of time from onset of infarction with the highest risk immediately after the onset of the chest pain and a diminishing risk thereafter. Therefore it appears reasonable to extend the principles of coronary care to the suspected victim of myocardial infarction before he reaches the coronary care unit and thus into the earliest moments after infarction when the risk of cardiac arrest is highest. Mobile coronary care units have achieved notable results with this approach, but such units are not available to the majority of patients sustaining acute myocardial infarction. Some of the principles of prevention of life-threatening arrhythmias, however, may be applied in the absence of the sophisticated electronics of the mobile coronary care unit.

The preceding discussions of ventricular tachycardia, premature ventricular contractions, and the bradycardia-hypotension syndrome in acute myocardial infarction have been primarily based on the assumption that such prophylaxis may prevent some deaths prior to arrival at a basic life-support facility. It now appears reasonable to extend this approach to include all patients with suspected myocardial infarction even in the absence of a detectable arrhythmia. Lidocaine may be given to all such patients (1 to 4 mg per minute as intravenous infusion, 150 to 300 mg intramuscularly) provided that the heart rate is above 60. If the initial rate is below 60, lidocaine carries the risk of suppression of "backup" idioventricular pacemaker foci, which might be needed if sinus arrest or complete heart block were to ensue. Atropine should not be administered prophylactically for bradycardia unless hypotension is also present, since atropine may increase the risk of ventricular fibrillation in patients with acute myocardial infarction.

QUESTIONS

Your 48-year-old opponent collapses while playing handball. He complains of crushing chest pain and a sense of impending doom. His pulse is regular at a rate of 110 per minute. Your medical bag is in your car outside the gym.

1. What is the most likely cardiac arrhythmia?
2. Should an antiarrhythmic drug be administered. prior to transporting the patient to a hospital? If so, what drug and why?
3. After an ambulance has been called, you observe 15 premature beats per minute while palpating his pulse. What would you do now?
4. Before you have had a chance to carry out your plan in response to question No. 3, your patient becomes ashen and his pulse is noted to be very weak at 160 per minute. Your medical bag has not yet been brought from your car. What is the most likely arrhythmia present?
5. What observations might help you differentiate the various possible arrhythmias?
6. Do you have time to wait for your bag to be brought in before treating? Why?

7. What might you do to terminate the arrhythmia?

Your response to question No. 7 is effective, and the pulse suddenly slows to 110 and becomes stronger. To reduce your patient's pain and apprehension prior to transport to the hospital you administer morphine. A few minutes later the patient complains of nausea, vomits, and again becomes very pale. His pulse is again observed to be weak but regular at a rate of 35 per minute.

8. What are the possible mechanisms of this new problem?
9. What drug would you try first in an attempt to correct this new problem?
10. The scenario is roughly the same, but your handball opponent is 21 years old, the chest pain is very mild, and the pulse initially is 190 and regular. How does this change your approach to the problem? What now is the most likely arrhythmia? What should you do to treat it?

PART FIVE

Emergencies involving environmental excess

CHAPTER 14

Heat emergencies

Partially because the various terms for heat emergencies are occasionally mis-used, it is important to differentiate at least three types of clinical situations result-ing from exposures to excessive heat: heat exhaustion, heat pyrexia, and heat cramps. Emergency care can be lifesaving, providing that the proper therapy is instituted.

HEAT CRAMPS

Heat cramps are characterized by severe muscle pains and cramps, particularly in the lower extremities and sometimes in the abdomen. The condition is, of course, more of a problem in a hot environment and in individuals who do a lot of sweating. Because heat cramps may progress to heat exhaustion, the systemic picture may in-clude faintness, dizziness, and a marked weakness.

Immediate aid involves replacement of sodium chloride. In fact, drinking large quantities of water may increase the severity of the cramps. Enteric-coated sodium chloride tablets given with water are usually sufficient. If a patient is brought to the hospital or is in the emergency room, an infusion of isotonic sodium chloride is the ideal treatment.

HEAT EXHAUSTION AND HEAT SYNCOPE

Heat exhaustion can be recognized by the clinical feature of general peripheral collapse, which is usually of a mild to moderate degree. The patient may complain at the onset of generalized weakness and lassitude and may even faint. Helpful in identifying heat exhaustion is the pale, clammy skin of the patient. The temperature of the skin may be either normal or decreased. In addition to profuse sweating, nausea and vomiting may be seen. There is a fast, weak pulse and blood pressure is ususally decreased. The pupils may be dilated.

The immediate care of a heat exhaustion victim dictates moving him to a cooler environment, if at all possible. Clothing should be loosened and the patient should be encouraged to drink fluids, particularly water with sodium chloride added.

If syncope has occurred, the patient should be placed in the supine position with the feet elevated. An intravenous infusion of isotonic saline solution hastens the patient's return to a more normal state. Coffee may serve as a beneficial stimulant, and aromatic spirits of ammonia may be helpful.

A patient suffering from heat exhaustion has a definite pallor, caused by the nature of his peripheral vasomotor collapse. This is in marked contrast to the reddish blush of the patient suffering from heat pyrexia or heat stroke.

Placing cold applications on the patient's body, especially around the forehead, is beneficial; the reduction in body temperature can be aided by an electric fan blowing over the patient.

Because heat exhaustion is characterized by the pooling of large quantities of blood in the skin, the reduced amounts of circulating blood can be partially corrected by elevating the legs well over the body and, if necessary, applying elastic bandages to increase blood return to the right side of the heart.

HEAT PYREXIA (HEAT STROKE OR SUNSTROKE)

In contrast to heat exhaustion, heat stroke, more effectively termed *heat pyrexia*, is an emergency of greater magnitude. Heat exhaustion occurs more commonly in women, and heat stroke is seen most often in men. Like heat exhaustion, heat pyrexia indicates poor acclimatization to excessive heat usually associated with high humidities. The individual is unable to adjust to the heat by the body's temperature-regulating mechanisms. Accordingly sweating ceases, causing a further rise in body temperature. Unlike the normal or slightly subnormal temperatures of victims of heat exhaustion, temperature elevations to more than 106° F may be found in patients with heat stroke. Such temperatures cannot be tolerated by the body's vital organs, especially the brain, and death may result. As previously mentioned, these patients have a reddish flush to the skin. Initially cardiac output is increased as reflected in the elevated blood pressure and the strong, bounding pulse.

There is a significant mortality associated with heat stroke. Death may claim as many as one fifth to two thirds of its victims; aged persons and those with previous cardiac difficulties are particularly susceptible.

The cardinal signs of heat stroke, in addition to a history of exposure to a combined elevated temperature and humidity, are hot, dry, reddish skin, agitation, coma, and hyperpyrexia. At the onset the patient may experience dizziness, headache, and marked dryness of the mouth. Unconsciousness may quickly ensue.

In addition to the cardinal signs, early symptoms of heat stroke may include lethargy, dizziness, confusion, vomiting, diarrhea, abdominal and muscular cramps, polydipsia, polyuria, and cerebellar dysfunction. The systolic blood pressure may soon fall with the pulse becoming rapid and shallow. The respirations are usually rapid, either panting or irregular in type. Although the skin of most patients is hot and dry, occasionally a patient continues to sweat freely. Some patients may have a seizure.

Immediate measures demand as rapid a fall in body temperatures as possible. If emergency treatment is delayed until the reddish flush of the skin turns to a grayish color, the prognosis becomes increasingly worse. All possible measure should be utilized to reduce the body temperature. These may include placing the patient in a tub of ice cold water or continued washings with rubbing alcohol. Wrapping the patient in cold, wet sheets while an electric fan is blowing on the patient is an effective measure. Of all the measures used to rapidly reduce the body's temperature, ice bath immersion is the fastest, and it is preferred over sponging. Drugs such as phenothiazine are also less effective measures.

During cooling one can counteract the induced vasoconstriction with vigorous massage. Increased surface evaporation is aided by fanning the patient. Repeated small doses of chlorpromazine or diazepam control shivering and make the ice treatment more tolerable for the patient who is awake.

Frequent recordings of the temperature are indicated inasmuch as it may again rise after an initial fall if continued efforts to cool the patient are not maintained. Unlike the heat exhaustion patient, the patient with heat stroke should be placed in a head-up or partially reclining position. Immediate efforts to reduce body temperature should not cease until the temperature has been reduced to less than 102° F.

All patients with heat pyrexia should be hospitalized.

Oxygen should be given to the patient once the emergency room is reached or during transportation to the hospital in the ambulance.

In addition to reducing the body temperature as rapidly as possible to diminish the stress and injury imposed by the hyperthermia, one should support the increased cardiovascular demand produced by the hyperthermia. The majority of heat stroke victims have an almost doubled cardiac index and marked hypotension as well as considerable peripheral vascular dilatation. Plasma volume is reduced by considerable loss of body fluids; therefore intravenous fluid administration is indicated. Ringer's lactate solution should be used.

If the patient's blood pressure continues to be dangerously low, a beta adrenergic stimulation of the myocardium is indicated. Isoproterenol may be given at the rate of 1 μg per minute. One should not make the mistake of giving an alpha adrenergic agent, which would not increase the cardiac output.

After the initial treatment of rapid immersion in an ice water bath and administration of isoproterenol, if indicated, consideration can then be given to use of a diuretic. Mannitol as a 12.5 gm bolus may be administered if there is concern that tubular flow has been reduced during marked renal vasoconstriction. An additional dose of 12.5 gm per liter of intravenous fluid can be added.

As soon as time permits, the bladder should be catheterized to monitor urinary output.

Intravascular coagulation accompanied by hemorrhage may occur at a later stage. The physician must be alert for this complication and be prepared to administer heparin to inhibit the fibrinolytic mechanism by competitively inhibiting plasminogen activation.

The patient's return from unconsciousness to a well-oriented mental state may take as long as several hours after body temperature has been reduced to a near-normal state. If immediate care of the patient has been deficient or slow in arriving, permanent brain damage or disabling neurologic deficits may persist.

Under normal conditions in a man who consumes 3,000 calories per day 65% of heat loss is by radiation, convection, and conduction. Thirty percent is lost by evaporation of water from the skin and lungs and 3% is used to warm the cooler air he breathes. Two percent is lost through excretion.

Heat stroke is seen under a variety of conditions, but it is often associated with athletic activity, such as long distance running and prolonged calisthenics. Heat stroke is frequently encountered by those in military service. Alcoholics are prone to be affected.

When the temperature-humidity index is more than 87, persons should be cautioned against vigorous exercise. When going to an environment with greater than normal heat and humidity, one should acclimate oneself gradually over a period of weeks. Fluid intake should be adjusted according to the fluid lost by sweating. This may require as much as 10 quarts of water a day.

The average individual can avoid the complications of excessive heat if he takes the time to allow acclimatization to increased heat. One should be careful to replace fluids and salts lost by excessive sweating and, of course, high temperatures and humidity during distance races warrant a reduction in physical activity.

Considerable experience with heat injuries has been obtained by sports medicine personnel. The American College of Sports Medicine recommends that distance races of 10 miles or more should not be conducted when the wet-bulb temperature-globe temperature exceeds 28° C (82.4° F). They recommend that runners be encouraged to frequently ingest fluids during competition and to consume 400 to 500 ml of fluid 10 to 15 minutes before competition. The early recognition of warning symptoms preceding heat injury may include piloerection on the chest and upper arms, chilling, throbbing pressure in the head, unsteadiness, nausea, and dry skin.

Persons with renal, pulmonary, and cardiac disorders are more subject to complications from temperature extremes.

Drugs that are likely to cause phototoxic reactions or enhance one's problems in excessive sun and heat conditions include the phenothiazines, the thiazides, the antihistamines, and the sulfonylureas, such as tolbutamide (Orinase) and chlorpropamide (Diabinese).

QUESTIONS

1. Discuss the early warning symptoms of environmental heat emergency.
2. Contrast the symptoms of the two conditions heat syncope and heat stroke.
3. Explain the role of positioning and other attempts to control the peripheral vasomotor collapse of heat exhaustion.
4. What is the role of stimulants in the treatment of heat exhaustion, heat stroke?
5. What is the expected mortality in the various environmental heat emergencies?
6. Discuss the relationship of sustained hyperthermia to attendant cardiovascular problems.
7. What treatment is given first priority in both heat stroke and heat exhaustion?
8. What particular efforts may be made to support the increased cardiovascular demand in heat emergencies?

SUGGESTED READING

O'Donnell, T. F., et al.: The circulatory abnormalities of heat stroke, N. Eng. J. Med. **287:**734-737, 1972.

CHAPTER 15

Lightning injuries

When a lightning bolt is discharged between cloud and earth following the development of a large charge at the bottom of a cloud, the current contained in such a bolt may vary between 12,000 and 200,000 amperes. Thus when a person is struck by lightning, he becomes highly charged. It is reasoned that the static electricity buildup in clouds results from the collision between particles of ice carried by updrafts and downdrafts. A large buildup of an electrical charge at the bottom of cloud is attracted to the opposite charge of earth, resulting in a lightning bolt.

The amount of current, the time of passage, and the resistance of the local body tissues all determine the ultimate degree of injury in the patient who is hit by a lightning bolt.

The number of deaths from lightning shock in the United States each year has been estimated at approximately 300. This number represents only one fourth of all persons struck by lightning. Most injuries from lightning do not result from the mainstream of the bolt but are caused by current flowing through the victim from direct contact with the charged ground. Many of the injuries from lightning result from the fires it causes. Approximately 75% of all reported farm fire losses originate from lightning, and more than 80% of all livestock losses from accidents are a result of lightning.

Often as many as a dozen individuals are knocked to the ground by a bolt of lightning. In such a situation the rescuer should avoid the general axiom that first aid efforts should be centered on the living rather than the apparent dead. If an individual shows signs of life, the chances are good that he will survive. On the other hand, many of those individuals who are apparent fatalities can be revived if cardiopulmonary resuscitative efforts as outlined in Chapter 12 are followed.

Metabolic activity, as well as heart action and respiration, stops almost instantly when a person is struck by lightning. The heart may start again in sinus rhythm. The onset of degenerative changes is apparently delayed by the sudden cessation of metabolic activity to the extent that successful resuscitation may be achieved in the victim who has apparently been dead for longer than 4 minutes. Therefore vigorous efforts at resuscitation following lightning shock are often rewarding.

An amazing variety of clinical findings may be present immediately following lightning shock even though the patient appears to be only stunned by the lightning. The patient may be unable to move his extremities. Deafness or blindness may be present. There is often an intense vasoconstriction. If the victim is pregnant, fetal maceration may occur. Fortunately many of the complications are only transient, but the victim should be transported to the nearest medical center where definitive care can be administered.

Whereas some individuals may be only momentarily stunned following a lightning shock, others require cardiopulmonary resuscitation. Artificial respiration, as described in this book, as well as closed-chest cardiac massage, should be administered immediately. Cardiopulmonary resuscitation may be necessary during transportation to the hospital, and respiratory depression may be such that artificial maintenance of respiration should be continued for several days. In addition, cardiac defibrillation may be required in a certain percentage of patients. Originally it was believed that most patients fibrillate following a lightning shock; however, additional evidence now suggests that a majority have simple asystole.

In the management of a lightning injury cardiopulmonary resuscitation becomes the item of top priority. General supportive measures including fluid resuscitation with low molecular dextran or osmotic diuresis may be indicated. Tetanus prophylaxis should be administered. Large volumes of fluid, digitalization in many instances, diuresis, and careful monitoring of vital signs, intravenous pressure, and urine output are essential. Early central nervous system manifestations after lightning injury may include coma, convulsions, hysteria, and amnesia. Cataracts may be a late sequela.

One should assume that multiple skeletal injuries may have followed the tremendous repulsive force. The skull and extremities should be checked by the rescuer for the possibility of fractures. Temporary paraplegia may be caused either by the effect of lightning on the central nervous system or by spinal cord injury.

The rescuer should be prepared for the victim to complain of deafness, blindness, and other neurologic deficits. Fortunately most of these are temporary. Post-lightning shock psychosis has been reported.

A word concerning prevention is always in order. To the golfer in an electric storm the advice is to get rid of his clubs, get away from trees or golf carts, and lie down on the ground in the area of greatest depression. A thick woods is a relatively safe spot.

During an electric storm an automobile with a metal top is one of the safest spots. Certainly one should avoid being in a swimming pool, near a single tree, near horses or cattle, or on the top of a hill or mountain. One should always avoid either being the tallest object or being near the tallest object in a given vicinity. One should *never* raise an umbrella over his head in an electric storm.

QUESTIONS

1. What variety of clinical findings may be present immediately following lightning shock?
2. What should one do or not do in an electric storm?

SUGGESTED READING

Apfelberg, D. B., Masters, F. W., and Robinson, D. W.: Pathophysiology and treatment of lightning injuries, J. Trauma 14:453-460, 1974.

CHAPTER 16

Frostbite

A relatively simple approach is required in the immediate treatment of a portion of the body subjected to freezing temperatures for a sufficiently prolonged period to produce severe vasospasm and the even cessation of circulation. If the extremities, for example, have progressed from an initial tingling and painful condition to that of numbness and total anesthesia, the sequelae of the frostbite may require prolonged definitive care. To reduce the time of the cold exposure, efforts should be made at once to rewarm the affected area. Moderately rapid rewarming is now preferred to earlier concepts supporting gradual rewarming. Placing the frozen extremities in a water bath heated to approximately 110° F provides rapid rewarming. Attempts should not be made to improve circulation or to rewarm by massaging the affected part because this may increase the tissue damage.

Any constricting garment or dressings should be removed. Blisters should not be opened, and only gentle manipulation should be attempted. If pain is severe, an analgesic may be administered. Smoking should be denied the victim. The victim should not be allowed to walk or bear weight on the affected area.

Obvious contamination should be avoided. Although various modalities of definitive therapy may be used later, the individual administering immediate care should specifically note whether or not tetanus toxoid or tentanus antitoxin has been administered. Tetanus prophylaxis is essential. Prophylactic antibiotic therapy may be administered as a part of the initial definitive therapy. In any event the patient should be admitted to the hospital if definitive therapy is required.

QUESTIONS

1. How long should one wait before rewarming the affected area of a frostbite victim?
2. Should rapid rewarming be employed?
3. Why should attempts not be made to improve circulation? Explain.
4. What other treatment should specifically *not* be employed in frostbite?

CHAPTER 17

Decompression sickness and air embolism

JEFFERSON C. DAVIS

Until recently, barometric pressure-related emergencies were the sole province of a limited group of physicians working in support of commercial or military deep-sea diving, tunneling, bridge building, or high-altitude or space operations. Developments within the past few years have made it mandatory that all physicians, regardless of specialty, become familiar with the life- and function-threatening consequences of sport as well as commercial exposures to these environments.

The availability of excellent quality self-contained underwater breathing apparatus (scuba) has made diving one of the world's fastest growing individual sports. Scuba diving has been considered to be limited to seacoast and resort areas, but a weekend visit to almost any body of water in the United States quickly proves that notion to be erroneous. Scuba divers can be found in every city; besides diving in local lakes, a common practice is for a group or club to charter an aircraft, fly to a popular diving area, dive, and then fly home. In either event any physician could be faced with the clinical manifestations of decompression sickness or air embolism at any time. Definitive therapy is specific and requires expeditious immediate management and coordinated emergency transfer to the nearest recompression chamber.

Similar clinical manifestations requiring comparable diagnostic acumen, emergency management, and definitive therapy can result from exposure to high altitudes in nonpressurized aircraft or sudden loss of cabin pressurization in a pressurized aircraft flying at a high altitude.

The numbers of people exposed to these environments with their attendant risks have reached a significant level, but presently we are only on the threshold of vast expansion in both areas.

TERMINOLOGY

The following terminology includes most of the effects of changes in barometric pressure:

    I. Mechanical effects (Boyle's law)
        A. Barotitis ("ear squeeze," "ear block")
        B. Barosinusitis ("sinus squeeze," "sinus block")

C. Barodontalgia ("tooth squeeze," "tooth block")
D. Trapped gastrointestinal gas expansion (ascent to altitude)
E. Pulmonary problems
1. "Lung squeeze" (breath-hold diving)
2. Pneumothorax
3. Pneumomediastinum
4. Air embolism
II. Decompression sickness (Henry's law)
A. Bends
B. Chokes
C. Neurologic decompression sickness
D. Vasomotor collapse (shock)
E. Skin manifestations
F. Aseptic bone necrosis

This chapter concerns pneumothorax and those disorders requiring emergency use of the recompression chamber: air embolism and the first four manifestations of decompression sickness listed above.

The basic principle of scuba is to constantly regulate inspired air pressure so that intrapulmonic pressure always equals water pressure at any depth. So long as these pressures are equal, there is little danger of a pulmonary overpressure accident. However, it is important that the diver and his physician realize the following factors:

1. Barometric pressure changes tremendously even in shallow depths of water (with each foot of seawater pressure increases by 0.445 pounds per square inch).
2. A pressure differential of only about 80 mm Hg is sufficient to force air bubbles across the alveolar-capillary membrane.
3. Shallow depths are most dangerous for breath-holding ascents because of greater Boyle's law volume expansion and alveolar pressure rise. For example, the volume change during ascent through the 33 feet of water from 99 to 66 feet is equal to the volume change from only 11 feet to the surface.
4. Pulmonary overpressure accidents have been reported during breath-holding ascent from as little as 5 to 7 feet of water.

PNEUMOTHORAX AND PNEUMOMEDIASTINUM

If pulmonary overpressure results in rupture through the pleura, a pneumothorax can occur. If this occurs while the diver is still ascending under water, it amounts to a tension pneumothorax. Treatment is by standard thoracocentesis, and a compression chamber is not required.

If the alveolar rupture introduces pulmonary interstitial gas, it dissects along bronchi to the mediastinum and usually migrates to neck subcutaneous tissue, resulting in pneumomediastinum and subcutaneous emphysema. Management is conservative with bed rest and observation only, unless the chest x-ray film shows attendant pneumothorax or there are neurologic manifestations suggesting cerebral air embolism. The latter manifestation, which requires the use of a recompression chamber as soon as possible, is discussed in detail.

AIR EMBOLISM
Etiology

Cerebral air embolism is the result of breath-holding ascent from depth by a scuba or surface-supplied diver. It has also occurred rarely in breath holding during rapid decompression of a pressurized aircraft cabin. Expansion of the volume of gas trapped in the lungs by a closed glottis as barometric pressure decreases accounts for distension. If the tensile strength of the lung is exceeded, air is introduced directly into pulmonary veins through lung rupture.

Clinical manifestations

The most significant feature in the diagnosis of cerebral air embolism is the sudden onset of neurologic symptoms during or immediately following decompression from a dive with scuba or surface supply of air or other gas mixture. The neurologic pattern may be most confusing in that many small bubbles may occlude arterial supply to diverse areas of the brain. Commonly the first manifestation is seizure activity, either focal or generalized. The patient may be suddenly rendered unconscious, show visual field defects or blindness, or have any imaginable combination of other sensory or motor deficits. Shock and death may occur if the volume of bubbles is great and if recompression facilities are not immediately available.

Treatment

The overriding factor in management of the cerebral air embolism patient is to get him to a recompression chamber as rapidly as possible. During transportation the patient must be kept in a Trendelenburg position, preferably tilted 15 degrees to his left side. If oxygen is available, it should be administered by mask to achieve as near 100% inspired concentration as possible. An intravenous infusion of dextran or lactated Ringer's solution should be started. It is reemphasized, however, that there should never be a delay in transportation to a recompression chamber to institute any other therapy. The *one* determining factor in the outcome of the case is the time delay between onset of symptoms and recompression therapy. Every minute lost decreases the chances of complete recovery, or at best prolongs cerebral ischemia and cellular hypoxia with resulting tissue edema, and leads to a difficult course of therapy. A recent case illustrates this problem.

A 19-year-old man was being given "free ascent" training at a lake. In this portion of scuba training, the student and his instructor descended normally to a 30-foot depth. The student removed his mouthpiece and ascended with the instructor to the surface, exhaling all the way. All was normal until immediately after surfacing, when the student became rigid and lost consciousness. He was rescued by the instructor, and on the shore he remained comatose with clonic jerking of the entire left side. A helicopter was dispatched to fly the patient at low altitude, to avoid bubble expansion, to the nearest recompression chamber, 80 miles away. Recompression therapy was begun 2 hours after onset. At the chamber, examination revealed response only to noxious stimuli, plantar Babinski reflex on the right, and extensor reflex on the left. Corneal reflexes were absent; pupils were equal and reactive. The left lower extremity was rigidly extended. He was treated in the recompression chamber according to U.S. Navy Treatment Table VIA for air embolism. This treatment includes

30 minutes at an air pressure equivalent to 165 feet of seawater (6 atmospheres absolute [ATA]) to achieve maximum bubble volume reduction. This was followed by prolonged intermittent oxygen-air breathing at 60-foot and 30-foot equivalents in the chamber to provide not only slow decompression but also hyperbaric oxygenation to hypoxic tissues.

During the treatment he recovered orientation, and rigidity of the left lower extremity disappeared. However, despite repeated and prolonged therapy, vision did not return for 12 hours apparently because of the 2-hour delay in reaching the chamber. Besides hyperbaric oxygen, dexamethasone and intravenous mannitol were used to combat cerebral edema. The patient had fully recovered 24 hours following the incident.

This case is important in suggesting another etiologic mechanism for cerebral air embolism during decompression. Despite the fact that the patient did exhale during ascent, air was apparently introduced into the pulmonary veins. It is considered most likely that localized air trapping in blebs or bullae accounted for lung rupture into vessels.

Another case illustrates the danger of breath holding at shallow depths. A 19-year-old man was on his first scuba dive of the day. On reaching 50 feet he decided to surface after only a short time and experienced difficulty breathing at a depth of 10 feet. He held his breath and ascended to the surface, where he immediately lost consciousness, was rescued, and was taken aboard the boat. He was positioned on the left side with the head down at an angle of 20 degrees and given 100% oxygen. Intravenous administration of low molecular weight dextran was started. He was flown at sea level cabin pressure to the recompression chamber, arriving 8 hours after onset. On arrival he was somewhat improved but still had 50% weakness of the right upper and lower extremities and an extensor right Babinski reflex; he was alert and oriented. After only 6 minutes at 6 ATA in the compression chamber, he recovered fully, and the treatment according to the U.S. Navy Treatment Table VIA was successfully completed. This case further points out that although it is obviously important to get the patient to a recompression chamber as soon as possible, one should never consider the chamber too distant to try to reach.

Prevention

With a satisfactory air supply divers simply breathe normally during ascent from depth. If an equipment malfunction or depletion of air supply at depth makes this impossible, the diver must exhale continuously during ascent to vent the increasing volume of air in his lungs. Any evidence of obstructive pulmonary disease, pulmonary blebs, cysts, or bronchial asthma should disqualify a candidate for scuba instruction. During rapid decompression in an aircraft, normal breathing is all that is required.

DECOMPRESSION SICKNESS
Etiology

Despite the fact that decompression sickness resulting from too-rapid ascent from compressed air environments has been known since the development of the caisson in the mid-1880's, many features of basic etiology are still unclear. Synonyms for this disorder include "caisson disease" and "compressed air illness." Inasmuch as patients seen by a physician who does not specialize in diving medicine are generally sport scuba divers, this section concentrates on this population, and thus considers the breathing medium to be compressed air.

As previously mentioned, to balance the linear increase in water pressure as the scuba diver descends, the breathing regulator is designed to provide air pressure equal to water pressure at any depth. As the alveolar air pressure increases at depth, the partial pressure of inspired gases increase. For example, at 99 feet of seawater (or 4 ATA), the absolute barometric pressure is 3,040 mm Hg. Approximately 79% of this pressure is nitrogen (2,400 mm Hg, compared to 600 mm Hg inspired nitrogen partial pressure [pN_2] at sea level breathing air). This results in an alveolar nitrogen pressure of approximately 2,360 mm Hg. This alveolar pressure is rapidly reflected in arterial blood and is presented to all tissues. A highly complex set of variables including differences in tissue perfusion and solubility factors results in a family of tissue nitrogen uptake curves throughout the body. Tissue nitrogen saturations achieved in diving then are a function of depth and time.

U.S. Navy and other decompression schedules are based on calculations and testing of ascent methods to avoid exceeding safe rates of decompression after diving. The tissues can tolerate a certain degree of supersaturation, but if barometric pressure is lowered beyond a critical level of nitrogen supersaturation that can be held in the tissues, it comes out of solution as bubbles. The result is a series of events caused by bubble embolization of various tissues, agglutination of platelets caused by the intravascular bubble foreign bodies, tissue ischemia, and hypoxia resulting in edema. Venous bubbles are swept through the pulmonary artery to produce pulmonary embolism, and possibly bubbling occurs de novo in tissues. The resulting symptoms and signs constitute the family of disorders known as decompression sickness.

Clinical manifestations

Bends. Mild to severe deep, dull pain usually located in or around joints may occur immediately after surfacing from a dive or may begin as long as several hours later. Any area may be involved, but most commonly pain is in the knees, ankles, shoulders, or elbows. Usually no objective findings are present, although occasional patients have shown some edema around affected joints. There may or may not be tenderness in the involved areas. In some cases, local pressure as with a blood pressure cuff gives temporary relief if applied directly over the joint. Although bends itself is not life threatening, it indicates that bubbles have formed. Some patients progress to more serious manifestations if left untreated. Bends is by far the most common type of decompression sickness.

Chokes. Chokes is a much more serious form of decompression sickness characterized by burning substernal pain, dyspnea, and a nonproductive cough. The exact pathophysiology is not clear, but animal studies have shown great volumes of bubbles or foam in the pulmonary artery, right ventricle, and atrium following unsafe decompression. It is considered likely that chokes actually represents massive bubble pulmonary embolism. Patients with this rare form of decompression sickness may progress rapidly into profound shock or may develop neurologic forms of decompression sickness.

Neurologic decompression sickness. In both diving and altitude-induced decompression sickness, some patients proceed through a pattern of bends, chokes (with or without vasomotor instability), and neurologic manifestations. Others develop one form only as an isolated event without any of the other forms. When this is neurologic decompression sickness, the event may be confusing in that embolism may occur at any level of the brain or spinal cord. The diver is likely to develop spinal cord lesions apparently as a result of congestive infarction that is caused by massive bubble formation in the epivertebral venous system. This is heralded by the onset (soon after decompression) of severe, girdling, abdominal pain either with or without sensory and motor impairment of lower extremities accompanied by loss of bowel and bladder control according to the level and extent of embolization. In altitude decompression sickness, neurologic involvement is more likely to result from single or multiple arterial emboli in the brain. Because many bubbles of varying sizes may result in involvement of diverse brain areas, the neurologic examination can be somewhat confusing and could erroneously indicate hysteria. There may be scintillating scotomata, visual field defects, blindness, aphasia, vertigo, patchy sensory or motor losses, loss of consciousness, and focal or generalized seizures. With neurologic manifestations a shock picture may supervene; therefore vital signs must be carefully monitored.

Vasomotor decompression sickness. A small percentage of persons develop severe shock with hemoconcentration. The precise mechanism is still not clear, but it is considered most likely that bubble embolization, ischemia, hypoxia, and bubble-induced changes in blood elements result in loss of fluid from the intravascular to the extravascular spaces. Shock may also occur secondary to the massive pulmonary embolism of chokes described previously. Although adequate fluid replacement is important, experience has shown that decompression sickness patients often respond poorly until recompression therapy is instituted.

Treatment

Of paramount importance is a high index of suspicion. Unfortunately sport scuba divers are often unable to give precise times and depths of their diving, so that the physician must take the history of diving and then proceed to manage the patient according to his clinical picture.

It is important to do a complete physical examination if possible, but again, as with cerebral air embolism, in the serious cases transportation to a recompression facility is the overriding consideration. It must be remembered that a patient who has a chief complaint of simple bends pain or a seemingly minor neurologic manifestation may have a more serious neurologic deficit demonstrable on complete examination.

As a first aid measure and during transportation to a recompression chamber, the administration of 100% oxygen by mask is indicated. The major purpose of oxygen administration is to wash out nitrogen, so anything less than 100% oxygen is not as effective. An anesthesia mask or aviator's breaking mask is suggested to achieve this goal. Because of the known platelet agglutination and hemoconcentration secondary to bubble embolization, it has been suggested that dextran and lactated Ringer's solution be used as an adjunct to recompression therapy, and it may be started before transportation.

It is important that all physicians and emergency room staff members know the location of the nearest civilian or military hyperbaric or recompression chamber and how to contact it immediately in an emergency. This information should be as readily available in the emergency room as is poison control center data. Time is of the essence in treatment of decompression sickness, as it is in air embolism.

Transportation to the chamber must be made by the most expeditious means available. During transportation oxygen administration and intravenous fluids should be continued and the patient should be placed in the Trendelenburg position. If the recompression chamber is not within easy access of surface transportation, movement by air ambulance must be considered. In both decompression sickness and air embolism, it is crucial that the patient not be exposed to significant increases in altitude that may cause the bubbles to enlarge as a result of a decrease in air pressure. It is preferable to move the patient in an aircraft with a pressurization system capable of maintaining sea level equivalent pressure, although unpressurized helicopter movement at low altitude has been successful.

It is beyond the scope of this chapter to discuss details of definitive treatment in recompression chambers. The basic mechanisms of action are to reduce bubble volume throughout the blood and other tissues, restore normal perfusion, eliminate excess nitrogen, and provide hyperbaric oxygenation of hypoxic tissues. All adjunctive measure are continued or they may be instituted in the chamber. Recompression chambers adequate to treat these disorders are generally steel vessels pressurized with meticulously clean compressed air. The patient and at least one attendant go into the chamber together and are pressurized to the treatment depth. At pressures equivalent to 60 feet of seawater (2.8 ATA) and shallower, the patient breathes 100% oxygen by mask intermittently on prescribed treatment schedules. The treatment of cerebral air embolism requires an initial "dive" in the chamber to at least 165 feet of seawater (6 ATA) followed by the intermittent oxygen-air treatment described previously. Clinical results in early cases are dramatic, and success may be achieved even in late cases; therefore movement to the nearest recompression chamber is always indicated even if the delay may be great.

QUESTIONS

1. Why is the scuba diver at greatest risk of pulmonary overpressure while breath holding during ascent at very shallow depths?
2. List the major clinical manifestations of cerebral air embolism.
3. What is the immediate care of the cerebral air embolism patient?
4. Why is bronchial asthma a definite contraindication to diving?
5. Decompression sickness is initiated by inert gas bubbles evolved from solution in blood and other tissues. List three secondary effects of intravascular gas emboli.
6. What is the most likely mechanism of chokes?
7. Describe the clinical manifestations of the spinal cord lesions of decompression sickness.
8. What is the purpose of 100% oxygen inhalation as a first aid procedure for decompression sickness?
9. In transporting a patient with decompression sickness or air embolism to a recompression chamber, what major precaution must be observed?
10. What are the four major mechanisms of action of the recompression chamber in the treatment of decompression sickness and air embolism?

SUGGESTED READINGS

Bennett, P. B. and Elliott, D. H.: The physiology and medicine of diving and compressed air work, ed. 2, Baltimore, 1975, The Williams & Wilkins Co.

Erde, A., and Edmonds, C.: Decompression sickness: a clinical series, J. Occup. Health **17:**324-328, 1975.

Hallenbeck, J. M., Elliott, D. H., and Bove, A. A.: Decompression studies in the dog. In Lambertsen, C. J., editor: Underwater physiology: fifth symposium on underwater physiology, Bethesda, Md., 1975, Fedn. Am. Socs. Exp. Biol.

National oceanic and atmospheric administration diving manual, Washington, D.C., 1975, U.S. Government Printing Office. (Stock No. 003-017-00283.)

Rivera, J. C.: Decompression sickness among divers: an analysis of 935 cases, Milit. Med. **129:** 314-334, 1964.

CHAPTER 18

Critical burns

BOYD E. TERRY

The seriously burned patient deserves and requires maximum compassion from the physician. Unpleasant features of burns often elicit a defeatist attitude from those observing the burn. This attitude may explain why many burned patients receive minimal initial care that is often poorly suited to their needs. Transportation of the burned patient without initial care frequently ends in disaster.

Frequently the question is asked: Is there a method, such as immediate immersion in cold water, that can prevent a superficial burn from becoming a full-thickness burn? The answer is no, unless the physician is present and can douse the patient in cold water at the moment of the burn, when it may theoretically have some importance. In terms of initial physician care this is a helpful maneuver for the alleviation of pain in superficial burns. The critically burned individual, on the other hand, rarely complains of pain and is usually quite calm; therefore it is important not to treat one's own emotions by giving narcotics for anticipated pain. Deep burns actually destroy the nerve endings, and pain is absent.

Another puzzling observation is that the severely burned patient may frequently be ambulatory. One wonders how this could be possible in the patient with impending "burn shock." Such reasoning leads to the underestimation of the severity of burns. If the patient is given adequate initial fluid therapy, burn shock is rare because it is prevented before appearing in a diagnosable state. Burn shock does not occur as rapidly as does hemorrhagic shock but appears over a period of hours in the untreated patient.

AIRWAY

Of primary importance in initial care of the severely burned patient is the need to assure an airway. One might think that a severely burned patient would have burns into the bronchi of the respiratory tract, but this is rarely true except in burns incurred in a closed-room steam explosion. Reflex mechanisms ordinarily close the glottis to heat stimuli, thus protecting the lower respiratory tract; however, the pharynx, nasopharynx, and mouth may be burned. The damage to the lower respiratory tract from smoke inhalation ordinarily manifests itself several hours after the burn is initially seen. The hazard of upper respiratory tract obstruction is most easily circumvented by insertion of nasotracheal or orotracheal tube. The patient burned in the head and neck area generally has serious burns over the usual tracheostomy site. Tracheostomy is best avoided as an initial measure because it compounds the possibility of later pneumonia and sepsis from the extended burn wound.

Edema is of greatest concern in initial management, particularly in the infant and child. The subsidence of edema after 48 to 72 hours allows for the nasotracheal tube to be removed. Certainly if one is in the position to dictate transport of the patient who has been burned in the head and neck area, he must do this only with the assurance of adequate airway placement and care as the patient is transported. On rare occasion it is necessary to perform escharotomy of the circumferentially burned upper torso to allow expansion of the chest wall (see discussion on associated injury).

A major problem confronting the severely burned individual is acute gastric dilation, which may cause airway problems by aspiration of vomited gastric contents. Nasogastric intubation is important as a preliminary step to nasotracheal or orotracheal intubation to prevent aspiration. Well-intended large doses of narcotics (seldom needed in the severely burned patient) may be the factor that compounds an already severe airway problem.

EVALUATION

History and physical and general evaluation are singularly important in the initial care of the burned patient and are most frequently overlooked. The patient has obvious physical findings, but frequently there are associated injuries and conditions that affect the outcome of the burn. These must be determined early. Initially the burned patient is lucid and able to converse, whereas several hours later he may not be so because of delirium that frequently accompanies larger burns. The dictum that "burn patients die not of their burn but of the complications of the burn" serves to emphasize the importance of determining pertinent history and physical findings. It is evident that the evaluation of the cardiorespiratory and renal systems by history becomes valuable in the initial management. This allows for the anticipation of significant problems likely to be worsened by the burn.

Age, size of burn, amount of full-thickness burn, and general health are of greatest value as predictors of ultimate patient survival. Patients younger than 3 and older than 50 years have higher mortality. The "rule of nines," though a rough approximation, helps to estimate the size of burns (head 9%, each upper extremity 9%, each lower extremity 18%, and 18% for anterior and posterior trunk, respectively). A full-thickness burn is defined initially by absence of response to pinprick and ultimately by requirement of skin graft.

FLUID REQUIREMENTS

Early administration of resuscitative fluids to the burned patient is a preventive measure against burn shock. It is equally important to prevent another complication of the patient with severe burns: acute renal failure. Traumatic acute tubular necrosis is common in the burned patient. Hemolysis of red cells in damaged capillaries causes deposition of pigments in the renal tubules at a time when urinary flow in the tubules is low. Maintenance of adequate tubular urine flow prevents irreversible damage should tubular necrosis occur. Particularly in the patient with an electric burn (in whom myoglobin pigment is circulating in addition to heme pigment), it is important to ensure adequate tubular urine flow.

The essential fluid requirement can be satisfied with a balanced electrolyte solution such as Ringer's lactate. The administration of blood is contraindicated as a resuscitative agent unless there is blood loss from another injury. Intravenous solution is necessary for all burns of more than 20% and for many pediatric burns, which are smaller in area. Burns around the head and neck preclude early oral intake of fluid even though the burned surface area is small; they indicate the need for intravenous fluids. The route of intravenous fluid administration is important. Many times extremities cannot be used for giving intravenous fluid because of the burn, and particularly in the severely burned patient it may be necessary to give fluid through the subclavian vein by percutaneous puncture. Such entry through a cleansed area of the burn with subsequent changes of the catheter on a frequent basis is much safer than a cutdown through burn tissue or the use of lower extremities, which precludes the monitoring of central venous pressure.

Urinary output must be monitored on a hourly basis in the severely burned patient; placement of a Foley catheter becomes necessary as an initial event. This monitoring provides information as to the volume of urine produced and frequently indicates the presence of heme pigment. The use of intravenous mannitol may then be warranted to provide immediate tubular diuresis should there be a lag in the production of adequate urinary flow.

How much and what kind of fluid to be given can be decided in all burn patients by giving lactated Ringer's solution initially in such amounts as to produce urinary output in the range of 50 ml per hour in the adult and approximately 1 ml per kg per hour in the infant and child.

ASSOCIATED INJURY

Other injuries of the burned patient, particularly extremity ischemia and eye injury, are frequently obscured and must be assiduously sought by careful examination. The former is caused by edema with circumferential burns leading to distal ischemia, primarily in the extremities. Escharotomy is rarely necessary but is limb saving when there is vascular compromise. Escharotomy is performed by incising the skin to the level of the subcutaneous fat in a longitudinal direction on either side of the extremity.

Eye injuries are uncommon because of the very adequate protection the eyelids afford. In the occasional burn of the eyelids the primary requirement is immediate coverage of the cornea by tarsorrhaphy (suturing together of the upper and lower eyelids). Edematous lids swollen shut are good protection and rarely hide corneal damage. However, early examination is essential!

IMMEDIATE ACTION TO TREAT INFECTION

The burned patient is at risk from airborne and contact sources of contamination from the immediate environment and must be protected from infection. Tetanus toxoid, or tentanus immune globulin (human) in those who have not been immunized, is a specific requirement for burned patients. Removal of clothing, rapid cleansing of the burn wound with Betadine "scrub" solution, and removal of any loose dead tissue minimize contamination of the burn wound. The patient should be managed with clean, preferably sterile, technique. Once cleansed, the burn wound should be covered with sterile dressings or at least by a sterile sheet with provision for conservation of body heat with blankets. Elevation of the ambient temperature to 30° to 32° C with external heaters prevents shivering and adds to patient comfort. Caloric and vapor losses through the burned skin are very large and require particular attention in the infant and child.

Antibiotics are best withheld for the treatment of specific infection rather than being used prophylactically. Cultures of the burn wound should be obtained on initial inspection.

The use of topical agents on the burn wound should be deferred until definitive evaluation and care are rendered by the burn surgeon.

QUESTIONS

1. List several modalities of general emergency care that may need altering in considering treatment of the severely burned patient.
2. Discuss the particular significance of history taking in the burn patient.
3. Fluid and electrolyte balance is a critical factor in the case of the severely burned patient. Explain the rationale of this statement.
4. Of what therapeutic importance is determination of the extent of the burned area?
5. Discuss alternative routes of fluid administration in the severely burned patient.
6. What are the particular implications of burn damage to the control of pain? Discuss.
7. What may the initial care team usually expect to find in assessing airway damages that accompany the various degrees of thermal burns?
8. Discuss the implications of applying topical agents to the burn in the early stages of patient care.

CHAPTER 19

Animal and insect contact

HENRY M. PARRISH

SNAKEBITES
Snakes and their identification

Approximately 10% of the species of snakes native to the United States are poisonous. Pit vipers, of the family Crotalidae, comprise the bulk of these snakes, and they are responsible for most snakebite accidents. Pit vipers native to the United States include *Crotalus* (large rattlesnakes), *Sistrurus* (pigmy rattlesnakes and massasaugas), and *Agkistrodon* (moccasins—including copperheads and cottonmouths). Coral snakes (of the general *Micrurus* and *Micruroides*) are the only other native poisonous snakes. One or more species of poisonous snakes are found in every state except Alaska, Hawaii, and Maine.

It is important to identify the offending snake if at all possible. Emergency rooms should obtain pictures of venomous snakes to assist in their identification. Pit vipers have a characteristic pit located between the eye and the nostril on each side of their bodies. They also are identified by elliptical (catlike) pupils and two well-developed fangs that protrude from the maxillae when their mouths are opened. Rattlesnakes have rattles attached to their tails.

Frequently the snake has been captured or killed by the time the emergency vehicle paramedic or the emergency room physician sees the patient. Not infrequently the snake's head has been chopped off and left behind at the site of the accident. If so, the pit viper can be identified by turning the snake's belly upwards and noting a single row of subcaudal plates just below the anal plate. Harmless snakes have a double row of subcaudal plates.

The coral snake is a small, beautifully colored reptile with broad rings of scarlet and black separated by narrow rings of yellow—"Red next to yellow will kill a fellow." The snout is black. On rare occasions one may encounter an albino or a black coral snake. Several harmless snakes resemble coral snakes, but the yellow and red rings on their bodies are separated by black rings. Coral snakes have round pupils and lack facial pits. A pair of short, erect fangs protrude from their maxillae.

Diagnosis

A brief history is important. Was the patient bitten by a snake? Did he see the snake? Approximately how long was the snake and what color was it? Did the snake rattle before biting the patient? Was the snake captured or killed? If so, the snake, including the head, should be brought in for identification. (A word of caution: Recently killed or dying snakes have been known to inflict snakebite wounds. It is safer to kill the snake and put the parts in a bag or container; a stick or forceps should be used to handle the snake.) What was the activity of the patient at the time of the bite? It is appalling how many people are handling a snake when the bite occurs. What time of day did the bite happen? This is an important observation in following the progression of signs and symptoms of snake venenation. One should record when first aid was started. When was antivenin given? How much antivenin was given, and what route of administration was used?

The site of the bite should be inspected. Was the bite inflicted on bare skin or was there intervening clothing? Are fang or tooth marks present? Most textbooks incompletely describe snakebite wounds. One does not always find two fang puncture wounds. There may be one, two, three, four, or more fang punctures. Occasionally a patient is so stunned by a snakebite that he just stands still and is struck repeatedly by a snake. Also a snake may make an indirect strike and thereby inflict only a superficial laceration. Small tooth marks may be present. Is the bite wound painful? Any area of swelling around the fang punctures usually indicates that venom has been injected into the wound. Puncture wounds inflicted by coral snakes are small and may be difficult to see with the naked eye. I have found it useful to observe snakebite wounds through a 2 to 3 power magnifying glass. This may not be practical in the field.

Are signs and symptoms of venenation present? Pit viper venenation is diagnosed primarily by local signs and symptoms. Systemic manifestations are usually found only in more serious cases, and their onset may be delayed. Pit viper bites have the two "P's" (puncture wound and pain) and the two "E's" (edema and erythema). Systemic signs and symptoms include shock; nausea; vomiting; diarrhea; melena; numbness, tingling, and paresthesias in the extremities or around the mouth; muscular fasciculations in the bitten extremity; coma; convulsions; and motor or respiratory paralysis.

Immediate care

The patient should be reassured. Being bitten by a large snake can be a terrifying experience. It has been estimated that about 6,700 people are bitten by venomous snakes annually in the United States, but there are only about 14 to 15 deaths per year. The case fatality rate is about 0.21%. Approximately 27% of bites by venomous snakes result in little or no venom being injected into the wound.

The bitten part of the body should be immobilized. If possible, the patient should lie down. However, if one must decide between immobilization and seeking prompt medical attention, the latter should be sought. It is preferable to transport the patient to a vehicle by means of a stretcher or piggyback when no assistance is available. It is usually possible to walk on a bitten leg for several hours after a bite. As soon as a vehicle is reached, the snakebite victim should be driven to the nearest source of antivenin. In my experience, this indicates a hospital emergency room rather than a physician's office.

A tourniquet or constricting band should be lightly applied to the involved extremity several inches above the bite. The constricting band should be only tight enough to occlude the superficial venous and lymphatic flow. It should not occlude the arterial circulation, and it should be released every 10 minutes for 2 minutes. As the edema resulting from the venom spreads, the tourniquet should be advanced to keep just ahead of the swelling. One should not use a tourniquet for longer than 2 hours. The tourniquet helps impede the spread of venom until incision and suction can be used to remove the venom mechanically or until antivenin can be administered to neutralize the venom.

Incision and section should be used as soon as possible to remove the venom. It is most effective if used within the first 30 minutes following a bite, although I have removed venom as long as 60 minutes after the bite. If possible, the skin near the bite should be washed before incising the area. This may remove some of the snake venom. Incisions, linear or cruciate, ¼ inch long and ⅛ to ¼ inch deep, are made into the subcutaneous tissues over the fang punctures. Suction should be continued for about 1 hour. Snakebite cups, other suction apparatus, or even oral suction may be used for this purpose.

One may have to treat shock in the snakebite victim. Such shock may result either from the emotional trauma of being bitten by a snake or from the hypotensive effects of pit viper venom. The treatment of shock is discussed in detail in another chapter.

Hospital management of venomous snakebites includes the three "A's" (antivenin, antibiotics, and antitetanus prophylaxis). Antivenin *(Crotalidae)* Polyvalent (North and South American antisnakebite serum), produced by Wyeth Laboratories, is effective in treating the bites of all pit vipers indigenous to the United States. When confronted with a coral snake bite, one should use Antivenin *(Micrurus fulvius)* (North American coral snake antivenin), which is also manufactured by Wyeth Laboratories. Because antivenin is a horse serum product, one should obtain a history about past allergies. Even if a history of allergy to horse serum is negative, a skin test or a conjunctival test for horse serum sensitivity should be carried out before antivenin is administered.

HYMENOPTERA INSECT STINGS
Reactions to insect stings

Hymenoptera insects including honeybees, bumblebees, ants, and yellow jackets and other wasps, inflict stings that produce a variety of reactions in man including local reaction only, slight general reaction, moderate general reaction, severe general reaction, and delayed-type reaction only. Also one may observe generalized toxicity, including convulsions, from multiple Hymenoptera stings. By far the most feared reaction is the severe general reaction, or anaphylaxis. Hymenoptera insects were responsible for 40% of the deaths from venomous animals in the United States from 1950 to 1954. By way of contrast, poisonous snakes produced only 33% of the fatalities. The venom of Hymenoptera insects is injected into human beings by means of an ovipositor. It should be remembered that the honeybee's ovipositor is usually broken off in the victim and may continue to exude venom for several minutes. On the other hand, a wasp may sting a victim several times. In one study of 86 persons who died from Hymenoptera stings, 66 died within 1 hour, and 72 were dead within

5 hours. This finding emphasizes the gravity of Hymenoptera sting anaphylaxis and the necessity for prompt and effective therapy.

A nonallergic reaction to a sting may consist of local swelling, redness, and pain. A general or allergic reaction consists of signs and symptoms at a distance from the sting site. Allergic reactions may produce the following manifestations: urticaria, generalized itching, nasal congestion, sneezing, laryngeal edema, asthma, nausea, vomiting, shock, vascular collapse, tightness in the chest, a feeling of impending doom, and loss of consciousness. Symptoms may vary in frequency or intensity. Most severe reactions occur within 30 minutes following the sting. Symptoms of a delayed reaction or serum sickness include aching of the joints, fever, malaise, lymphadenopathy, pruritus, and skin eruptions.

Treatment of insect stings

Treatment of Hymenoptera stings should be carried out promptly. The stinger, should be removed if present, by flicking it out with a fingernail or a knife. One should not grasp and squeeze the stinger as this may enhance venom injection. A tourniquet should be applied between the sting and the heart for bites on an extremity. It should be applied tightly enough to obstruct the superficial venous and lymphatic flow but not tightly enough to obstruct an artery; the tourniquet should be released briefly every 5 minutes. An ice bag should be applied to the sting area. The patient should lie down and be kept warm.

Epinephrine hydrochloride, 1:1000 solution, is the drug of choice in treating systemic reactions to Hymenoptera stings. For an adult 0.3 ml should be injected subcutaneously at the site of the sting and 0.3 ml in an unaffected arm. Small children weighing 20 kg or less should be given 0.10 to 0.15 ml. For larger children a dose based on body weight between approximately 0.15 ml and 0.3 ml should be given. Epinephrine should be repeated in 20 minutes if there has been little or no response. Antihistamines, such as diphenhydramine hydrochloride (Benadryl), 50 mg administered intravenously, are useful for treating stings. If an oral preparation can be used, liquids are preferable to tablets.

If the patient is unconscious, is in shock, and has poor peripheral circulation, the epinephrine can be given intravenously. Also one should administer an intravenous drip of 500 mg of normal saline containing metaraminol (Aramine) or norepinephrine (Levophed). Hydrocortisone, (Solu-Cortef) 100 mg, may be added to the intravenous solution.

If largyngospasm is not relieved by epinephrine hydrochloride, one may have to give oxygen, insert a tracheal tube, or do a tracheostomy on the patient. Cardiopulmonary resuscitation may be needed. Some success in treating systemic reactions to Hymenoptera stings, including laryngospasm and bronchospasm, has been reported by using oral inhalation of epinephrine (Medihaler-Epi) bitartrate.

The patient should be transported to a hospital emergency room while treatment is being administered. After recovery, patients should be encouraged to see an allergist so that they can be hyposensitized, issued an emergency Anakit (Insect Sting Treatment Kit [Hollister-Stier]), instructed on how to prevent insect stings, and given an emergency identification bracelet or necklace.

SPIDER BITES
Identification of dangerous spiders

Although several species of spiders in the United States may inflict painful bites, the two species that are most dangerous and may produce fatalities are the black widow spider *(Latrodectus mactans)* and the brown recluse spider *(Loxosceles reclusa)*. The black widow spider is found in most states in the continental United States. The brown recluse spider is found primarily in Missouri and in other midwestern and southwestern states. Spiders bite their victims by means of horny fangs or chelicera that are attached to venom glands.

The female black widow spider is usually black dorsally with a crimson hourglass on the ventral side of the abdomen. Occasionally one sees two or more distinct triangles or only an irregular crimson marking.

The brown recluse spider is grayish brown in color and has a violin-shaped marking on the dorsal aspect of its cephalothorax.

Symptoms of spider venenation

Symptoms produced by brown recluse spider bites vary from quite minor to severe or even fatal. One may observe one, two, or more small puncture wounds with a small red papule. In moderately severe bites this may extend in 6 hours to a bluish gray discoloration around the bite area. After 24 to 48 hours a black area may form that is surrounded by signs of inflammation. This area of necrosis may become quite large. In severe or fatal cases the patient may also develop intravascular coagulation, hemoglobinemia, hemoglobinuria, coagulation defects, renal damage, fever, rash, and shock.

Black widow spider bites often occur while the victim is sitting in an outdoor privy. Bites on the genitalia or buttocks are common. The signs and symptoms of venenation by black widow spiders may include one or more of the following: small puncture wounds with or without surrounding signs of inflammation, local pain, severe cramping, pain in the muscles beginning within 15 to 60 minutes; a boardlike abdomen; difficulty in breathing; nausea; vomiting; excessive sweating; paresthesias; and hypertension. Death may result from cardiac or respiratory failure. This condition may be mistaken for an acute surgical abdomen.

Treatment of spider venenation

There is little evidence to support the use of tourniquet, incision, or suction as first aid measures for treating spider bites. In many instances the victim does not see or capture the spider that has bitten him. Therefore there may be a delay in diagnosis.

A horse serum antivenin, Antivenin *(Latrodectus mactans)*, is available for treating black widow spider bites. Early use of the antivenin is recommended. After the patient has been skin tested for horse serum allergy, one or more vials of the antivenin are diluted in normal saline and administered intravenously. In less severe cases the antivenin may be given intramuscularly. Methocarbamol (Robaxin), 10% calcium gluconate, and warm baths also may be used to alleviate muscle spasms and pain. The patient should be given tetanus immunization and a broad-spectrum antibiotic. Other measures that may afford relief are analgesics, corticosteroids, and antihistamines. However, when using these drugs, one should remember that black widow spider venom is a respiratory depressant.

At the present time there is no specific antivenin for brown recluse spider bites. This is an urgently needed pharmacologic agent inasmuch as recognized brown recluse spider bites are increasing while black widow spider bites are decreasing because of improved housing with indoor toilets and the demise of small farms. The treatment of brown recluse spider bites includes tetanus immunization, broad spectrum antibiotics, and corticosteroids. For severe bites, 100 mg of triamcinolone orally may be given daily. After several days this dose may be gradually reduced. Surgical excision of the skin lesion and a skin graft may become necessary. Supportive treatment includes intravenous fluids, analgesics, and sedatives. In rare instances renal dialysis may be required. Heparin may be used to counteract coagulation defects that may result from severe bites.

QUESTIONS

1. Is it possible for a venomous snake to bite a person and not cause venom poisoning?
2. Why should one administer a skin test before giving snake antivenin?
3. Is the same antivenin used for both pit viper bites and coral snake bites?
4. Are incision and suction still considered effective treatment for snakebites?
5. Why should one exercise caution in removing a bee stinger?
6. What is the mechanism of death following insect stings?
7. What is the single most effective drug in treating Hymenoptera sting allergy?
8. Is there an antivenin available for black widow spider bites?
9. What drugs relieve the muscle spasms that are associated with black widow spider venenation?
10. Do you think that appropriate antitetanus immunization should be used in treating venomous animal bites? Why?

SUGGESTED READINGS

Anderson, P. D.: What's new in loxoscelism?, Mo. Med. **70:**711, 1973.

Brown, H., and Bernton, H. S.: Allergy to the hymenoptera: clinical study of 400 patients, Arch. Intern. Med. **125:**665, 1970.

Horen, W. P.: Arachnidism in the United States, J.A.M.A. **185:**839, 1963.

Insect Allergy Committee of the American Academy of Allergy: Insect-sting allergy: questionnaire study of 2,606 cases, J.A.M.A. **193:**115, 1965.

Minton, S. A., Jr.: Venom diseases, Springfield, Ill., 1974, Charles C Thomas, Publishers.

Parrish, H. M.: Analysis of 460 fatalities from venomous animals in the United States, Am. J. Med. Sci. **245:**129, 1963.

Parrish, H. M.: Incidence of treated snakebites in the United States, Public Health Rep. **81:** 269, 1966.

Parrish, H. M. and Hayes, R. H.: Hospital management of pit viper venenations, Clin. Toxicol. **3:**501, 1970.

Thorp, R. W., and Woodson, W. D.: Black widow: Americas' most poisonous spider, Chapel Hill, 1945, The University of North Carolina Press.

PART SIX

Emergencies involving pharmacologic excesses

CHAPTER 20

Immediate care in the drug scene

GEORGE R. GAY

Man has an inborn craving for medicine. Heroic dosing for
several generations has given his tissues a thirst for drugs. The desire to
take medicine is one feature which distinguishes man, the animal,
from his fellow creatures.

Sir William Osler

For years we have seen and treated innumerable "OD's" (overdoses)—of almost
any conceivably bizarre combination of chemical agents—at the Haight-Ashbury
Free Medical Clinics. These unfortunates have often been dumped at our doorstep,
or sometimes an actual call for help from several doors, streets, or blocks away may
reach us. Resuscitation bag in hand, then we make the mad dash to help.

As our own experience and sophistication have evolved, we have developed
protocols of emergency technique with proven clinical efficacy that (perhaps most
important of all) are acceptable to our clientele. Our approach has remained one of
exclusive medical and psychosocial aid, and one of implicit confidentiality. To provide the assistance needed, we must remain flexible, dynamic, and—above all—
credible. Acceptance lies in credibility, and our particular nonpunitive and nonjudg-
mental approach has made us privy to (often lifesaving) histories and other information that are simply not forthcoming in a standard emergency room.

Initially, we compute all available information at hand: "Some dude's lying in
the middle of Haight Street—I think he shot-up." As our first guideline we implicit-
ly count on and expect what might be ordinarily considered the unusual if not out-
right grotesque. If we play it too cool or too slow, we will be filling out a lot of death
certificates.

There are several very practical rules of thumb in approaching the overdose
case, and for the purpose of our initial discussion we define the overdose victim as
a depressed, obtunded, or comatose individual (the "wired" sympathomimetic reaction to an overdose of speed and cocaine is discussed later).

1. Do not look for *pinpoint pupils*. This is a time-wasting activity that does not
   achieve anything, and this is the sign of the *amateur!* Hypoxia may cause dilatation, or mixed drugs may mask this sign of opiate intoxication and may cause the
   "pupil watcher" to misdiagnose and so to clinically misrespond or, even worse,
   to become a confused "nonresponder."

145

2. Do not look for intubation equipment. First, oxygenate this patient; breathe for him ("pink him up"), and leave intubation for later. Call for the intubation expert as time allows, but do not waste these initial vital moments in "on-the-job training."

3. Do not waste other precious moments in a pious needle-mark inspection. (They may be anywhere from the feet to the penis, and other places you would never think of looking.)

4. Do expect *multiple* drug abuse to have produced these cases of respiratory depression. Only (a) the true opiate-using novice or patient who has been "clean" (such as having been involuntarily detained in jail or the county hospital for detoxification purposes) *or* (b) the individual who is using multiple respiratory depressants concurrently is in danger of respiratory depression and death from the usual poor grade "stuff" (heroin) available on the streets of San Francisco (which may be 1% or less in purity). *Always* suspect that a young comatose patient who is hypo- or areflexic, with marked respiratory depression (from apnea to 2 or 3 shallow gasping breaths per minute), with a cyanotic, clammy pallor, and with a questionable or nonexistent history, to have a heroin (or mixed narcotic-sedative hypnotic) overdose.

5. Always suspect *alcohol* to not only contribute to an obtundation of protective respiratory reflexes but also to contribute to a stomach full of a potentially devastating mixture of particulate matter and acid pH.

INITIAL TREATMENT

To be effective treatment must be prompt, and proper measures are essential. Here, in simple outline form, is the method of emergency therapy that we have developed at the Haight-Ashbury Free Medical Clinics. Remember—*in this order*—the ABCD's of resuscitation:

A. Clean the mouth, and establish the *airway*.
B. *Breathe* for the patient if he is apneic, or assist his respirations if they are inadequate.
C. Assess the *cardiovascular system*, and give support when necessary (from a vigorous slap on the chest to external cardiac massage to intravenous or intracardiac stimulating drugs).
D. Administer *drugs* necessary to maintain the patient—cardiac stimulants, bicarbonate to reverse acidosis, or steroids or others—but only after A, B, and C are fully managed and under definite control.

Establish the airway

Clean the patient's mouth. (We use a quick wipe with a towel, handkerchief, or shirttail, while pulling the tongue forward.) Mucus, blood, vomitus, gum, or tobacco may be found with surprising regularity.

With the patient in the supine position, tip his head slightly up and back. Grasping the jaw at the angles of the mandible and at the point of the chin, draw his head back, chin high, to a "sniffing-like" position, being careful not to hyperextend his neck. (Think of the position in which you would hold your head to catch the fragrance of freshly baked bread as you walk past a bakery.) Ensure that the tongue is forward and not occluding the posterior oropharynx. A flaccid tongue is in every way analogous to a quarter-pound of loose hamburger flopping about in the posterior airway. (If reflexes are present, the patient will protect his own airway; so watch your fingers!) If oropharyngeal reflexes are absent, insert an oral airway; if one is not readily available, hold the tongue forward with your fingers. A simple maneuver to insert an oropharyngeal airway is to put it in "upside down," and then turn it upright when it is almost three fourths of the way in. This generally catches and pulls the tongue forward. (Check to make sure that the airway is open.) If available, a *soft* red rubber nasopharyngeal airway is quite handy. Use copious lubricant jelly and a soft tube, and never exert more pressure than will blanch the nail beds of your inserting fingers. Observe these rules and (1) you will have an airway less stimulating to partially obtunded upper airway reflexes, and (2) you will not have traumatically excised the middle turbinate bone with the resultant hemorrhage that you may then expect.

Breathe for the patient

Breathe for the patient if he is apneic or if he is breathing inadequately—mouth-to-mouth, or mouth-to-nose; or use an Ambu bag if one is handy—do not wait! If we consider room air to be composed of 20% oxygen, we can expect efficient mouth-to-mouth respiration to provide at least 15% oxygen for the patient. Make sure that air is entering his lungs and that his chest, not his stomach, is expanding. Listen for breath sounds with a stethoscope over both sides of the chest and over the stomach. (Air entering the stomach sounds much like flatus passed in the bathtub.) In the patient who may have a full stomach (that is, everyone) expect regurgitation. Usually a comatose patient about to vomit "swallows" or moves his neck muscles of deglutition once or twice just before the act.

If air is being forcibly blown into the patient's stomach, vomiting is virtually assured. You may or may not have a suction apparatus at hand, but even if you do, be ready to turn the patient to the left lateral decubitus position (being more vertical, the right mainstem bronchus is more vulnerable) as the patient vomits. A properly inserted cuffed esophageal tube is a real luxury and may be lifesaving in this situation.

Assess the cardiovascular system

Check the pulse for rate, rhythm, and deficit. Check the precordial, femoral, temporal, and radial pulses. Do not be lulled into complacency by the strong, full pulse of hypoxia because it may be premonitory to terminal arrhythmia and cardiac cessation. Remember if the patient arrives with a *heartbeat*, you can almost certainly save him.

If the heartbeat is absent, give a firm, full-handed slap over the precordium. If there is no immediate response, then begin external cardiac massage by placing the heels of the palms of your hands over the patient's lower sternum and depressing firmly 50 to 60 times per minute. Allow the airway partner of your team to take over for a full artificial inspiration after every fourth precordial compression. Determine the cardiac status and rhythm pattern with an electrocardiograph (if available). Institute appropriate action, such as defibrillation or intravenous pacing, if the facilities are available.

In severe cases of narcotic and other drug overdose, especially if long neglected, the patient's cardiovascular system may be so depressed that pulmonary edema may develop. In this case, intubation or tracheostomy—in addition to continuous positive pressure respiration—is literally lifesaving. *Think* of propoxyphene and alcohol (as well as of heroin and methadone) when you are faced with pulmonary edema.

Administer drugs

Administer such drugs as may be considered necessary as you continue the treatment previously outlined. If the patient has collapsed veins, as many addicts do, try the external jugular, the subclavian, or the femoral veins; in a dire emergency inject into the muscle mass at the base of the tongue—this flows directly into the superior vena cava. If this chapter could have but one message that would be remembered, it should be this: *Naloxone (Narcan) is your first-line drug in narcotic overdose!* Immediately give 2 to 4 ml intravenously (0.4 mg per ml). You may repeat the dosage at least twice at 5 to 10 minute intervals; the only limitation is failure of the patient to respond to this test—which is completely diagnostic for the presence of narcotics. Naloxone, a pure narcotic antagonist, is totally devoid of the agonistic effects that are seen with levallorphan (Lorfan) or nallorphine (Nalline). If there is any narcotic agent contributing to this depressant overdose, heroin, methadone, oxycodone (Percodan), codeine, propoxyphene, or others, you can reverse the effect and bring your overdose victim back to consciousness within seconds (almost literally one or two circulation times) for 20 to 40 minutes.

If you have good reason to suspect a recent overdose of respiratory depressant drugs, or if adequate (though depressed) respiratory effort is present, administer doxapram hydrochloride (Dopram) intravenously. The dosage is 3 to 5 ml (1 ml = 20 mg) administered by intravenous push; this may be repeated in 5 minutes and again in another 5 minutes. The beauty of this nonspecific respirogenic analeptic drug is in its inherent margin of safety (therapeutic index, 50:1). Physicians have classically feared the analeptics for their low margins of safety (ratio of effective dose to convulsive dose). Indeed with the clinical use of doxapram, although convulsions are not a generally feared consequence, the possibility of a metabolic acidosis (in the face of a general cardiovascular pressor response of 20% to 30% increase in heart rate and blood pressure seen with usual dosage) is very real. This unfortunately has limited the use of doxapram, a potent temporary respirogenic and general arousal agent. The treated comatose patient immediately "lightens," and his protective laryngeal and pharyngeal reflexes return with his general sensorium within a period of 3 to 5 minutes. He then tends to drift downward again, but never to his previous depth of anesthesia. Thus any young patient who has overdosed depressant drugs (of whatever nature) can be rendered at once more conscious and more able to protect his airway. (Remember the *temporary* effect, and never turn your back on such an apparently chemically resuscitated patient.)

We have now shown in a series of clinical trials (mainly in handling the multiple depressant overdose victim) that the cardiovascular pressor effects mentioned previously are totally ablated by concurrent administration of the beta blocker propranolol hydrochloride (Inderal). A dosage of 1 mg intravenously per minute to a total dosage of 8 mg (2 mg = 2 ml) is all that is generally needed. We therefore in doxapram plus propranolol have achieved an almost perfect analeptic protocol. Caveat emptor: Be aware of propranolol's contraindications—bronchial asthma and congestive heart failure. And also be aware of the 1° to 2° F temperature elevation that may be seen in overcrowded, underventilated areas with the use of doxapram as described. Plenty of ice and ice water should be kept handy—as well as intravenous fluids—to correct dehydration.

Stay with the patient until he is fully responsive. Observe him for several hours if at all possible. If he has used a long-acting narcotic, such as methadone hydrochloride (Dolophine), he may lapse back into coma and die from respiratory failure if the relatively short-acting narcotic antagonist naloxone is allowed to wear off and is not repeated. This situation allows you to utilize the services of the friend or friends (if any) who brought in the overdosed patient. These are "friends" in a very real sense because, being sophisticated in drug lore, they realize the chance they take in bringing him to you. They can be held legally responsible for their unfortunate companion's condition or for his possible death. If present, however, and if approached in a positive and friendly manner, these individuals can be utilized as the most knowledgeable and practical private duty nurses available for this particular medical problem.

If the patient fails to respond to the measure previously outlined, then follow routine and established emergency procedures. First, secure a route for administering intravenous fluids, preferably with a large-bore cannula. Begin the administration of a glucose-electrolyte solution. If moderate to severe acidosis is suspected, administer sodium bicarbonate in appropriate amounts. Draw blood for chemistries and secure a urine specimen for analysis. Always search for any possible nondrug etiology, such as evidence of head trauma, blood loss, diabetes, acute infectious processes, or increased intracranial pressure. Undress the patient and conduct a thorough body search for puncture or gunshot wounds.

If long-standing drug depression is suspected (for example, when an unresponsive patient is discovered unattended), be on guard for atelectasis, pulmonary edema, or pneumonia. In this event avoid the doxapram and initiate immediate hospitalization, vigorous pulmonary therapy, aggressive antibiotic treatment, and cardiopressor or steroid therapy when indicated.

What we see increasingly is the "smack head" who professes to disdain "downers" (or "reds" or "yellows") and alcohol, but who increasingly takes these drugs in addition to the poor grade "street junk" both to help him "get off" and to alleviate symptoms of withdrawal or carry him over until he can "score" again.

IDENTIFICATION OF TRUE NARCOTIC ADDICTION

To specifically identify true narcotic addiction, in this the era of the middle class junkie (or the invisible junkie), the following two tests are definitive, safe, and reliable:

1. For the *nontolerant* "pseudojunkie" (who may nonetheless be full of holes as a pincushion and have abscesses) try the "pseudojunkie," or Gay-Senay, test: Methadone, 15 to 20 mg, administered by mouth or subcutaneously, creates a somnolent, narcotized state within 30 to 40 minutes.
2. For the truly *narcotic-dependent* individual utilize the "Narcan test" of Blachley: Naloxone, 0.4 mg, injected intravenously or subcutaneously precipitates with-

drawal symptoms within 30 seconds to 30 minutes (depending on the route of administration).

BASIC GUIDELINES FOR THE PHYSICIAN

1. Remember that the major complications of drug abuse arise basically from four facets:
   a. Acute overdose ("downers" or "uppers")
   b. Idiosyncratic reactions
   c. Adulterants used
   d. Route of administration
2. Consider the possibility of drug abuse in every patient.
3. When you think of drug abuse think of *multiple drug abuse*, and always think of *alcohol*. Remember the marked potentiation of depressant physiologic effects that alcohol produces. Beware of the danger of alcohol-propoxyphene combinations (which cause *10* times more deaths than alcohol-codeine combinations). Always remember that nalaxone is effective as a propoxyphene antagonist.
4. Remember the unhygienic aspects of illicit drug use. Be knowledgeable of drug adulterants and substitutes.
5. If gunshot or knife wounds are present, think "drug lifestyle."
6. Recognize the various disease patterns that occur among drug abusers of various types.
7. Never fail to differentiate drug overdose and withdrawal patterns from other conditions, for example, diabetes, head trauma, or acute surgical abdomen.
8. Remain flexible and dynamic, and keep your head and senses open. Be ready and able to deal with the bizarre. Remember that there is nothing wrong with using snake oil if the snake oil works.

THE "ART" OF TREATMENT OF THE DRUG USER

Surely the physician who represents a pure "medical model" will fail to satisfy the demands of the young illicit drug user. Through the years we have evolved a workable, effective, and imminently humane approach that we abbreviate "ART."

A is for *acceptance.* By serving as intermediary you can help the drug user adapt to and regulate his environment as drug effects dissipate so that his reentry is much less deleterious to his personal psychological and physical cosmos.

R is for *reduction of stimuli, rest,* and *reassurance.* A quiet and nonthreatening environment and a gentle (though professional) approach generates gratitude and greatly diminishes both self-destructive and outwardly destructive behavior of drug emergence.

T is for our recognized therapeutically effective *talkdown technique.* Sincerity, concern, and a gentle manipulation of your patient's psychologic landmarks may well prove to be your most effective therapeutic approach in returning him to a safe and controlled perception of his situation and hence to the realities that he must face in the "straight" outside world.

SPECIFIC PATTERNS IN COMMONLY MISUSED DRUGS

We now have truly entered an era of self-experimental polypharmacy. If we hold in mind several basic tenets of current sociologic trend, we, as health pro-

fessionals. can at least maintain the flexibility necessary to continue to learn.
1. People use drugs, and the more potent the better.
2. Our species has attained a scientific expertise in chemistry that far outstrips its meager talents for self- or social control.
3. What people ingest or inject may not necessarily be found in the *Physician's Desk Reference* (PDR). With the mind-boggling emergence and widespread use of multiple psychotropic drugs, the physician must educate himself in entirely new disciplines of psychologic and medical therapeutics.

Marijuana

The category of marijuana includes the cannabinoids: *Cannabis* species, "hash-ish," and "hash-oil." With the exception of the foolish and overzealous psychic voyager who would self-inject a mulch of vegetable material containing leaves of the *Cannabis* species into his veins, it is absolutely safe to assume that you will never witness a death by marijuana overdose. Overuse via the inhalation (smoking) route may result in an occasional case of marijuana overdose consisting of nausea and vomiting. When a person with a very structured (rigid or inadequate) personal-ity (or psychologic "set") experiments with the drug in an improper physical setting, he may not be able to cope with feelings of "spaciness," depersonalization, or losing control and may thus experience an acute anxiety reaction. This may be seen in unsophisticated drug experimenters who ingest "Alice B. Toklas" ("hash") brownies. That is, they unwittingly overtitrate their degree of intoxication. The more experi-enced user usually takes just what he feels he needs as a "roach" is passed around a communal circle. Indeed he may experience a "social high," or "contact high," in proper company without any drugs.

Usually a calm and sympathetic counselor is all that is needed in these cases. The benzodiazepine antianxiety agents, such as chlordiazepoxide, 10 to 25 mg, or diazepam, 10 to 20 mg, given intramuscularly or by mouth, may completely relieve or prevent recurrence of any panic or anxiety reaction. The oral route is usually less threatening and produces markedly satisfactory therapeutic results within 30 to 40 minutes. The *talkdown technique*, especially when combined with gentle massage, usually works without the need for pharmaceutical intervention in approximately the same period of time.

When calm, the marijuana smoker and the LSD user appear strikingly similar: at ease, nonviolent, often offering "vibrations" of brotherhood and love to all who are in attendance. Indeed marijuana and LSD users are *not* violent individuals with one possible exception: when trapped with the drug that can mean a prison record and long years of legal harassment for them.

With the recent national trend to decriminalize personal use of marijuana (cou-pled with a deemphasis on "pot busts"), a generalized relaxation and fewer "marijua-na crises" are being seen in emergency situations. As "bad press" has mellowed out, marijuana "overdoses" have all but disappeared from the emergency room.

LSD

Lysergic acid diethylamide (LSD) and other psychedelic drugs (MDA, STP, DMT, psilocybin, mescaline, nutmeg, Mace, morning glory seeds, Hawaiian wood rose) are capable of producing abnormal psychic effects. A calm and sympathetic therapeutic atmosphere is vital in the emergency care of LSD-induced anxiety or paranoia. The patient should be taken to a supportive environment. This area must provide a "calm center" that excludes extraneous external stimuli. Quiet, sensitive music may be playing, and a mild, fragrant incense may be unobtrusively present. The patient should be talked to in a quiet, positive, yet sensitive and reassuring voice. Physical contact (touching hands) may be employed if it is not obviously uncomfortable to the patient.

It is amazing how rapidly a rational and sympathetic individual can calm the severely agitated LSD user. By all means avoid crowds and noises. Do not employ doctors, nurses, aides, or other attendants in *uniform*, and do not attempt immediate aggressive physical measures. One such patient, as a nasogastric tube was being placed in a legitimate effort to empty her stomach, cried out in panic, "My God, they're trying to put a snake in me!" Approach the psychedelic user mentally and emotionally, and employ physical restraint only when the patient threatens his own or your physical well-being.

Again, the LSD "bummer" has probably been caused by an improper environmental setting, or the patient simply may possess a "set" that is too rigid or too inadequate for a "good trip" in any circumstance.

This is an ideal situation in which to employ the "ART" technique. We firmly believe, as well, that chlorpromazine hydrochloride (Thorazine) and other phenothiazines are almost always contraindicated. Aside from the psychologic implications of the needle, the LSD "trip" may thereby be pharmacologically "aborted" and may become subconsciously subverted. This material may later reappear in the form of flashbacks and cause severe anxiety and even suicidal impulses to appear in the susceptible or inadequate personality. In addition, a combined anticholinergic effect may prove life threatening from a pharmacologic standpoint. Therefore with adverse LSD reaction, be gentle, be rational, and be sympathetic. Do not be overly cynical or clinical. If you can "flow with" the trip, so can (and will) your patient.

If LSD flashbacks occur after a "bummer" (or afer mismanaged medical intervention), again the best treatment is by reason and reassurance.* If the patient is acutely agitated, the benzodiazepines (diazepam, 10 mg, or chlordiazepoxide, 25 mg, given orally 3 times a day) may be of value. Flurazepam (Dalmane), 30 to 60 mg given at bedtime, may offer a restful sleep with minimal REM (rapid eye movement). Avoid needles and syringes whenever possible in these rare situations.

Occasionally you may be called on to treat a baby or a child, yet unable to talk, for LSD ingestion. As with prescription medication, psychedelics may be left within a child's access. The treatment is to love and fondle the child. Offer continuous physical contact and love for at least 8 hours. The child is in no physical danger and often responds immediately to your close attention, stroking, and reassuring voice.

Amphetamines ("speed")

Methylphenidate (Ritalin) and phenmetrazine (Preludin) are surrogates of "speed." As a physician, you will probably not be called on to treat a "speed freak"

---

*The true *flashback*, as originally described, has proved to be largely another exaggerated reaction of overzealous antipsychedelic reporting. With the exception of a rare and truly psychologically disturbed individual, the flashback phenomenon has all but disappeared from emergency rooms.

during a "run." Should this occur, however, he is not hard to spot. He looks like Rasputin: wild-eyed and woolly, undernourished, unkempt, and unwashed. He looks as if every nerve ending in his body were being continually stimulated. If the speed freak should seek your care for symptoms of acute amphetamine psychosis (full blown with paranoia and auditory and visual hallucinations) he may well require hospitalization.

The same paranoia attendant to large-dose amphetamine abuse in most instances also keeps this patient away from the doctor's door. Be happy of this, too. The amphetamine abuser (who has rewritten the pharmacology books by sometimes "shooting" as much as 5 gm per day) may develop a pharmacologic paranoid psychosis and may often be prone to violence, so be sure that you have the proper "muscle" around before you take on an aroused "speed freak." Physical contact is to be avoided here; the patient may interpret any physical contact as hostile—and these folks are often armed.

Although not physically addicting in itself, "speed" eventually "burns itself out"; that is, the user "crashes." The pattern is one of prolonged sleep that is followed by ravenous hunger and then deep depression—at which time he turns to barbiturates, heroin, methaqualone, meprobamate, alcohol or other "downers" to allow his body some rest. You concern as a physician is, first, is he violent and paranoid and therefore dangerous to himself or others? Then, is he near an exhaustion phase? Finally, is this problem compounded by other drugs such as, barbiturates or heroin?

Treatment consists of three phases: (1) initial detoxification, (2) initial abstinence, and (3) long-term aftercare. Our concern is initial detoxification, and the classic treatment for the "speed freak" is "C and C": *chloral hydrate* 1,000 to 1,500 mg given by mouth, and *closet*—or a quiet place to sleep without undue noise or visitors. If the diagnosis is uncertain as a result of the other medications described previously, you will need flexibility to determine your next move. Basically the question you must determine and act on is this: Is he or she on the way "up" or "down?" Intravenous drugs are to be avoided, but a good sedative regime for the pure "speed freak" is diazepam, 10 to 30 mg; chlordiazepoxide, 10 to 25 mg; or phenobarbital, 60 to 200 mg. These drugs should be given by mouth or intramuscularly and titrated to the individual's needs.

Cocaine

Cocaine is the prototype of the stimulant drug that is capable of producing euphoric excitement and, in high dosage, hallucinatory experience. These properties rank cocaine high in the esteem of the experienced drug abuser and lead to the highest degree of psychic dependence.

In the current drug subculture hierarchy, cocaine has become the "champagne of drugs" both because of its expense and its high esteem as an enhancer of social and sexual poise. The "coke" user looks down on other drug types and indeed represents the upper class. The "rich man's" drug, cocaine may be purchased illegally for $500 to $1,500 an ounce. Depending on the source, it is usually diluted, or "stepped on", by the street peddler about 7 times. Pure wholesale cocaine is sold to medical institutions for approximately $25 an ounce. Recently with the influx of cocaine into the Hollywood elite and other upper economic classes, the practice of "snorting" or "sniffing" (a process by which a "line" of cocaine is inhaled into a nostril, often through a rolled high denomination bill) has been revived and has to some extent supplanted intravenous use. Cocaine has been inhaled more recently through a red, white, and blue McDonald's milkshake straw. Wavy Gravy has called cocaine "the thinking man's Dristan."

One of the complications of sniffing is the not infrequent perforation of the nasal septum by necrosis secondary to the vasoconstrictive effect of cocaine. "Sniffers," "snorters," or "snarfers" are also prone to infection of the mucous membranes. A "reactive hyperemia" (clogging of nasal airways by engorged membranes) occurs as the vasoconstriction wears off, accounting for the dyad carried by chronic cocaine sniffers: (1) the "paraphernalia," such as spoon and snuffbox, and (2) the nose drops.

Systemically cocaine stimulates the central nervous system from above downward. The first recognizable action is on the cortex. In man this is manifested by definite euphoria, garrulousness, restlessness, and excitement. There is some evidence that perceptual awareness and cognitive speed are increased. There may also be an increased capacity for muscular work, probably because of a lessened sense of fatigue. Headache may be reported. After small amounts of cocaine, motor activity is well coordinated. But as the dose is increased, stimulation of lower motor centers causes tremors and convulsive movements.

If overdose occurs, the victim may report depression, confusion, dry throat, and dizziness. Hyperreflexia is noted, and eventually clonic-tonic convulsions appear. Such acute reaction, when accompanied by cardiovascular and respiratory collapse, constitutes the typical "caine reaction" and demands immediate supportive medical intervention.

Cocaine potentiates response to epinephrine and norepinephrine of organs that are supplied by sympathetic nerves and appears to slow the normal uptake of these neurohumors. A direct effect is increased gastrointestinal motility with a cathartic response and an occasional explosive result.

The action of cocaine on the medulla results in an initial increase in respiratory rate, but the depth of respiration is soon diminished to a rapid and shallow pattern. As depression follows stimulation, irregular or Cheyne-Stokes respirations may appear, and death may then occur as a result of central respiratory depression. The vasomotor and vomiting centers may also share in the stimulation, and sweating and vomiting are not uncommonly noted. A dangerous elevation in body temperature may result from the drug's effect on the heat-regulating center in the diencephalon. Vasoconstriction, increased muscular activity, and reduced heat radiation also occur. Hyperpyrexia and hypermetabolism may contribute directly to convulsion and this extreme situation requires immediate and most aggressive intervention. Other than purely supportive respiratory measures, resuscitative efforts should be carried out by experts *only* in controlled situations (ambulance or hospital) as follows:

1. Administer oxygen by positive pressure and artificial respiration if necessary. First, be assured that an open airway is present.
2. Use the Trendelenburg (head down) position. Wrap arms and legs, if needed, to increase blood flow to the head.
3. Inject small amounts of short-acting barbiturates, for example, thiopental (Sodium pentothal), 25 to 50 mg, if convulsions are present. This may be repeated, but gently. Do not force a general depressant effect to the point of no return.

4. Initiate administration of intravenous fluids.
5. Keep the patient cool and keep crowds away. Beware of hyperpyrexia; use ice or ice water sponging.
6. Give general muscle relaxants if necessary, such as succinylcholine, to facilitate intubation and administration of positive pressure oxygen.
7. Continuously monitor vital signs.

Although less dramatic, the situation far more likely to confront the emergency physician is that of the chronically "wired" "coke head." This individual may have rather profound sympathomimetic overstimulation with sometimes frightening cardiovascular pressor effects.

The treatment is quite similar to that of the "speed freak." Our experience has demonstrated an excellent response to the "ART" technique with the use of the benzodiazepines as adjunctive therapy. Through experience at providing medical coverage for large outdoor music festivals, we have determined that the specific use of propranolol hydrochloride given intravenously provides an almost instantaneous reversal of hypertension and tachycardia, and (reflexly) tachypnea. The treatment consists of 1 mg propranolol given intravenously at 1-minute intervals. We have not found more than 8 mg to be necessary for completely effective therapy in any of more than 200 patients so treated. Continuous cardiopulmonary monitoring reveals a reversal of cardiopressor effects almost immediately in addition to some degree of alleviation of anxiety. The patient often reports that he is still "high" at this point, and it should be noted that the central emetic effect is not obtunded. The propranolol regime appears to offer a dramatic therapy for protecting these patients from the dangers of cerebrovascular accident, death from cardiac arrhythmia, or from high-output congestive heart failure.

The adulterants of many of the drugs casually used in such settings must be recognized. Lidocaine, which is often used to adulterate cocaine, may indeed offer some protective influence on the heart. Likewise in the cocaine user who has been self-administering this drug for some period of time, a tachyphylactic reaction may be lifesaving.

In cases in which complete reversal of the dopaminergic effect is desired (reversal of "high"), we have utilized the butyrophenone haloperidol (Haldol). The dosage is 10 to 25 mg of haloperidol by mouth immediately, followed by 25 mg by mouth each day for 1 week thereafter. Because of the likely extrapyramidal effects—ataxia, torticollis, oculogyric crisis—it is necessary to supplement this treatment with specific daily administration of either benztropine mesylate (Cogentin), 2 to 8 mg per day, or diphenhydramine hydrochloride (Benadryl), 50 to 200 mg per day.

PCP

An illicit street drug of major concern is PCP or phencyclidine. The widespread use of this drug was noted throughout the country in 1977 and 1978. PCP is also known as "elephant," "hog," "beast," "animal tranquilizer," "the peace pill," or "angel dust." PCP is commonly encountered in doctored cigarettes as "crystal joints," or "dusters." Originally synthesized as a general anesthetic in the 1950s, this agent was shortly relegated to veterinary anesthesia (Sernyl, Sernylan) because of the commonly encountered unpleasant subjective dissociative effects in humans.

One "stick" (or cigarette) containing PCP may retail on the street for $2.00 or more. PCP is also "snorted" or "horned" as a powder. The sought-after effect of intoxication is a mild dysphoric state, but all too often the user takes "one toke over the line," which may cause a comatose trance to appear as a rigid catatonia. A true hypermetabolic crisis state may also be attendant. Such an afflicted person may prove extremely frustrating to the uninitiated health professional.

Treatment in these cases is generally symptomatic; mild intoxication may be handled by conservative close observation and monitoring of vital signs. The airway is generally not a problem in the PCP overdose victim; the spastic toxicity of the neck muscles tends to maintain a patent breathing passage and respiration is generally adequate. Close attention must be directed toward maintaining normothermia, however, and fluid balance should be managed by intravenous infusion. In our clinical experience, when hypermetabolism (and hyperthermia) ensue, the PCP overdose victim will respond quite favorably (and dramatically) to the cocaine overdose protocol previously outlined. Muscle spasms and tonic rigidity may be well managed both by massage and by judicious intramuscular administration of benzodiazepines (diazepam, 10 to 20 mg, or chlordiazepoxide, 10 to 25 mg). The application of the science of "ART" is of special value, and the spaced-out PCP victim is often thus restored to contact with his particular reality within 30 to 60 minutes.

Close observation is mandatory, however, because aid-station facilities may not be adequate for a victim who has ingested a large quantity of the drug. When in doubt, the patient should be hospitalized.

PCP is closely related to the general anesthetic ketamine, and indeed this latter agent is now achieving a small but recognized potential for abuse.

Barbiturates

Other "downers" or "dopers" include methaqualone (Quaalude) and glutethimide (Doriden). The pure "doper" is easy to spot. He dresses sloppily, has poor personal hygiene, burns holes in his clothing with his cigarettes, and talks at the speed of 33⅓ rpm. He is ataxic and exhibits sustained horizontal nystagmus. If he is in this toxic state, there is little to do but observe him for adequate respiration and try to get him properly hospitalized for evaluation and detoxification. As he "comes off" the various downers, convulsions or even hyperpyrexia and death are likely to occur. However, few "barb freaks" take only barbiturates, so beware of the superimposed pharmacology of additional drugs. (Always think "alcohol.")

Many of our acclimated young drug users accept convulsion as part of "coming down" off barbiturates. If possible, however, hospitalization should be arranged. (As few as six secobarbitals taken over a 30-day period can cause convulsions on withdrawal. See Table 20-2.)

Grouped pharmacologically with the barbiturates are glutethimide (Doriden), methaqualone (Quaalude), meprobamate, and alcohol. Watch for a combination of these.

The benzodiazepines—diazepam and chlordiazepoxide—although generally classed as sedative-hypnotics, possess a much lower physiologic addiction potential (to cause addiction it takes truly heroic doses) and possess as well a much higher margin of safety or therapeutic index.

The datura and belladonna alkaloids

In addition to the standard depressant, stimulant, or hallucinogenic drug problems, the physician may be challenged by a variety of miscellaneous adverse drug reactions such as scopolamine delirium because scopolamine and other similar drugs are widely available in nonprescription, over-the-counter sleeping medications. Scopolamine in therapeutic dose causes drowsiness, euphoria, amnesia, and dreamless (restless) sleep. Indeed, scopolamine (henbane) is an anesthetic of classic literature, and scopolamine and morphine have been used for the "twilight sleep" used in delivery. Excess dosage, however, may cause hallucination, excitement, and delirium. Reports of stramonium poisoning from jimsonweed tea date back to 1676. Treatment of belladonna delirium may be a high-risk task: if the physician administers the wrong medication (such as a phenothiazine tranquilizer), he may produce an additive reaction (anticholinergic) that may prove fatal. We recommend supportive treatment for scopolamine intoxification while holding in ready reserve the use of physostigmine for treatment of anticholinergic drug–induced delirium and coma.

Diacetylmorphine (heroin, "smack")

The average heroin addict "shoots up" three to four times a day with the "junk" he procures on the street. Aside from the hepatitis caused by the dirty needle, he may show up in your office with the racking chills of "cotton fever" (either acute septicemia or an allergic response to the multitude of foreign material that he injects into his veins daily).

The average heroin habit in the Haight-Ashbury is roughly $40 per day (money usually tabulated "on the margin," that is, in bartered goods, services, or "dealing"). This equals to four $10 ("dime") glassine bags or "balloons" (material held in dime-store toy balloons) and weighs as much as 400 mg of purchased "junk." If the "junk" is 1% heroin, it contains 4 mg heroin, and 20% good "Mexican brown" contains 20 mg heroin. The remainder of the "material" (cooked up to dissolve in tap water and filtered through cotton to remove impurities) consists of the following:

1. A major filler substance, usually the common sugars or starch, talc, or baking soda may be present; on rare occasion strychnine may be added for an intended lethal "hot shot."
2. Quinine, a common adulterant on the East Coast, is not usually seen in California.
3. Also present are a vast array of common and, surprisingly often, exotic organisms. These consist largely of *Staphylococcus, Streptococcus, Meningococcus, Clostridium, Corynebacterium,* mixed mouth flora, fungi (often *Candida*), and various other parasites including the organisms that cause malaria.
4. Of particular interest and concern to the attending physician are the *gram-negative* organisms to be found in abundance including *Escherichia, Pseudomonas, Salmonella, Klebsiella, Proteus, Shigella, Serratia, Haemophilus, Enterobacter,* and *Bacteroides.*

One may roughly estimate that these adulterants (in addition to the intrinsic depressant effect of heroin) account for one fatality for each 200,000 injections. Thus we could hypothesize with good statistical backup that if there are 150,000 individuals in New York City "shooting up" four times a day, the death rate is three per day.

THE BATTERED FLOWER-CHILD SYNDROME

These overdose victims may be dumped at your doorstep like the morning paper, or they may be accompanied by one or two frightened and reticent friends. These people may provide an all-important history of what has occurred and can serve as private duty aides by sitting with their friend as he is recovering after your ministrations. The vital point is not to turn these young people away or to underestimate their street knowledge.

Remember that you, as a physician (not to be trusted) and as being older than 30 (*certainly* not to be trusted), are the court of last resort for these young people. They will have previously instituted their own street methods of resuscitation before consulting you. Not only must you then deal with narcotic reversal, specifically naloxone, or with multiple drug depression, but you must also further deal with the possible adverse consequences of these methods of street resuscitation. Briefly, your problem may be any of the following.

"Boxer's mouth"

"Stimulation" is the common form of street resuscitation. This may consist of walking the overdose victim around, putting him in a cold shower, applying ice to his testicles, slapping him vigorously (hence possible blood, mucus, or broken teeth in the mouth), or squeezing sensitive areas such as the testicles or nipples.

The "speed" reversal

The pharmacologic knowledge of the street recognizes that depressant overdose may respond to amphetamines. Hence your client may have recently been "shot up" or "dosed" with "speed." This *really* muddies the waters, and in the hypoxic, acidotic, or comatose patient, it may cause convulsions.

"The heavy salt trip"

The mythology of the street says that table salt "takes up" or "binds" heroin, thereby nullifying its depressant effects. Therefore a like volume of salt to the amount of heroin used (for example, 1 spoonful) is diluted with tap water and injected intravenously. This strongly hypertonic solution in the presence of an already severely depressed cardiovascular system may well contribute to pulmonary edema. Perhaps some basis for perpetuation of the salt injection theory lies in the not uncommon occurrence of missing the junkie's sclerosed veins and injecting the solution subcutaneously. The intense pain attendant to such a procedure certainly would then have an arousal effect on the overdose victim.

"The milk run"

The "street-wise" (although not necessarily smart) drug user also nurtures a common myth that milk given intravenously reverses the overdose. In actuality a lipoid pneumonia may be the sad result of this practice.

"Cotton fever"

Acute septicemia or allergic reactions ranging upward to anaphylactic shock and death may follow injection of unknown foreign material by infected "outfits."

Less immediate problems such as malaria or syphilis transmitted by unsterile syringes, abscesses, bacterial endocarditis, or bacterial emboli may be watched for, but these complications are within the experience of the emergency physician. It is rather the hidden, self-inflicted injuries of the criminalized drug-using counter-culture—the battered flower-child syndrome—of which we must be increasingly wary.

DETOXIFICATION AND WITHDRAWAL

Table 20-1 indicates clinically used dosages of various analgesic drugs and their relative values in relieving surgical pain. All of these drugs are specifically and effectively reversed by naloxone.

Table 20-2 gives sedative and dependence-producing dosages of the common sedative-hypnotics.

Table 20-1. Dosages of analgesic drugs

Agent	Dosage	Route
Raw opium	0.3-0.6 gm	Oral (ingested or smoked)
Morphine	8-16 mg	IM or SC
Codeine (methylmorphine)	15-60 mg	Oral, IM, or SC
Heroin (diacetylmorphine)	2-5 mg	IM or SC
Dihydromorphinone (Dilaudid)	1-4 mg	IM or SC
Meperidine (Demerol)	50-150 mg	IM or SC
Oxycodone (Percodan)	1-2 tabs	Oral
Methadone (Dolophine)	10-20 mg	Oral, IM or SC
Propoxyphene hydrochloride*	65-130 mg	Oral
Propoxyphene napsylate*	100-200 mg	Oral
Pentazocine (Talwin)*	50-100 mg	Oral
	30-60 mg	IM or SC

*Recommended dosages; not generally considered equivalent in analgesic dosage.

Table 20-2. Common sedative-hypnotics and their abuse potential

Drug	Oral sedating dose (mg)	Dependence-producing dose (mg)	Time needed to produce dependence (days)	Convulsions in withdrawal
Secobarbital	100	800-2,200	35-37	Within 2-3 days
Pentobarbital sodium	100	800-2,200	35-37	Within 2-3 days
Chlordiazepoxide	25	300-600	60-180	Within 5-8 days
Diazepam	5-10	80-120	42	Within 5-8 days
Meprobamate	400	1,600-2,400	30	Within 5-8 days
Chloral hydrate	500	3,000-4,000	30	Within 5-8 days
Glutethimide	250	1,500-2,000	30	Within 5-8 days
Methaqualone	150	1,800-2,400	30	Within 3-5 days

Signs and symptoms of acute withdrawal

Opiates. The following are signs and symptoms of withdrawal from the opiates (drugs that are like morphine in their pharmacologic activity).

Adult	Newborn of addicted mother
Symptoms of "superflu"	Generally premature by weight (less than 2,500 gm)
Anxiety	Irritability
Rhinitis	Hyperactivity
Dilated pupils	Tremulousness
Abdominal cramps	Vomiting
Diarrhea, vomiting	Poor food intake
Shaking chills	Diarrhea
Profuse sweating	Fever
Sleep disturbances	High-pitched cry (once heard, easily identified)
Generalized aches and pains	Major seizures

In adults, withdrawal is extremely debilitating, but not generally life threatening. Withdrawal symptoms appear 6 to 8 hours after the last "fix," reach a maximum in 24 to 36 hours, and usually subside after 5 days. In infants, withdrawal may cause death.

Detoxification technique

Opiates. To treat withdrawal, titrate to a baseline maintenance dosage. Then maintain *or* withdraw the drug in a stepwise manner. If detoxification is to be your choice, the symptomatic regime in Table 20-3 is recommended as effective and (rela-

Table 20-3. Short-term opiate detoxification

Symptom complex	Treatment
Pain (or expressed somatic discomfiture)	Propoxyphene napsylate (Darvon-N), 200-300 mg; propoxyphene hydrochloride (Darvon), 130 mg; or pentazocine (Talwin), 100 mg, every 4-6 hr. Pentazocine within 12 hours of a "fix" may produce narcotic antagonism, creating "instant cold turkey" and thus reducing the medication's analgesic effect.
Sleeplessness	Flurazepam (Dalmane), 60-120 mg at bedtime; chloral hydrate, up to 2.5 gm at bedtime. At the Haight-Ashbury Detoxification Section we avoid use of the short-acting barbiturates, glutethimide, or methaqualone.
Nervousness	Phenobarbital, 30-60 mg; diazepam (Valium), 5-10 mg; or chlordiazepoxide (Librium), 10-25 mg every 6-8 hr.
Gastrointestinal distress	Belladonna leaf extract, phenobarbital (Belphen No. 1), oxyphenonium bromide and phenobarbital (Antrenyl-phenobarbital), or dicyclomine hydrochloride (Bentyl), 2 capsules every 4 hr. For pronounced nausea and vomiting, prochlorperazine (Compazine), 5-15 mg every 4 hr orally or 10 mg by rectal suppository.

tively) safe. Severe symptoms (even to individuals with a demonstrated low tolerance for discomfort) may be noted to subside within 5 days. Diazepam or flurazepam or both may be continued for an additional 21 days when (hopefully) the external life situation of the patient has improved.

In infants, gradual withdrawal should be carried out over the first 7 to 21 days of life, utilizing (minute) diminishing daily doses of narcotic substances.

Common sedative-hypnotics. Signs and symptoms of withdrawal from the sedative-hypnotics are equivalent to the delerium tremens of alcoholism. They are as follows:

Anxiety	Postural hypotension
Sleep disturbances	Delirium
Irritability	Hyperpyrexia
Restlessness	Major motor seizures
Abdominal cramps, diarrhea, vomiting	Death may ensue

Sedative-hypnotics. Begin with initial maintenance and then, if desired, a gradual phenobarbital substitution can be used in withdrawal.

For sedative-hypnotic–dependent individuals the following formula can be used to accurately calculate the dosage of phenobarbital necessary to initiate and carry out withdrawal:

$$\frac{\text{Amount of drug reported taken daily}}{\text{Regular oral hypnotic dose}} \times 30 \text{ mg phenobarbital} =$$

Total daily phenobarbital dose needed to initiate withdrawal

Ascertain the number of pills that the patient has been taking per day (for example 12 "reds" or secobarbital tablets per day) and give him twelve 30 mg phenobarbital tablets in three or four divided doses for the first day. Then begin tapering one or two 30 mg doses per day. Give care and attention to signs of both intoxication (nystagmus, slurred speech, ataxia) and incipient delirium or prodromata to seizure activity (in which case the dosage may be increased). This is shown in the following example:

Patient is taking 1,200 mg secobarbital per day.
1,200 = 12 × 30 = 360 mg phenobarbital needed to start treatment (three or four doses divided over 24 hours).
If signs of intoxication (nystagmus, slurring, ataxia) appear, cut the dose of phenobarbital by one half.
If signs of withdrawal continue, increase phenobarbital by increments of 30 mg, every 3 to 4 hours until stable.
If advanced signs (tremors, weakness, hyperreflexia, postural hypotension) occur, immediately administer phenobarbital, 200 mg intramuscularly. When the patient is stable, reduce phenobarbital by 30 mg per day.

In this example, complete (and comfortable) detoxification should occur within 10 to 12 days. Mild tranquilizers and/or flurazepam or chloral hydrate may be continued at the therapist's judgment.

THE DRUG USER REQUIRING HOSPITALIZATION

One of the greatest skills that can be acquired as an emergency physician is the (unfortunately often mostly instinctive) knowledge of when to hospitalize. Although your effectiveness depends to a great extent on the ability to quickly mobilize the patient and return him to his friends and family (and not to the police), there are those inevitable cases in which hospitalization is mandatory.

Several clues and rules of thumb can contribute to your effectiveness as the staff physician for such a patient:

1. When faced with the decision to "withdraw" rather than "maintain" a physiologically addicted patient, choose to "maintain." (It cuts down on those 3 AM calls that report, "Doctor, your patient is convulsing!")

2. In almost all instances the safest drug on which to maintain a patient is the drug that he was taking previously (obvious limitations, such as heroin, pertain here).

3. Recognize that with the tremendous increase in the percentage of *female* drug abusers, you will be dealing with some specific physiologic complications of women. (Approximately one third of all patients now seen in drug treatment programs are women, whereas 10 years ago it was one in six or seven.)

4. Recognize what seems to be an inordinately low pain threshold as well as an increased tolerance to analgesics, sedatives, and hypnotics in these patients. Do not undermedicate from fear of overdose or whatever personal reasons you may have. Their pain is very real; it is best approached by a rule of titration: Give a small dose "on demand"; when no more "demand" is forthcoming, you have reached the baseline level—a very important point for you to keep in mind.

5. Do not expect "drug-seeking behavior" to disappear once the patient is hospitalized. A careful analysis of his own personal "stash," and a careful search of visitors for supplemental drugs may well save you from the problem of in-hospital overdose. (A daily urine check may prove enlightening as well.) What we are talking about here is a tricky road to tread; it is essential that you seem to be a healer and not as a policeman to this patient, and his recovery depends in no small degree on this factor. This involves putting yourself in the middle as go-between and protector, a job that is not well suited to all conventionally trained physicians.

6. Recognize specific problems in the drug user who may require surgery. These include preanesthetic hypertension or hypotension, difficulties with anesthetic induction (a high tolerance), sudden signs of congestive heart failure or pulmonary edema without evidence of fluid overload, adrenal exhaustion in the "speed freak" or "coke head," postoperative ileus, and potentially lethal seizures postoperatively if alcohol, barbiturate, or other sedative-hypnotic addiction is not recognized.

7. The two-pack-a-day smoker has fourfold pulmonary problems postoperatively. Utilize aggressive pulmonary therapy during the postoperative period.

8. Recognize drug-related illnesses requiring hospitalization. White reported on 200 consecutive hospital admissions for drug-related illnesses, as shown in Table 20-4.

9. Recognize the vast array of complications that may occur in the drug user. (See outline.)

Table 20-4. Drug-related illnesses requiring hospitalization

Disease	Percent of admissions
Acute hepatitis	30.5
Infection	27.5
Detoxification	11.5
Diabetes mellitus	7.5
Pulmonary disease	6.0
Overdose	5.0
Cardiovascular disease	4.0
Gastrointestinal disease	3.5
Venereal disease	3.5

10. Realize that the patient who has been detoxified in the hospital is at double jeopardy for decreased tolerance and increased possibility of overdose following discharge.
11. Recognize the distinct differences presented by the patient who requires hospitalization while receiving daily methadone. With 80,000 individuals now in registered methadone programs in the United States, we have seen a steadily increasing morbidity and death rate from overdose in methadone addicts. In truth the new "hard-core" addict in the United States is the methadone addict who daily receives a government-inspected and approved narcotic. In comparison the street junkie who is using 1% to 4% heroin might be thought of as analogous to the person who is trying to get drunk on 3.2% beer!

Clinical complications that result from abuse of various drugs

Dermatologic complications

A. Local
   1. Skin tracks, shooting tattoos
   2. Pop scars, excoriations
   3. Abscesses, ulceration (seen with all intravenous drug use; most marked with the more excoriating—high pH—barbiturates)
   4. Thrombophlebitis (septic)
   5. Hand edema, sphaceloderma (gangrene)
   6. Camptodactylia
   7. Bullae, bullous impetigo
   8. Pigmentary disorders
   9. Pseudoacanthosis nigrans
   10. Tourniquet pigmentation
   11. Cheilitis
   12. Contact dermatitis
   13. Cigarette burns (seen with use of the depressants after "nodding out")

    14. Dental and gingival disorders (most often seen in the "cotton mouth" of the chronic amphetamine or cocaine user)

    15. Perforated septum (may be seen in the chronic cocaine "sniffer")

    16. Nasal congestion (cocaine)

B. Systemic
    1. Serum sickness–like reactions
    2. Fixed drug eruption
    3. Eyelid edema
    4. Urticaria, pruritus
    5. Purpura
    6. Jaundice
    7. Thromboembolic phenomena (petechiae, Osler's nodes)

C. Psychogenic
    1. Excoriations
    2. Acne excoriae
    3. Self-induced tattoos
    4. Wrist scars
    5. "Battered child syndrome" (seen in families that are psychologically erratically balanced as a result of drug abuse)

Cardiac complications

A. Endocarditis (suspect in presence of fever of undetermined origin, septic pulmonary emboli) may include tricuspid, and multiple valvular involvement. Especially seen are *Staphylococcus, Pseudomonas, Enterobacillus,* and *Candida.*

B. Toxic myocardial disease

C. Pulse, blood pressure changes, electrocardiographic abnormalities

D. Acidosis, hypoxia, hypercapnea, hypotension, hypertension

Vascular complications

A. Septicemia ("cotton fever") (especially *Staphylococcus aureus, Candida, Enterococcus,* gram-negative organisms; also *Clostridium tetani*); leukocytosis; malaria

B. Thrombophlebitis, arteritis, arterial occlusion

C. Metastatic lesions of bone, brain, lung, and kidney

D. Sequelae of vascular injection (vasospasm, ischemia, arteriovenous fistulae)

E. Mycotic aneurysm

F. Angiothrombotic pulmonary hypertension

G. Necrotizing angiitis

Pulmonary complications

A. Pneumonitis (aspiration)

B. Pulmonary embolism (air, dried blood, other foreign material)

C. Pulmonary edema (especially with heroin, methadone, propoxyphene)

D. Pulmonary infections (with unusual bacteria)

E. Talc contamination
    1. Chronic pulmonary fibrosus (may greatly decrease compliance and vital capacity; may lead to "stiff lung syndrome")
    2. Foreign body granulomas
    3. Pulmonary hypertension (may lead to secondary cardiac failure, cor pulmonale)

F. Increased incidence of tuberculosis

Hepatic complications

A. Acute or chronic hepatitis (may be transmitted by saliva, fecal-oral routes) (elevated transaminases, presence of hepatitis antigens)
B. "Junk" hepatitis
C. In alcoholism, nutritional cirrhosis and possibly hepatic carcinoma

Neurologic complications

A. Noninfectious
  1. Depressant overdose
    a. Increased intracranial pressure, convulsion, cerebral edema
    b. Sequelae: delirium, chronic organic dysfunction, postanoxic encephalopathy
  2. Stimulant overdose
    a. Massive sympathetic stimulation: sweating, dilated pupils, tachycardia, hyperactivity, confusion, delirium, hyperpyrexia, arrhythmia, convulsion
    b. Sequelae: toxic psychosis, paranoia, adrenal exhaustion
  3. Cerebrovascular accident: thrombotic and occlusive phenomena
  4. Acute transverse myelitis, paraplegia
  5. Peripheral nerve lesions
    a. Plexitis
    b. Neuropathy
    c. "Saturday night elbow," peripheral "pressure" nerve injury
B. Infectious and postinfectious
  1. Bacterial meningitis
  2. Brain (subdural, epidural abscesses)
  3. Peripheral nerve or muscle damage
  4. Tetanus (especially in "skin popping" young females)
  5. Embolic phenomena: central nervous system dysfunction (blindness and deafness)

Complications of muscle, bone, kidney, and connective tissue

A. Acute rhabdomyolysis, myoglobinemia, myoglobinuria
B. Unilateral "crush syndrome"
C. Chronic fibrosing myopathies
D. Arthralgia, arthritis
E. Pyogenic osteomyelitis
F. Nephrotic syndrome (glomerulonephritis, oliguria, anuria)
G. Acute, chronic renal failure
H. Connective tissue disorders (hyperimmune reactions)
I. Intervertebral disc space infection (*Staphylococcus aureus, Pseudomonas*)

CHANGING PATTERNS IN DRUG ABUSE

Drug patterns, particularly among adolescents and alienated youth (but ranging through persons of all ages) have changed dramatically in the last 20 years. In the accepting and somnolent 1950's, patterns were relatively constant and predictable. "Illegal" drugs were confined to certain racial, ethnic, and philosophic minorities most often submerged within black, Puerto Rican, Mexican-American, and rarely Oriental urban ghettos. The dominant culture—our great "silent majority"—confined itself to relatively traditional and legal agents of abuse such as alcohol, cigarettes, and certain prescription psychotropic drugs. Through the dissatisfied, violent 1960's, however, and into the confused and turned-off 1970's, contemporary drug patterns have shifted so dramatically that at the present time one can predict with certainty only change itself. These everchanging patterns of drug misuse present disturbing new challenges to the health professional at every level, particularly in the management of acute drug reactions. The physician must keep abreast of the societal dynamics of our drug-oriented society (which first heeded Tim Leary's proselytizing of "turn off, tune in, drop out") and must suddenly accept the role of therapeutic expert knowledgeable about a vast assortment of chemical agents. Our current philosophy of "better living through chemistry" is daily reinforced through a variety of channels from physician overprescription of amphetamine-like diet pills to television ads that say, "Take 'Sominex' and sle-e-ep."

In addition to an exploding availability of psychoactive drugs of every type, we see a growing contempt for years of misdirected "scare" drug education (analogous to the old venereal disease movies of World War II). Potential drug experimenters mistrust traditional sources of drug education given by parents, church groups, or the kindly old general practitioner. Unfortunately much of our current drug information gap was created by the dishonest presentation of facts on marijuana by those who have for generations espoused the "killer weed" philosophy, just as we have created our own credibility gap by intimating that the good guys are still *us*, and the bad guys are still *them*. We view ever more skeptically the proffered lists of good drugs and "bad" drugs: Aspirin and penicillin are good (unless, of course, an overdose of aspirin promotes gastric bleeding or penicillin produces an allergic response and possibly death); alcohol and cigarettes are, if not good, at least legal; while marijuana and LSD are bad, and heroin is not even to be discussed anymore. We have literally "wished it away"—back into the ghettos—"where it (classically) belongs." Meanwhile, the American Medical Association and the Food and Drug Administration confuse and frighten us with their squabbling, contradictions, and apparent lack of any coherent direction.

In truth drugs are neither good nor bad. Drugs can make sick people healthy and healthy people sick. In varying doses drugs can produce neutral, beneficial, or adverse psychopharmaceutical effects on different individuals in different sets and in different settings.

Through a mixture of miseducation and our everpresent puritanical reliance on law, order, and punishment to legislate morality in medical situations, the individual drug user has come to be viewed (and, not coincidentally, to view himself) as a criminal and not as a patient. Further there is a romantic element involved here. The antihero criminal aspects (the "hustling," the paraphernalia, and the semireligious ethic of this underground lifestyle) offer, at least initially, an exciting and invigorating alternative to boredom. Whatever the new wide-ranging sociologic patterns, a large percentage of all of us—from subteen to geriatric junkie—will experiment with illegal drugs because of (a) almost universal drug availability and (b) attendant peer-group pressure.

These two variables have interacted in coordinated lockstep. Peer pressure has always been with us, but never before has there been available the astonishing assortment of drugs, manufactured both legally and illegally, that is now to be found on every street corner, in every schoolyard, and in every medicine chest. It is perhaps not surprising that our population has become more sophisticated in its practical drug information than are our general physicians. In years past a huffing paternalism and an unflappable authoritarianism secreted the physician behind his wall of ignorance. If he was punitive and moralizing, he somehow had our best interests at heart. The drug user of today is reluctant to seek medical or psychologic help in traditional in-patient medical facilities until his pain is unbearable or until he is literally carried in unconscious.

QUESTIONS

1. Cleveland Clyde took 200 acid trips in 1967. In 1968 he shot speed in 1- or 2-week "runs." In 1969 he sniffed or shot cocaine at least once a day. In 1970 he shot smack for 2 months (every day). During this time span, he was *physiologically addicted* to how many drugs?
   a. 1   c. 3
   b. 2   d. 4

2. Helen the Hooker got strung out on smack in 1970. The "new junkie" (hooked since 1967) consists of what percent females?
   a. 10%   d. 50%
   b. 15%   e. 75%
   c. 33%

3. Haight Street Omar was used to drinking white port, but he overdosed on "the rich man's drug." He took:
   a. Cocaine (Peruvian)
   b. Owsley acid
   c. Panama red
   d. Saigon smack

4. Ron the Speed Freak is grinding his teeth and needs some sleep. He tries some:
   a. Window pane   d. Acapulco gold
   b. Coke   e. Smack
   c. Peyote

5. Fat Freddy takes his welfare check and scores a lid of "good grass" from Dealer McDope. It turns out to be 10% THC. (Everyone knows that Dealer McDope deals only in "the finest imported and domestic weed.") He:
   a. Got burned, as usual
   b. Made a good deal for once

6. Wayne the Wino drinks one fifth of tequila, takes 15 "Mexican reds," and then snorts some PCP. The doctors who see him at San Francisco General Hospital are *most* concerned with:
   a. Dehydration
   b. Aspiration pneumonitis
   c. Respiration
   d. Hypokalemia
   e. Halitosis (which beats no breath at all)

7. Fat Freddy goes out again, this time to score some "barbs." He brings back some No. 4 red gelatin caps, each filled with 190 mg of white (bitter) powder for which he trades $15 in food stamps. He:
   a. Got burned, as usual
   b. Scored good Lilly Seconals
   c. Scored lousy Mexican reds
   d. God knows

8. Joe the Junkie scores a "quarter" bag of 1% smack. He has how many milligrams of heroin?
   a. 1 mg   c. 4 mg
   b. 2 mg   d. 20 mg

9. Marvin the Needle Freak shot up 5 "Mexican reds." They did not look like the picture in the PDR—each one contained 20 mg secobarbital, 10 mg strychnine, and 170 mg lactose. Marvin got:
   a. Abscesses   c. "Off"
   b. A headache   d. "Offed"

10. Andy the Android is snarfing "angel dust" again. He is likely getting:
    a. Oregano   c. PCP (Sernyl)
    b. LSD and grass   d. Catnip

Bonus

11. The Nose that Knows snorted 5 lines of what was sure to be quality Peruvian coke and failed to "get off," but the most sensitive part of her body (that is, her *nose*) went to sleep. She was most likely sniffing:
    a. Peruvian sunshine
    b. Procaine (Novocaine) plus amphetamine
    c. Lidocaine (Xylocaine)
    d. Powdered Erythroxylon coca

ANSWERS

1. a. If we consider a true physiologic addiction as one that demonstrates the development of tolerance on repeated dosage and physical signs of withdrawal on cessation of use, then he was addicted to only one drug, "smack."

2. c. Fully one third of the "new junkie" popu-

lation are females. Ten years ago, it was only one out of six or one out of seven.

3. a. The "rich man's drug," or "the gift from the sun god," is cocaine.

4. d or e. Ron would probably try Acapulco gold (marijuana) or, if he had access to it, smack (the ultimate downer). Certainly window pane (acid) is not conducive to sleep, neither is cocaine or peyote.

5. b. Fat Freddy made a good deal for once. Grass with a 10% THC content would be beyond Fat Freddy's fondest dreams.

6. c. Respiration, of course. Aspiration pneumonitis must be suspected but is integral to the entire respiratory picture. Blood pressure certainly might be lowered and supportive measures should be instituted.

7. d. Fat Freddy cannot really be blamed this time. Not enough information is given here.

8. c. Figuring 400 mg in a "quarter," or $25, bag of smack, 1% heroin would equal 4 mg.

9. d. "Offed." Marvin has joined his ancestors after exceeding 30 mg of strychnine in one intravenous dose.

10. c. Andy is snarfing PCP (Sernyl), although all of the others have been sold on the street as "angel dust."

11. c. Lidocaine (Xylocaine). If amphetamine were present, The Nose That Knows might also have gotten a systemic "rush."

SUGGESTED READINGS

Carveth, S. W., Burnap, T. K., et al.: Training in advanced cardiac life support, J.A.M.A. **235:** 2311-2315, 1976.

Carveth, S. W., Reese H. E., and Buchman, R. J.: Stadium resuscitation (a life support unit). In Stephenson H. E., editor: Cardiac arrest and resuscitation, ed. 4, St. Louis, 1974, The C. V. Mosby Co.

Chambers, C. D.: Some considerations for the treatment of non-narcotic drug abusers. In Brill, L., and Lieberman, L., editors: Major modalities in the treatment of drug abuse, Boston, 1970, Little, Brown & Co.

Cohen, S.: The drug dilemma, New York, 1969, McGraw-Hill, Inc.

Cooper, J. R., Bloom, F. E., and Roth, R.: The biochemical basis of neuropharmacology, ed. 2, New York, 1974, Oxford University Press, Inc.

Dole, V. P., and Nyswander, M.: A medical treatment for diacetylmorphine (heroin) addiction, J.A.M.A. **193:**646-650, 1965.

Dole, V. P.: Detoxification of methadone patients and public policy, J.A.M.A. **226:**780-781, 1973.

Eckenhoff, J. E., Helrich, M., Hege, M. J. D., et al.: Respiratory hazards of opiates and other narcotic analgesics, Surg. Gynecol. Obstet. **101:** 701-708, 1955.

Eddy, N., Halbach, H., Harris, I., and Seevers, M.: Drug dependence: its significance and characteristics, Psychopharmacol. Bull. **3:**1, 1966.

Einstein, S.: The use and misuse of drugs, Belmont, Calif., 1970, Wadsworth Publishing Co., Inc.

Gabel, R. A.: Cardiopulmonary resuscitation, Am. Fam. Physician **7:**68-75, 1973.

Gay, G. R., Matzger, A. D., et al.: Short term heroin detoxification on an outpatient basis, Int. J. Addict. **6:**241-264, 1971.

Gay, G. R., Winkler, J. J., and Newmeyer, J. A.: Emerging trends of heroin abuse in the San Francisco bay area, J. Psychedelic Drugs **4:** 53-64, 1971.

Gay, G. R., Smith, D. E., Wesson, D. R., and Sheppard, C. W.: Outpatient barbiturate withdrawal using phenobarbital, Int. J. Addict. **7:** 17-26, 1972.

Gay, G. R., Senay, E. C., and Newmeyer, J. A.: The pseudo-junkie: evolution of the heroin lifestyle in the non-addicted individual, Anesth. Analg. **53:**241-247, 1974.

Gay, G. R., and Inaba, D. S.: Treating acute heroin toxicity, Anesth. Analg., 1976.

Gay, G. R., Inaba, D. S., Sheppard, C. W., Newmeyer, J. A. and Rappolt, R. T., Sr.: Cocaine: history, epidemiology, human pharmacology, and treatment. A perspective on a new debut for an old girl, Clin. Toxicol. **8:**149-178, 1975.

Gay, G. R., and Trantham, J. G.: Medical-surgical complications of drug abuse, Int. Surg. **60:** 327-331, 1975.

Hekiman, L. H., et al.: Characteristics of drug abuser admitted to a psychiatric hospital, J.A.M.A. **205:**125, 1968.

Inaba, D. S., Gay, G. R., Newmeyer, J. A. and Whitehead, C.: Methaqualone abuse: lucking out, J.A.M.A. **224:**1505-1509, 1973.

Interim report of the commission of inquiry into the non-medical use of drugs, Le Dain Commission, Ottawa, 1970, Crown Copyrights.

Isbell, H., and Chrusciel, T. L.: Dependence liability of non-narcotic drugs, Geneva, 1970, World Health Organization.

Jaffe, J. H.: Methadone maintenance and the national strategy. In Proceedings of the Fourth National Conference on Methadone Treatment, 1972.

Jaffee, J. H.: Drug addiction and drug abuse. In Goodman, L. S., and Gilman, A., editors: The pharmacological basis of therapeutics, ed. 5, New York, 1975, Macmillan, Inc.

Jude, J. R.: Cardiopulmonary resuscitation, J.A.M.A. **193**:678-679, 1965.

Kramer, J. C.: Controlling narcotics in America, Drug Forum, Part I, **1**:51-69, 1971; Part II **1**: 153-167, 1972.

Kersh, E. S., and Schwartz, L. K.: Narcotic poisoning: an epidemic disease, Am. Fam. Physician **8**:90-97, 1973.

Lingeman, R. R.: Drugs from A to Z: a dictionary, ed. 2, New York, 1974, McGraw-Hill, Inc.

Loomis, T. A.: Essentials of toxicology, Philadelphia, 1968, Lea & Febiger.

Louria, D. B., and Wolfson E. A.: Medical complications of drug abuse, Drug Therapy pp. 35-44, August, 1972.

Musto, D. F.: A study in cocaine: Sherlock Holmes and Sigmund Freud, J.A.M.A. **204**:125, 1968.

Newmeyer, J. A., and Gay, G. R.: The traditional junkie, the aquarian age junkie, and the Nixon era junkie, Drug Forum **2**:17-30, 1972.

Preble, E. and Casey, J.: Taking care of business: the heroin user's life on the street, Int. J. Addict. **4**:1-24, 1969.

Poisons: emergency treatment, Safety Promotion Committee of the Canadian Government, Ottawa, 1972, Information Canada.

Sheppard, C. W., and Gay, G. R.: The changing face of heroin addiction, Int. J. Addict. **6**:17-26, 1971.

Smith, D. E., and Gay, G. R.: It's so good, don't even try it once: heroin in perspective, Englewood Cliffs, N.J., 1972, Prentice-Hall, Inc.

Standards for cardiopulmonary resuscitation (CPR) and emergency cardiac care (ECC), J.A.M.A. **227**:833-868, 1974.

Thompson, D. S.: Emergency airway management, Am. Fam. Physician **11**:146-153, 1975.

Weil, A.: The natural mind, Boston, 1973, Houghton Mifflin Co.

White, A. G.: Medical disorders in drug addicts: 200 consecutive admissions, J.A.M.A. **223**: 1469-1491, 1973.

Yablonsky, L.: Synanon, the tunnel back, New York, 1965, Pelican Books, Inc.

Young, A. W. Jr., and Sweeney, E. W.: Cutaneous clues to heroin addiction, Am. Fam. Physician **7**: 1973.

CHAPTER 21

Poisonings

GEORGIA B. NOLPH

APPROACH TO THE PATIENT

One should find out as soon as possible the "3 W's"—who, what, and when. *Who* should include the patient's name, age, approximate weight, and telephone number. If a telephone caller states that someone has been poisoned, these data can be elicited at the time of the call so that records can be obtained, and everything can be prepared by the time the patient arrives. Time is important; therefore the patient must be brought to the facility with the necessary equipment for treatment. While talking, one should find out *what* has poisoned the patient (if one is not familiar with the symptoms of toxicity and the treatment, this gives an opportunity to look it up), *when* the patient was poisoned, and how long a period of time has elapsed. Finally, the container, plant, or other involved object should be brought in with the patient.

SURFACE-ACTING POISONS

The patient should be drenched immediately and thoroughly with a steady stream of water while his clothing is being removed; the skin should then be cleansed with water. Eye contamination also requires immediate washing of the eyes with a gentle stream of running water while holding the eyelids open. Chemicals should not be used in washing the eyes!

INHALANTS

All doors and windows, should be opened and the patient should be carried to fresh air immediately. Tight clothing should be loosened, and the patient should be wrapped in blankets, and kept quiet. Alcohol should not be given to the patient. If convulsions occur, the patient should be kept in bed in a semidark, quiet room. The patient's respirations must be watched; if they should become irregular or stop, artificial respiration should be started.

INGESTANTS (ANTIDOTES)

Antidotes are used to delay absorption of the poison and to buy added time to transport the patient to a place where further emergency treatment and then definitive treatment can be given. The universal antidote, consisting of activated charcoal, magnesium hydroxide, and tannic acid in proportionate parts of $2:1:1$, is obsolete

Table 21-1. Antidotes

Poison	Antidotes	Dosage	Side effects
Acids	Milk or water	For patients 1 to 5 yr, 1 to 2 cups; for those older than 5 yr, up to 1 quart	
Alkalis	Milk of magnesia	1 tablespoon in 1 cup water	
	Milk or water	For patients 1 to 5 yr, 1 to 2 cups; for those older than 5 yr, up to 1 quart	
	Vinegar	Diluted 1:4 with water	
Organic phosphate insecticides (parathion, TEPP, HETP)	Atropine	1 to 2 mg IM	
Morphine	Naloxone	0.4 mg as IM bolus, 0.8 mg 3 min later	
	Nalline	5 to 10 mg IV	Blocks central nervous system, depressive effects
Alkaloids, atropine, strychnine, nicotine, quinine, morphine, physostigmine	Potassium permanganate, 1:10,000 solution, or tannic acid, 0.5% solution	For gastric lavage	
Mercury, copper, gold, arsenic, antimony, lead	BAL (2, 3-dimercaprol, British anti-Lewisite); less effective for silver; ineffective if there is extensive tissue damage; not to be used for cadmium or iron poisoning	For severe intoxication: 3 mg per kg every 4 hr for 2 days, every 6 hr on third day, then every 12 hr for 10 days or until recovery For mild intoxication: 2.5 mg per kg every 4 hr for 2 days, every 12 hr on third day, then daily for 10 days	Lacrimation, salivation, nausea, vomiting, increased temperature, decreased blood pressure, pulmonary edema (may be diminished by previous administration of ephedrine)
	Cuprimine	Children and adults, 250 mg by mouth, 3 or 4 times daily; infants, 250 mg daily in fruit juice	
Snakebites	Antivenin		

and should not be given. Activated charcoal (Norit-A, Darco G-60, Nuchar C, and Requa) is a potent adsorbent that inactivates many poisons and is effective for virtually all chemicals except cyanide if given early. Neither the pH of the poison nor the pH of the gastrointestinal tract reduces the potency of this adsorption. The dosage of activated charcoal is 1 to 2 tablespoons in an 8-ounce glass of water. Activated charcoal should *not* be given before, or simultaneously with, syrup of ipecac as the charcoal inhibits the emetic action of the ipecac.

Table 21-1 lists some of the more common antidotes. Using an antidote may do more harm than good unless extreme caution is used.

EVALUATION

The evaluation of the patient must be tendered with consideration of how much time has elapsed since the ingestion or exposure. With this in mind the classification suggested by Teitelbaum is most useful:

	Asleep	Can be aroused	Will answer questions	Comatose	Does not withdraw from painful stimuli	Reflexes absent	Respiratory or circulatory depression
Class 0	X	X	X				
Class 1				X			
Class 2				X	X		
Class 3				X	X	X	
Class 4				X	X	X	X

TREATMENT

Emergency care consists of the basic triad of maintaining an airway, emptying the stomach, and giving a cathartic. In any patient, an airway must be maintained by one means or another. Thick or profuse secretions may require suctioning. An oral airway or an endotracheal tube may be needed to assist the patient in breathing. Cough or gag reflexes should be checked in all patients, even those who are awake. Anoxia should be avoided; oxygen must be given under pressure for pulmonary edema, and the shock, which results mainly from an increased venous space caused by dilation, not myocardial failure, should be treated. A central venous pressure catheter should be placed, and effective circulating blood volume must be restored.

Emesis

One must decide *whether* emesis should be induced. To induce emesis, a finger or the blunt end of a spoon should be placed at the back of the patient's throat after precautions are taken to prevent the patient from biting the finger. The best method is the use of syrup of ipecac, 20 ml with 2 to 3 glasses of water for a child and 30 ml with 2 to 3 glasses of water for an adult. (This corresponds to 4 teaspoons for a child and 2 tablespoons for an adult.) Syrup of ipecac should be in the armamentarium of every household with children. A patient in whom emesis is being induced should be in a face-down position with the head lower than the hips to prevent aspiration of vomitus.

Anything that will cause more damage on the way up and that can be neutralized in the stomach should be left there. Contraindications to emesis include an unconscious or comatose patient; convulsions; ingestion of corrosive poisons with symptoms of severe pain, vomiting, or burning in the mouth and throat; acids and acidlike products such as toilet bowl cleaners (sodium acid sulfate), rust removers (hydrofluoric acid), iodides, and silver nitrate (styptic pencils); and alkalis and alkali-like substances such as drain cleaner (sodium hydroxide, lye), washing soda (sodium carbonate), ammonia water, and household bleach (sodium hypochlorite).

The ingestion of petroleum distillate products such as kerosene, gasoline, or lighter fluid is no longer considered to be an absolute contraindication to induction of emesis by all physicians involved in treating this ingestion. This has become a new area of controversy: Some think that it is safer to induce emesis following petroleum distillate ingestion by children than it is to put a lavage tube down a struggling child.

All products of emesis should be saved and sent to the laboratory for identification and quantification of ingestants.

Gastric lavage

Gastric lavage allows some quantification of the material removed and also an entry for antidotes and cathartics. Lavage should be performed within 3 hours of ingestion unless large amounts of milk, cream, or enteric-coated drugs have been ingested. These delay absorption and thereby make lavage feasible after a longer period of time has elapsed. Small nasogastric tubes may be easier to put into place, but they limit the amount and particle size of the material that can be removed. Therefore a No. 24 French tube should be selected for children and No. 34 French for adults. Chilling and applying lubricating gel to the tip facilitate its passage. The end of the tube should be positioned under water; if air bubbles are seen leaving the tube, it should be repositioned to make certain it is in the stomach and not a bronchus. The patient should be placed on his left side with his head supported but lower than his hips to increase drainage and minimize aspiration.

Generally, isotonic or half-isotonic physiologic saline may be used. Activated charcoal added to the saline increases adsorption. The choice of a specific lavage solution is as important as the manner in which it is used. Small amounts (50 ml) should be used repeatedly, rather than larger amounts less often, to decrease the passage of poison into the intestine.

Table 21-2 lists specific lavage solutions. The tannates formed when tannic acid is used as a lavage fluid may later redissolve and subsequently hydrolyze. Therefore they should not be allowed to remain in the stomach. Potassium permanganate is rarely used in present therapy. It is a very strong irritant in itself; if used, it must be well diluted so that no undissolved particles come in contact with the stomach or other tissues. Magnesium oxide or magnesium hydroxide may be used to neutralize acidic substances because they do not release the carbon dioxide that distends the stomach. The depressant effect of magnesium on the central nervous system is aborted if the material is not allowed to remain in the stomach.

Lavage should be continued until the return is clear; then activated charcoal in

Table 21-2. Lavage solutions

Solution	Concentration	Effective against
Activated charcoal	15 to 30 ml per 250 ml water	All chemicals except cyanide
Tannic acid	30 to 50 gm per 1,000 ml water	Alkaloids, certain glucosides, many metals, apomorphine, hydrastine, strychnine, veratrine, cinchona alkaloids, and salts of aluminum, lead, silver
Potassium permanganate	1:10,000 or 0.1 gm per 1,000 ml water	Alkaloids, quinine, strychnine, nicotine, physostigmine
Magnesium oxide or magnesium hydroxide	25 gm per 1,000 ml water	Acetylsalicylic acid, oxalic acid, sulfuric acid, other mineral acids and alkaline hypochlorite
Sodium bicarbonate	5%	Ferrous sulfate
Calcium lactate or calcium gluconate	15 to 30 gm per 1,000 ml water	Fluoride and oxalates
Ammonium acetate or dilute ammonia water	4 ml per 500 ml water	Formaldehyde
Normal saline	0.8% or 4 ml per 500 ml water	Silver nitrate
Iodine	15 drops tincture per 125 ml water	Lead, mercury, silver, quinine, and strychnine
Starch	75 to 80 gm per 1,000 ml water	Iodine (lavage until no blue returns)
Milk	Fresh or evaporated	Copper sulfate, croton oil, chlorates, thioglycolic acid

water and a cathartic should be given via the tube to promote rapid passage of the poison through the intestine. Three recommended cathartics are magnesium sulfate, Fleet Phospho-Soda, and sodium sulfate. Cathartics are contraindicated when the poison causes dehydration secondary to severe diarrhea and shock.

SPECIFIC CARE

Specific care depends on the category of substances ingested: foods, plants, heavy metals, drugs, or household products.

Food poisoning

Food poisoning can be traced to either a chemical or a bacterial source. Two variables are the dosage of the toxin or organism and the resistance of the individual. Some of the common food poisons are analyzed and shown in Tables 21-3 and 21-4.

Poisonous plants

Poisonous plants or parts of plants so completely surround us in our everyday living that we tend to minimize their dangers, often through indifference or ignorance.

Table 21-3. Chemical sources of food poisoning

Chemical	Source	Symptoms	Incubation
Antimony	Gray enameled utensils	Vomiting	Minutes to 1 hour
Cadmium	Acid liquids placed in cadmium-plated ice cube trays, pitchers, etc.	Cramps, diarrhea	15 to 30 minutes
Sodium cyanide	Silver cleaner	Weakness, coma, respiratory failure	Few minutes
Sodium fluoride	Cockroach powder (mistaken for baking powder or soda)	Gastrointestinal upset, convulsions, paresis	Minutes to 2 hours
Zinc	Acid foods cooked or stored in galvanized iron utensils	Pain in mouth, throat, and abdomen; diarrhea	Few minutes
DDT	Animals exposed to it	Unknown	Unknown

Table 21-4. Bacterial sources of food poisoning

	Botulism	Salmonella	Staphylococcus	Other
Source	Home-canned vegetables, preserved meats and fish Type A common in western states Type B common in eastern states Type E common in Alaska and Great Lakes area; commonly transmitted by fish products	Rat and mouse urine and feces, infected meat, duck eggs, unpasteurized milk and cheese, housefly and human carriers	Airborne droplets or skin infection, milk, mayonnaise, cream, salads, custard, cream-filled pastries, mincemeat, salted meat, tenderized ham Type A commonest cause of staphylococcal food poisoning	1. *Clostridium perfringens:* meat, especially beef and turkey 2. *Bacillus cereus:* foods made from corn flour 3. *Vibrio parahemolyticus:* shellfish
Incubation period	2 hr to 8 days, usually 12 to 48 hr	Usually 12 to 24 hr; can be 7 to 72 hr with 6 to 8 hr minimum	2 to 3 hr; may be from 1 to 6 hr	

Continued.

The inedible mushrooms or toadstools produce two types of poisoning: muscarine and peptide toxins from the phallotoxins and amatoxins. Muscarine poisoning, which affects the organs innervated by postganglionic and cholinergic fibers of the autonomic nervous system, produces violent symptoms within minutes of ingestion. The patient with muscarine poisoning has excitability, signs of confusion, profuse sweating, salivation, lacrimation, acute nausea, vomiting, diarrhea, bradycardia, and often

Table 21-4. Bacterial sources of food poisoning—cont'd

	Botulism	Salmonella	Staphylococcus	Other
Symptoms	Headache, dizziness, diplopia, constipation, diarrhea, abdominal pain, drooping lids, difficulty in swallowing, aphonia, respiratory paralysis, weakness, vertigo Nausea and vomiting typical of type E, rare in types A and B	Septicemia or gastrointestinal symptoms or both, abdominal pain, chills, fever, diarrhea, vomiting	Sudden violent nausea, vomiting, diarrhea, cramps, acute prostration (recovery within 1 to 3 days)	Diarrhea most prominent
Treatment	Treatment of respiratory failure; botulism trivalent antitoxin IV in 2 vials, repeated in 2 hr; cleansing enemas; lavage; IV fluids; catheterization	Maintenance of hydration and electrolyte balance; paregoric or morphine for pain and diarrhea	Nonspecific; maintenance of hydration; pain reduction with meperidine, 100 mg IM; propantheline bromide, 15 mg by mouth or IM; prochlorperazine for nausea and vomiting; paregoric, kaolin, pectin, or diphenoxylate (Lomotil) for diarrhea	1. As for *Staphylococcus* 2. As for *Staphylococcus* 3. As for *Staphylococcus* plus tetracycline, 250 mg every 6 hr
Comments	Two thirds of cases in USA are fatal; prevented by properly canning foods in pressure cooker, boiling foods for 15 minutes before eating, noting odor of toxin when opening container		Toxin heat stable, has no odor or taste, is not destroyed by boiling for 30 min or by refrigeration for 67 days	

dyspnea secondary to a marked increase in bronchial secretions. Death can ensue within hours. The specific antidote for the muscarine type of poisoning is intra-musclar injection of atropine, 0.65 to 1.0 mg, repeated every 30 minutes for the control of symptoms. The patient should also be hospitalized for intravenous re-placement of fluids; barbiturates should be given for the excitability and morphine should be given if needed for the severe abdominal pain.

The patient who incurs poisoning by the peptide toxin presents with symptoms occurring within 6 to 24 hours after ingestion of the mushrooms. The symptoms (violent abdominal pain, rapid dehydration with thirst, and diarrhea that can become bloody) are caused by the phallotoxins that act by poisoning the endoplasmic reticu-lum and mitrochondria of the cells. The amatoxins primarily affect cell nuclei and are therefore responsible for necrosis of liver cells and renal tubule cells as well as the fatty degeneration of striated muscle and brain cells. There is no specific anti-dote for the peptide toxins. Supportive and symptomatic treatment is aimed at correcting the dehydration, relieving the pain through use of morphine or other opiates, and hourly evaluation of urine output. Mannitol diuresis to prevent renal failure may be considered. Early hemodialysis is helpful because the small peptide toxins readily pass through the membranes. Dexamethasone (15 mg per day, intra-muscularly) or prednisone (100 mg per day, intramuscularly) may be given if neces-sary to control shock. The combination of penicillin, chloramphenicol, and sulfa-methoxazole is thought to help block the toxicity of amanitin by binding the toxin to serum albumin, and thereby, hastening its excretion. The intravenous enzyme cytochrome c is thought to possibly improve respiratory function in amanitin-dam-aged cells and has therefore been recently advocated.

The leaf blades of rhubarb plant are very toxic. With the exception of good tubers the entire plant of the potato, including raw sprouted potatoes, is in the same cate-gory. Among the poisonous garden flowers are the foxglove (flowers, leaves, and seeds); lily-of-the-valley (leaves, roots, fruit, and flowers); delphinium, larkspur, and staggerweed (seed and young plants); monkshood (flowers, leaves, and roots); and the bulbs of the narcissus, daffodil, and jonquil. Elderberry and black locust are among the poisonous trees and shrubs, whereas the rhododendron, rose bay, azalea, oleander, mountain laurel, and yellow jasmine are poisonous plants that are considered ornamentals. One should be wary of the leaves and roots of the cala-dium, the seeds and leaves of the castor bean, the stems and leaves of the dumbcane, and the berries of the lantana. Perilous wild plants include the bloodroot, baneberry, Jack-in-the-pulpit, marsh marigold, water hemlock, false hellebore, nightshade, poison hemlock, pokeweed, and jimsonweed. The number of plants mentioned illustrates the necessity of identification of any plant eaten, and the part and the amount of the plant ingested. Symptoms usually occur within 4 to 12 hours after ingestion of plants, mushrooms are the exception because onset may be greater than 12 hours. If the patient is seen within 4 hours of ingestion of a plant, if there are no symptoms, and if the toxicity of the plant is questionable, 15 ml of syrup of ipecac should be given; if the patient has not vomited, this should be repeated in 15 minutes. The patient should be observed for 12 hours. Jimsonweed and other plants containing atropine produce the symptom complex of increased temperature, dilated pupils, decreased respirations, and shock.

Heavy metals

Heavy metal poisoning is usually caused by ingestion of bichloride of mercury or by ingestion, inhalation, or absorption of lead via the skin. Symptoms of mercury poisoning include a metallic taste, gastrointestinal upset including bloody diarrhea, foul breath, sore gums, excessive salivation, progression to circulatory and respiratory failure, and severe renal tubular degeneration. The earlier the treatment is administered, the more effective it will be. Therefore first the patient should ingest raw eggs or milk to inactivate the mercury. (This can be done before the patient is brought to the physician.) Copious lavage is followed by the administration of BAL (British anti-Lewisite), according to the dosages recommended in Table 21-1, or Cuprimine (a penicillamine derivative), an oral antidote that is effective against mercury. The dosage of Cuprimine is 250 mg 3 to 4 times per day for adults and children and 250 mg per day in fruit juice for infants.

Symptoms of lead poisoning include anorexia, vomiting, abdominal pain, constipation, irritability, drowsiness, incoordination, convulsions, coma, weakness, or paralysis. Signs include an increased blood pressure, papilledema or optic atrophy or both, and paralysis of one or more cranial nerves. Treatment is begun with gastric lavage using a 1% sodium sulfate solution followed by administration of a saline cathartic, such as 30 gm of magnesium sulfate. Milk or a demulcent may be given as needed for the colic that follows; severe pain may be treated with morphine sulfate, 15 to 30 mg given subcutaneously for adults; the maximum dose for children is 1 mg per 10 pounds of body weight. Further treatment with BAL and edetate disodium calcium should be done to remove lead from bone tissue but only with hospitalized patients.

Drug intoxication

Symptoms of salicylate or aspirin intoxication are rapid, deep, pauseless breathing secondary to a direct central nervous system effect that decreases the carbon dioxide content of the blood, producing a respiratory alkalosis. Bicarbonate is then excreted by the kidney in a compensatory action. In addition, the patient may vomit and thereby lose chloride and water. Other symptoms include extreme thirst, profuse sweating, fever, and confusion or delirium followed by peripheral circulatory collapse, coma, convulsions, oliguria or anuria, and hemorrhage. Salicylate increases metabolic rate and prothrombin time and blocks utilization of ketones. Therefore what began as a respiratory alkalosis progresses to a metabolic acidosis. Children younger than 3 years of age develop the ketosis so rapidly that the respiratory alkalosis is rarely seen.

Treatment of salicylate poisoning is aimed at correcting the metabolic imbalance as quickly as possible. Thus the first step is to give syrup of ipecac (preferably at the site of ingestion before the patient is moved), 15 to 20 ml, followed by a large amount of water for a patient older than 1 year. This may be repeated in 30 minutes if emesis has not occurred; if this too is ineffective, gastric lavage must be done even 4 to 6 hours after ingestion. The half-life of salicylate in serum is 200 hours at urine pH 5.0, but it is 4 hours at urine pH 7.5. The rate of salicylate excretion in alkaline urine (pH 7.5) is fortyfold that in less alkaline (pH 5.0) urine. Therefore to facilitate excretion of the salicylate, the urine is alkalinized by using either sodium bicarbonate or potassium citrate of acetazolamide (Diamox). At the same time administration of intravenous fluids overcomes the dehydration and increases the urine flow. Because there is the danger of hypernatremia, hypokalemia, and hypocalcemia developing during the course of treatment, care must be exercised in following urine, blood pH and electrolyte levels. Therefore to facilitate urine alkalinization by rapid infusion of sodium bicarbonate, give 2 mEq per kg in concentrated solution (3.5% to 7% of which gives 45 to 90 mEq per 100 ml) while continuing hydration. For mild intoxication hydration may be maintained by intravenous fluids given at 20 to 40 ml per kg of body weight for several hours before slowing the rate. For moderate to severe intoxication dehydration deficits are approximately 50 mEq sodium chloride, 25 mEq sodium bicarbonate, and 20 to 25 mEq potassium acetate per liter of fluid in 5% dextrose solution, given at 1½ to 2 times the maintenance replacement rate. Hemodialysis can be utilized for patients with renal failure or oliguria in lifethreatening situations, but it is difficult with children. Peritoneal dialysis using 5 gm salt-poor serum albumin per 100 ml of dialysis fluid (such as 1½% Peridial) has also been reported. Fever may be lowered with cold or tepid sponges. Vitamin K decreases the bleeding tendency. Glucose decreases ketosis and increases blood sugar, which tends to fall by an unknown mechanism. Oxygen may be needed. When starting the intravenous therapy, blood should be drawn to determine the serum salicylate level, serum pH, and electrolyte levels. Six hours after ingestion, the patient may be discharged if the serum salicylate level is 40 mg per 100 ml or less. If the level is 40 to 50 mg per 100 ml, there is mild to moderate intoxication; 60 to 80 mg per 100 ml indicates moderate to severe intoxication, while more than 80 mg per 100 ml indicates severe salicylate intoxication.

Ammoniated mercury ointment, camphorated oil, methyl salicylate (oil of wintergreen), and boric acid are all dangerous and useless drugs that have no place in the family medicine cabinet. One teaspoon of methyl salicylate contains the equivalent of the salicylate found in twelve 5-grain ASA tablets. Boric acid intoxication is often the result of its indiscriminate use on large areas of broken skin or mucous membranes. Symptoms are erythema and exfoliation of skin (the "boiled lobster"), vomiting, inanition, dehydration, and convulsions. Treatment consists of the removal of as much boric acid as possible, intravenous fluids, barbiturates to decrease convulsions, and peritoneal dialysis of critically ill children.

Overdosage of headache remedies such as acetanilid or acetophenetidin produce methemoglobinemia, whereas the pyrazolon analgesics (for example aminopyrine) occasionally produce an agranulocytosis and aplastic anemia. Symptoms include cyanosis, chocolate-colored blood, severe anemia, and renal damage resulting from precipitation of methemoglobin in kidney tubules. The decrease in hemoglobin causes respiratory difficulties, and vascular collapse ensues, secondary to anoxia and central nervous system depression. One should lavage with magnesium oxide or magnesium hydroxide. One should also give enemas and laxatives, keep the patient warm, administer 5% dextrose in water intravenously, and place the patient in the oxygen tent or use artificial respiration as needed. Although the use of methylene blue, intravenously or orally, has been recommended in the past, it must be used with extreme caution, and only under the direction of those who are qualified and experienced in administering it.

Sniffing of glue, gasoline, and Freon is usually treated with fresh air or oxygen and a 5% carbon dioxide mixture. Alcohol taken with other drugs can produce an intoxication of the mixture and may appear as too much of either the drugs or the alcohol. Digitalis intoxication is usually caused by therapeutic measures but may result from intentional overdosage. Symptoms are anorexia, nausea, vomiting, abdominal pain, drowsiness, dizziness, visual disturbances, mental confusion, emotional disturbances, hallucinations, delirium, tremors, and convulsions. Cardiac signs vary from sinus bradycardia to ventricular tachycardia to ventricular fibrillation, cardiac arrest, and death. Treatment includes lavage and keeping the patient warm and sedated. The cardiac disorder should be monitored and treated with the appropriate medications. Phenytoin is effective in correcting some arrhythmias; its use has been recently questioned, and at this time the matter is unsettled. Intravenous sodium ethylenediamine tetraacetic acid (EDTA), a chelating agent, obviates the toxic symptoms of digitalis by decreasing the serum calcium level.

Iron poisoning is being seen more frequently as more women are taking iron preparations. As little as 1 gm is dangerous, and 2 gm can be fatal to a small child; it diffuses through the gastrointestinal tract so quickly that it overwhelms the iron-binding capacity. Shock ensues within 20 to 48 hours with corrosion of the gastrointestinal tract and hemorrhagic periportal necrosis of the liver. Vomiting, epigastric pain, diarrhea, a weak rapid pulse, pallor, cyanosis, and finally coma and respiratory damage may occur. Milk, magnesium oxide, or bismuth subcarbonate should be given immediately and followed with gastric lavage using a sodium phosphate solution. Plasma, blood, and glucose-saline intravenous solutions may be given for shock and dehydration. Deferoxamine (Desferal), a chelating agent, has been used. British anti-Lewisite (BAL) should not be used because it is harmful in this situation. Lipotropic agents and B-complex vitamins are recommended for prevention of liver damage. Although iron is reported to be nondialyzable, dialysis does seem to help at times.

Poisoning with atropine, belladonna, and stramonium (found in jimsonweed, stinkweed, or thorn apple) all have symptoms and signs of burning and dryness of the mouth, flushing, fever, intense thirst, visual disturbances, widely dilated pupils that do not react to light, weakness, giddiness, staggering gait, mental confusion, excitement, and delirium. Treatment consists of withdrawal of the causative agent and, in severe cases, lavage with 4% tannic acid solution with a residual of activated charcoal to adsorb the atropine remaining in the stomach after the lavage. In addition to other symptomatic treatment, pilocarpine, 10 to 15 mg, or methacholine, 10 to 30 mg, may be given to relieve the oral and visual symptoms.

Patients with morphine intoxication have a decreased rate and depth of respiration. The pale, cold skin becomes cyanotic, and circulatory failure follows. Depression of the central nervous system usually occurs, although meperidine (Demerol), codeine, and thebaine cause excitement and convulsions. Pupils are initially constricted. Strong black coffee may be given if the patient is conscious. The treatment of choice for a narcotic overdosage is naloxone (Narcan), the only drug available for the specific therapy of pentazocine (Talwin) intoxication. Naloxone is a narcotic antagonist devoid of any intrinsic respiratory or cardiovascular depressive action. Naloxone can cause tremor and hyperventilation associated with the abrupt return to consciousness in these patients. Dosage is 0.4 mg bolus given intravenously followed by 0.8 mg 3 minutes later. If Naloxone is unavailable, nalorphine (Nalline) or levallorphan (Lorfan) may be used. Supportive and symptomatic treatment is also required.

Successful drug suicides are most often accomplished with barbiturates (80%). The symptom complex of barbiturate intoxication includes excitement and hallucination leading to mental depression, stupor, coma, decreased respiration and blood pressure, decreased renal excretion, and shock. These signs and symptoms are treated by supporting the respiration and circulation in the Trendelenburg position by the use of artificial respiration containing 95% oxygen and 5% carbon dioxide if needed, pressor amines, blood transfusion, and hydration with 5% to 10% glucose solutions for shock. When the vital signs are stable and renal function is adequate, osmotic diuresis with intravenous urea, large amounts of fluids, and alkalinization of the urine may be undertaken. If the serum phenobarbital level is 20% or if the intermediate barbiturate serum level is 7%, dialysis should be performed.

When taken in too great an amount, ataractic or tranquilizing drugs are safer than the barbiturates but they must be recognized and treated in a specific manner. The symptoms are a deep sleep or coma or extrapyramidal signs, such as motor restlessness, parkinsonian syndrome, or some types of dyskinesias. The phenothiazine derivatives produce an initial sedation, then restlessness followed by tonic-clonic convulsions, deep respiratory depression, and a precipitous drop in blood pressure. These patients should be lavaged immediately and intravenous fluids should be given. Methylphenidate (Ritalin) (not amphetamines) and norepinephrine (not other pressor amines because they further decrease the blood pressure) may be used. **Epinephrine should not be used.** Glutethimide (Doriden) intoxication causes ataxia, nystagmus, mydriasis, drowsiness, and coma. The respiratory rate is normal, but the ventilation is poor, the pulse is increased, and the blood pressure is decreased. Treatment includes thorough gastric lavage, leaving 30 to 60 ml of castor oil in the stomach, and supporting the respiration. One should use caution in the administration of fluids to these patients because they can easily be overhydrated. If the blood level of glutethimide is 1.0 to 2.5 mg per 100 ml, the patient should be treated with adequate ventilation, pressors, and central nervous system stimulation. If there is no response to this treatment or if the blood level is more than 3 mg per 100 ml, the patient should be dialyzed. The dialysis equipment should be kept in place until the blood level fails to rise in a period of several hours during which no dialysis has taken place.

Household agents

With respect to the categories of household products and insecticides, the best sources of aid include current textbook of toxicology, the annual review of poisons and their dialyzability in the *Transactions of the American Society for Artificial Internal Organs*, and the resources of the nearest poison control center.

In treating patients with intoxication from one of the chlorinated hydrocarbon insecticides (benzene hexachloride [Lindane], chlordane, chlorophenothane [DDT], difluoro-diphenyl-trichloro-ethane [DFDT], dieldrin, heptochlor, methoxychlor, and Toxaphene among others), from phosphorus in rat or roach poisons or fireworks, and from moth repellents, oily or fatty substances such as milk, cream, oil purgatives, or demulcents should not be given because they increase absorption of these substances.

CARBON MONOXIDE POISONING

HUGH E. STEPHENSON, Jr.

Carbon monoxide, an odorless and colorless gas, is responsible for death in a variety of circumstances. In some large city hospital emergency rooms it is second to alcohol as the most common cause of poisoning death.

Newspapers carry accounts of carbon monoxide poisoning almost daily. Carbon monoxide may result from any fire in a closed space. Faulty exhaust pipes and worn-out mufflers or manifolds often lead to carbon monoxide leakage into the closed automobile. An idling automobile engine doubles its rate of carbon monoxide exhaust. Children have been fatally poisoned in closed cars while waiting for parents in grocery stores or on other errands. The heater takes in exhaust fumes from the car in front, and the carbon monoxide level within the car increases rapidly. During the spring and summer birds build nests that often plug flues, which in turn may produce carbon monoxide poisoning to the members of the household in the fall. A flue plugged with soot may do the same thing.

It is dangerous to move a barbecue grill into a closed garage in case of inclement weather. The use of the grill may provide an excellent opportunity for the accumulation of carbon monoxide within the closed, unvented garage. Guards in tunnels and workers in kilns are subjected to high levels of carbon monoxide inhalation. Drivers on crowded roadways often creep along bumper to bumper for a considerable distance. The carbon monoxide that is drawn into the car from the car in front may be sufficient to produce a dangerous level of carbon monoxide poisoning in the driver. This may be responsible for faulty judgment on the part of the driver. Unfortunately carbon monoxide gas has no odor, but its presence should be suspected whenever an unconscious patient is found in a garage or inside a closed building.

The *subjective complaints* experienced by the patient include headache, vertigo, irritability, frequent yawning, ringing in the ears, a feeling of tightness at the forehead, weakness, dimmed vision, aching limbs, a throbbing heart, a feeling of lethargy, vomiting, collapse, and unconsciousness.

The patient may not have the pathognomonic cherry red color at the onset but may be somewhat dusky in color. Muscular twitching, a rapid pulse, hyperreflexia, warm skin, dilated pupils, and Cheyne-Stokes respirations may be evident. Coma and unconsciousness may be evident when the patient is first seen.

The hypoxia and poisoning of tissues by carbon monoxide results from the special affinity of hemoglobin for carbon monoxide. This affinity is 200 to 300 times greater than that which hemoglobin shows for oxygen. Carbon monoxide and hemoglobin combine to form carboxyhemoglobin. Respiratory enzymes have a greater affinity for carbon monoxide than oxygen. There is evidence that carbon monoxide acts directly on cerebral tissue and causes brain damage, particularly in the area of the globus pallidus.

Obviously the treatment of carbon monoxide poisoning is of an urgent nature. Although permanent brain damage may have occurred before treatment is begun, one cannot, of course, be immediately aware of this fact. First, one should remove the victim from the environment contaminated with carbon monoxide. Artificial ventilation must be started at once; mouth-to-mouth respiration is a satisfactory approach. It is important that patients with carbon monoxide poisoning are given oxygen under high pressure, even more so than patients who have nearly drowned or who have been exposed to electric shock. Pure oxygen under 2.5 atmospheres of pressure reduces blood carboxyhemoglobin by 50% in approximately 40 minutes. With room air the same reduction would take 250 minutes. The high oxygen pressure chambers are ideal for carbon monoxide poisoning, but unfortunately they are not readily available to most patients in this country.

Morphine sulfate is not indicated with carbon monoxide poisoning. Respiratory stimulants are of little value. Whole blood transfusions have been advocated by some but are of questionable value. Methylene blue is no longer used. If considerable cerebral anoxia is suspected, it may prove helpful to put the patient in a hypothermic state as soon as the hospital is reached.

The question of giving carbon dioxide is often debated. The British Medical Council has voiced an affirmative vote in favor of the 5% mixture of carbon dioxide. Those who advocate a carbon dioxide mixture believe that a high level of carbon dioxide increases the ventilation, helps carboxyhemoglobin dissociation, and may serve to raise the oxygen pressure. On the other hand, the respiratory center may have already experienced excessive carbon dioxide exposure, and by giving carbon dioxide one decreases the amount of oxygen that can be delivered. In summary the question of the use of carbon dioxide in carbon monoxide poisoning has not been clearly resolved.

QUESTIONS

1. What information should you obtain when you receive a telephone call that someone has been poisoned or has taken an overdose?
2. Differentiate syrup of ipecac from tincture of ipecac and state the reasons why this distinction is important.
3. Classify a sleeping patient brought to you in an emergency room with a history of possible poison ingestion. Can he be aroused to answer questions? Classify in terms of the reflexes, withdrawal from painful stimuli, and other signs of respiratory or circulatory depression.
4. What are the contraindications to induction of emesis?
5. How does activated charcoal work as an antidote or in a lavage solution?
6. Why is tap water dangerous to use as a lavage solution?
7. What is the antidote for muscarine poisoning?
8. Why is alkalinization of the urine helpful in treating salicylate poisoning?
9. Why is iron poisoning dangerous, especially to children?
10. What is the treatment of choice for narcotic overdosage?
11. What are the basics of symptomatic and supportive treatment in the patient with poisoning or overdose?

SUGGESTED READINGS

Arena, J.: Poisoning: toxicology, symptoms, treatment, ed. 3, Springfield, Ill., 1974, Charles C Thomas, Publisher.

Arena, J.: Clin. Symp. **18:**1, 1966.

Beisel, W. R.: Recognizing and treating common food poisoning, Drug Therapy 4:72-75, 1974.

Coleman, A. B.: Current concepts, accidental poisoning, N. Engl. J. Med. **277:**21, 1967.

Dreisbach, R. H.: Handbook of poisoning: diagnosis and treatment, ed. 7, Los Altos, Calif., 1971, Lange Medical Publications.

Knepshield, J. H., Schreiner, G. E., Lowenthal, D. T., and Gelfand, M. C.: Dialysis of poisons and drugs: annual review, Trans. Am. Soc. Artif. Intern. Organs 13:590-633, 1973.

Roe, R. L., and Becker, C. E.: Poisoning and its treatment, Primary Care: clinic in office practice 1:69-86, 1974.

Teitelbaum, D. T.: Initial management of poisoning, Emerg. Med., 1970.

CHAPTER 22

The alcoholic patient

ALBERT B. LOWENFELS

Alcoholism, our most prevalent chronic illness, has been estimated to afflict almost 10% of all hospitalized patients. Although moderate social drinking is pleasurable and safe, anyone consuming more than a pint of whiskey or its equivalent per day is likely to develop serious medical or surgical complications under the following circumstances:

1. If heavy drinking has damaged a vulnerable organ, such as the liver or the pancreas.
2. If there is a coexisting acute illness or an accident. A good example is the intoxicated patient who sustains a head injury.
3. If regular consumption of alcohol is so great that nondrinking causes withdrawal symptoms.

Alcoholism is so prevalent that every physician will have frequent contact with both acutely and chronically alcoholic patients.

INITIAL EVALUATION

Because his habits are irregular and unpredictable, the acutely ill alcoholic patient usually seeks medical care in an emergency room—often at an inconvenient time. How difficult it is to maintain a professional attitude when the phone rings at 3 AM: "Doctor, please come down to see Mr. _____ in the emergency room. He is complaining of pain in his hip." . . . "Yes, he's drunk again."

The first goal should be to diagnose and treat the immediate medical problem. A second, equally important objective is to help the patient deal with his problem of alcoholism. If he is approached honestly, and if the patient is urged to make use of available community resources, such as Alcoholics Anonymous, alcoholism can be treated effectively.

The history

Every patient must be questioned about alcohol consumption. No one is protected against alcoholism by wealth, social status, or education, therefore as a rule all patients should be asked about their drinking habits. Questions should be as specific as possible. Does the patient drink a daily cocktail or two? What is the maximum amount that he might drink on a weekend? Is there a history suggestive of blackout spells or withdrawal syndrome? Clear, unambiguous questions are important: "How much do you drink during a day?" "Oh, three or four cans of beer." Eventually the patient admitted that at *night* he drank an additional seven or eight shots of whiskey!

Family, friends, police officers, and ambulance attendants can give valuable information about the unconscious or the uncooperative patient. Question these informants carefully before allowing them to leave the emergency area.

The physical examination

An alcoholic odor to the breath; erratic, unpredictable, belligerent behavior; altered sensorium; flushed skin; and tachycardia suggest acute alcoholism. Positive physical findings may be absent; thus the best confirmatory test is the blood alcohol determination.

In the absence of liver impairment it is difficult to detect chronic alcoholism. Many chronically alcoholic patients are malnourished and have prominent jowls and a red nose. Any overt evidence of liver failure such as jaundice, vascular "spiders," hepatomegaly, splenomegaly, ascites, caput medusae, gynecomastia, sparse pubic hair, or liver palms should intensify the search for underlying alcoholism.

Laboratory procedures and x-ray films

Helpful laboratory procedures for evaluating the alcoholic patient include the following:

1. Blood alcohol determination. The availability of this test varies from hospital to hospital, and in its absence the osmolality of the plasma may be helpful. Unless the patient has hyperglycemia, an elevated plasma osmolality is most likely due to alcohol.
2. Routine blood count and urinalysis.
3. Blood sugar determination. Acute alcoholism and hypoglycemia often coexist.
4. A serum amylase determination is essential whenever the patient has abdominal pain.

Helpful radiologic procedures include a chest film and skull films for the comatose alcoholic patient or the patient who has a head injury. If possible, skull films should be postponed until the patient is sober enough to hold his head still during the examination.

INDICATIONS FOR HOSPITALIZATION

Hospitalization of the alcoholic patient should be considered when:

1. The patient has any medical or surgical illness for which hospitalization is indicated.
2. There is evidence of an alcohol-related disease requiring treatment, such as pancreatitis or alcoholic hepatitis.
3. The patient is unconscious or there is a history of recent loss of consciousness following an injury.
4. There is evidence of an acute withdrawal syndrome, such as a convulsion or extreme agitation.
5. The patient is febrile without obvious cause.

6. There are impelling social reasons.

Patients who exhibit severe depression, anxiety, or uncontrollable behavior without evidence of organic disease should be evaluated by a psychiatrist.

ALCOHOL AND TRAUMA

Alcoholism is closely linked to all forms of injury, as can be clearly demonstrated by spending a few hours in any emergency room. A linear increase in the blood alcohol level results in a geometrical increase in the chances of causing an accident. The association between alcohol and automobile accidents is particularly strong; it has been estimated that approximately one-half of all automobile accident fatalities are related to alcoholism.

Fracture problems

The alcoholic patient is a poor historian, and therefore even if he denies a recent fall or injury, it is wise to consider that his painful, swollen, or deformed extremity might be broken.

In addition to diagnostic problems, treatment of fractures in an alcoholic patient can be vexing. For example, it is nearly impossible to use traction on the acutely inebriated person. A wise plan is to splint the patient's injury until the symptoms of acute intoxication or withdrawal have diminished; then definitive treatment should be started.

The withdrawal syndrome can be confused with the symptoms of a fat embolus because both cause fever and agitation. Fat droplets in the urine, a petechial skin rash, and a low arterial Po_2 favor the diagnosis of fat embolism.

Head injury

Approximately one third of all patients hospitalized following head injury are alcoholics; their management demands great skill to avoid confusing the signs and symptoms of acute alcoholism with a serious intracranial injury. Subdural hematomas are especially treacherous lesions because they develop slowly and insidiously. One should consider hospitalizing the alcoholic patient with a head injury when the patient:

1. Is or was unconscious or there is a history of probable or possible loss of consciousness.
2. Has a definite or suspected skull fracture.
3. Has a minor head injury or scalp laceration, and extracranial injuries.
4. Is confused or amnesic.
5. Has a minor head injury, but there are extenuating social circumstances. For example, if the patient lives alone or far from the hospital, or if his ability to care for himself is in doubt.

If the decision is made *not* to hospitalize, arrangements for adequate follow-up care must be made. Also, the patient or a member of the family should be given printed instructions that include a list of precautions.

ALCOHOLISM AND ABDOMINAL PAIN

Abdominal pain, another common and serious emergency problem in the alcoholic patient, can baffle the most experienced observer. Table 22-1 lists the various causes of abdominal pain that were found in a group of heavy drinkers admitted to a surgical service. Eighteen patients eventually died, and surprisingly the most common cause of death was intestinal obstruction from previous abdominal surgery.

Inability to obtain an accurate history from the acutely ill alcoholic patient greatly increases the diagnostic difficulties. For example, in a group of six alcoholic patients with rupture of the spleen, only one remembered any injury.

Delay in obtaining help significantly increases morbidity and mortality. When stricken by abdominal pain, the alcoholic patient commonly seeks temporary relief by having a few more drinks. Many hours later he arrives in the emergency room smelling of drink, belligerent, uncooperative, and unable to give a coherent history. Then further delay often ensues because the examining physician fails to recognize the serious nature of the underlying disorder.

Of the various abdominal disorders commonly found in alcoholic patients, pancreatitis is undoubtedly the most puzzling. To the intense embarrassment of the unwary doctor, it can simulate cholecystitis, appendicitis, myocardial infarction, perforated ulcer, or even a ruptured aortic aneurysm.

Elevated serum amylase does identify most patients with pancreatitis, but it also can be elevated in other abdominal disorders. The urinary and the peritoneal amylase levels are useful as well as the recently described amylase clearance test. Occasionally it is impossible to differentiate pancreatitis from other disorders and in these cases it is clearly preferable to settle the issue in the operating room rather than in the morgue. Laparotomy does not seem to increase the mortality rate in acute pancreatitis.

It is clearly unsafe to assume that abdominal pain in the alcoholic patient must be related to alcoholism. A patient was recently encountered who had severe abdominal pain, smelled strongly of liquor, and had a mildly elevated serum amylase. Yet the true cause of his pain was a ruptured aortic aneurysm! Regrettably alcoholism does not confer immunity against any of the causes of abdominal pain.

Abdominal paracentesis

Abdominal paracentesis is often used as a diagnostic aid in the alcoholic patient. It is helpful when:
1. An internal injury is suspected, but the findings are puzzling or the patient cannot give a clear history.

Table 22-1. Causes for abdominal pain in alcoholic patients

Illness	Number of patients
Lesions of pancreas	33
Gastroduodenal, esophageal lesions	24
Small bowel obstruction (adhesions)	10
Abdominal trauma	9
Liver, biliary tract disorders	8
Colorectal lesions	8
Miscellaneous	8
TOTAL	100

2. The patient is unconscious and there are vague signs suggesting abdominal injury. An abdominal tap is especially valuable for studying the hypotensive, head-injured patient. Inasmuch as head injury rarely produces shock, one must search for an extracranial injury, such as a ruptured spleen.
3. Finding an elevated peritoneal amylase can be informative if pancreatitis is suspected in equivocal cases.

A single, subumbilical tap performed with a plastic catheter is preferred; however, the procedure is dangerous when the intestines are distended. Other precautions include emptying the bladder and avoiding any scars or masses. Because air may enter the peritoneal cavity during the tap, it is wise to obtain flat and upright abdominal films before doing the procedure.

PREOPERATIVE PREPARATION

Both the chronic inebriate and the acutely intoxicated patient require special care if surgery is to be carried out safely. The following points have been helpful:
1. One should avoid operating on the acutely intoxicated patient unless a true emergency exists. When the patient is being prepared for an emergency operation, the stomach should be emptied with a large tube. Aspiration of gastric contents is the major anesthetic risk confronting the acutely intoxicated patient.
2. Because cessation of heavy drinking often leads to withdrawal syndromes, it is advantageous to defer elective surgery in heavy drinkers to allow for a 48-hour period of detoxification.
3. If either the history or the physical examination suggests alcoholism, the preoperative workup must include tests to ascertain nutritional status and liver function. If time permits, a needle biopsy of the liver should be done.
4. If there is evidence of liver damage, a careful evaluation of the coagulation mechanism should be included. The patient should be questioned about previous bleeding episodes. Examination should be done to ascertain an enlarged liver or spleen, or both. A complete blood count and platelet count should be done and both a partial thromboplastin time and a prothrombin time should be included.

WITHDRAWAL SYNDROME

Withdrawal symptoms are common when a heavy drinker enters the hospital and discontinues his usual daily intake of alcohol. Although the exact cause is unknown, alcohol is a cerebral depressant; therefore it is hardly surprising that abrupt sobriety leads to cerebral irritability. Withdrawal symptoms are especially frequent in patients who have been drinking steadily for at least 2 weeks or longer in excess of a pint of whiskey per day. Tremor, hallucination, seizures, extreme agitation, sweating, tachycardia, hyperactivity, fever, and dilated pupils may accompany withdrawal from alcohol. The most severe form of alcohol withdrawal has been termed delirium tremens. Approximately 10% to 15% of heavy drinkers develop serious withdrawal symptoms when they stop drinking.

Although various regimes have been used for managing the withdrawal syndrome, it is a self-limited process from which patients with mild cases recover promptly without use of drugs. The administration of alcohol either for prophylaxis or treatment of the withdrawal syndrome is not advised; safer and more effective agents are available. Furthermore giving alcohol lends tacit support to the patient's addiction.

Rest, hydration, correction of underlying medical or surgical problems, and supportive care by a sympathetic professional team are effective methods for managing the withdrawal syndrome. If drugs are necessary, "how much" is just as important as "which one." Just enough medication should be given to make the patient manageable without producing severe depression. Small, repeated doses are preferable to a single large dose. Chlordiazepoxide, a widely used agent in managing the withdrawal syndrome, can be injected parenterally to help calm the disturbed patient. Thereafter further medication can be given orally. Propranolol is undergoing evaluation and may prove effective in managing milder withdrawal states. Phenytoin, phenobarbital, or diazepam may be used to control the convulsions accompanying alcohol withdrawal, which are usually self-limited and do not require long-term anticonvulsant therapy.

QUESTIONS

1. Careful questions about alcohol usage should be part of the history because:
   a. If the patient is an alcoholic, he is ineligible for insurance benefits.
   b. Alcoholism is extremely prevalent and has serious medical and surgical consequences.
   c. If the patient is a heavy drinker, he should be allowed to take a shot or two of whiskey every day in the hospital.
2. In a 24-hour period the hospital emergency room sees 200 patients. How many are likely to be alcoholics?
3. A 48-year-old man is brought to the emergency room immediately after a fall from a train. He is semiconscious. Initial evaluation shows that his breath has a strong odor of liquor. There is a small laceration over the occiput. The pulse rate is 120, and blood pressure is 80/60. Both pupils are equal and react sluggishly to light. The abdomen seems somewhat tense.
   a. What additional tests or procedures might be helpful?
   b. List the order in which they should be performed.
   c. What do you think is the cause for the hypotension?
4. Most alcoholics are easily identifiable because they are unemployed, ill-kept, "skid-row" individuals. True or false?
5. Which of these patients should be hospitalized if they come to your emergency room?
   a. A 55-year-old man, moderately intoxicated, whose car was involved in an auto accident comes in after a brief period of unconsciousness. He feels all right now, and is anxious to go home. The reflexes are equal, and skull x-ray films are negative.
   b. A 72-year-old man has been on a week's binge. He now has pain in the epigastrium, vomiting, and fever of 39° C.
   c. An acutely intoxicated, belligerent man comes in with a painful hypertrophic scar over his abdomen.
6. A convulsion in a recently hospitalized patient might mean that:
   a. The patient has had an unrecognized head injury and is developing increased intracranial pressure.
   b. The patient is an alcoholic, and the convulsion heralds the onset of withdrawal symptoms.
   c. The patient is an epileptic, and you have forgotten to order anticonvulsant medication.
7. A 49-year-old woman, a known heavy drinker, develops periumbilical pain, bilious vomiting, and distention. She has had an appendectomy. She cannot tell whether the pain is steady or crampy, and on examination the abdomen is somewhat tender all over with no masses. Serum amylase level is 300 Somogyi units.
   a. What are the diagnostic possibilities?
   b. How would you confirm your suspicions?
   c. You decide to observe the patient, but the next day her condition has obviously deteriorated. The pain is more severe and the abdomen more distended. How should you proceed?

8. Any of the following might be found in a patient with delirium tremens *except:*
   a. Convulsions
   b. Agitation
   c. Tremulousness
   d. Sweating
   e. Hallucinations
   f. Elevated blood alcohol level

ANSWERS

1. b.
2. Approximately 20.
3. a, b, c. The patient probably has an extracranial source of bleeding, because head injury rarely causes shock. Search should be made for occult bleeding, as from a ruptured spleen.
4. False.
5. a, b.
6. All three answers are correct.
7. Initial diagnosis might be pancreatitis and/or intestinal obstruction. Because the condition fails to improve and the abdomen becomes more distended, exploration would be indicated.
8. f.

SUGGESTED READINGS

Bourne, P. G., and Fox, R., editors: Alcoholism—progress in research and treatment, New York, 1973, Academic Press, Inc.

Lowenfels, A. B.: The alcoholic patient in surgery, Baltimore, 1971, The Williams & Wilkins Co.

Lowenfels, A. B., Rohman, M., and Shibutani, K.: Surgical consequences of alcoholism, Surg. Gynecol. Obstet. **131:**129-138, 1970.

Ranson, J. H., Rifkind, K. M., Roses, D. F., Fink, S. D., Eng, K., and Spencer, F. C.: Prognostic signs and the role of operative management in acute pancreatitis, Surg. Gynecol. Obstet. **139:**69-81, 1974.

Robinson, A. G., and Loeb, J. N.: Ethanol ingestion—commonest cause of elevated plasma osmolality? N. Engl. J. Med. **284:**1253-1255, 1971.

Seixas, F. A., Williams, K., and Eggleston, S., editors: Medical consequences of alcoholism, Ann. N.Y. Acad. Sci. **252:**1-399, 1975.

Warshaw, A. L., and Lesser, P. B.: Amylase clearance in differentiating acute pancreatitis from peptic ulcer with hyperamylasemia, Ann. Surg. **181:**314-316, 1975.

PART SEVEN

Emergencies resulting from physical trauma

CHAPTER 23

Hand injuries

JOHN P. ADAMS

A great deal of time and effort in reconstructive hand surgery is devoted to the care of hands with disabilities that could have been prevented or substantially reduced if initial care had been adequate. The data on disabilities of parts of the body indicate that a great many disabilities involve the hand. Actually the total of combined injuries to the upper extremity indicates that it is the most frequently injured part of the body.

DIAGNOSIS

Care of the hand within the first few hours after injury often determines the degree of the patient's future physical impairment. The injured hand should be considered a surgical emergency and should receive prompt treatment, particularly if the wound is open. Treatment of any injury, but particularly one that involves an organ system as complex as the hand, wrist, and upper extremity, requires an accurate diagnosis at the onset. Such diagnosis can be made by an examination that embraces the basic components of this organ system:

1. The integumentary system
2. The intactness of the nerve supply
3. The motor function, as reflected in joint motion
4. The skeletal system
5. The ligamentous system

The initial examination should include inspection to ascertain the general nature of the wound, the degree of gross contamination, and whether the wound was produced by an avulsing or crushing type of injury. The wound should be covered with a well-applied, clean (perferably sterile) compression dressing. If hemorrhage is a problem, it can normally be controlled by a sterile compression dressing and elevation. Other than superficial inspection of the wound, no examination should be carried out through the wound itself. After the dressing has been applied, a detailed examination can be conducted, always distal to the site of injury. Sensation should be carefully assessed in the autonomous zone of the ulnar nerve in the pulp space the little finger, of the median nerve in the pulp space of the index finger, and of the radial nerve in the small area in the dorsal skin overlying the web space between the thumb and index metacarpals. Motion is determined by having the patient move individual joints. Despite severe injury, if the digit is properly supported the patient should be able to perform specific function; this can be ascertained and recorded. Possible fractures or joint subluxations or dislocations can be confirmed by adequate roentgenologic examination that should include x-ray films taken on at least three planes: anterior-posterior, lateral, and oblique. For specific suspected injuries, a single digit may be outlined in more detail. The vascular status can be assessed by the blanching characteristics of the nailbed and the general color and temperature of the extremity.

IMPORTANCE OF FULL HISTORY

Initial care obviously should include a careful history of the accident. It is important to know whether a wound was caused by a sharp object, such as a knife, in which crushing of tissues is not apt to occur, or whether a laceration was caused by a fall on a broken bottle or some blunt object. It is also important to determine whether heat was applied to the wound through friction or any other external cause.

Information should be obtained as to wound contamination by possible noxious agents (such as tear gas) or chemicals (such as turpentine, paint, or grease). The position of the hand at the time of injury should be ascertained, if possible, to accurately determine the levels of tendon laceration, such as in the palm and finger. For example, if the laceration occurs with the fingers in full extension, then the skin and tendon lacerations correspond to the same level; however, if the hand is in flexion, such as in grasping a knife, then the tendon laceration is always distal to the skin laceration when the fingers are placed in their anatomic position. Injuries caused by human or animal bites are in a special category to be considered later.

IMMEDIATE CARE

Wounds that involve open fractures, tendon lacerations, nerve lacerations more severe than digital nerve laceration, or wounds in which avulsion of the skin is part of the primary injury, require hospitalization and definitive care in the operating theater. As a general rule no definitive surgery to any deeper structures should be carried out in the emergency facilities unless there are unusual circumstances. The minor lacerations may be sutured in the emergency room; however, major wounds require hospital admission for adequate care. In many instances definitive care must be deferred for several hours for reasons ranging from a full stomach, other injuries, and inability to secure skilled surgical personnel to unavailability of operating room space. In such instances open wounds should be thoroughly irrigated with copious amounts of saline, or if saline is not available, tap water should be used for initial debridement of the wound, and then a sterile dressing must be reapplied. Once the wound has been covered with a sterile dressing, the emergency nature of the injury has been altered to a semielective nature. Definitive surgery, if indicated, may be carried out several hours later without increasing the complication rate.

There is a tendency in initial care of hands to do too much too early. When in doubt, one is better off doing too little: Incised wounds that are not severely contaminated should be cleaned. Suturing can usually be done immediately after irrigation and cleansing. The soft tissue is best supported in a firm compression dressing or in a splint with the wrist and hand placed in the position of function—

that is, with the wrist placed in neutral position, the fingers flexed at least 45° at each joint, and the thumb held in abduction and opposition. (The patient should be instructed in elevation of the part to reduce edema.)

Patients who have initial wound suturing in the emergency room must be seen promptly by the physician who will give aftercare. Even with minor injuries fingers tend to stiffen, and permanent disability may ensue. When major injuries are present and initial care is not available in the vicinity, the best treatment is to thoroughly irrigate the wound. If the wound is of a suitable type, it should be sutured (if infection is imminent, the wound should be left open), covered with a compression dressing, and placed in a supportive position with the wrist and hand as near to the functional position as possible. The patient should be transferred to a facility that provides definitive care. Certain types of wounds contaminated by foreign material such as tear gas, paint, grease, turpentine, or paint solvents require thorough cleansing as early as possible in whatever facility is available. In these circumstances the wound should remain open and no further definitive care should be given at that time.

BURNS

Hand burns can usually be classified in one of three categories: thermal, chemical, or electrical. Of the three, the electrical burn has the poorest prognosis. Initial care in the emergency room of any burn to the hand is normally a sterile dressing supported with a splint, and hospital admission is required if the burn is obviously greater than first degree. Definitive care of deep second- or third-degree burns should not be given in the emergency room setting. Initial inspection of most thermal burns easily distinguishes between first degree (redness), second degree (blistering), and third degree (full-thickness skin loss with possible loss of deeper structures). One exception is the burn produced by hot liquid, in which case skin injury may be minimal while injury to deeper structures may be severe. Electrical burns also tend to show more deep tissue injury than is apparent from superficial inspection.

BITES

Human and animal bites are a common type of acute hand injury that must be considered separately. Human bites are rarely, if ever, made by a rabid individual; therefore the primary concern is assessment of skin and deeper tissue damage. Wounds in the area of a joint must be suspected of having penetrated the joint. The local treatment is debridement and thorough irrigation. Local cauterizing agents should not be used. Lavage with antibacterial agents, such as 1% neomycin solution, may be indicated if the patient is seen within 1 hour after injury. After cleansing, the wound should always be left open and should be closed secondarily. Systemic antibiotics may be indicated.

An injury similar to a human bite is the penetration of the hand or finger by materials used in orthodontia. The wires and other appliances may penetrate deeply and may produce a closed-space infection.

Pets are the most common source of animal bites, and the general management is the same as management of human bites. Because the possibility of rabies is high in cases of bites by animals such as bats, the use of rabies antisera may be essential.

Snake bites should be excised. A venous tourniquet may be applied if the patient is seen immediately after the bite. Appropriate antivenom may be given in select cases but not routinely.

PSYCHOLOGIC EFFECTS

The psychologic effect of hand injuries is great. This is not surprising when one realizes that much of the information placed in our brains gets there because of activities of the hand. Therefore any hand injury is a threat to the livelihood of either the working person or the professional. The psychologic reaction is much greater than that of injury to any other part of the body with the possible exception of the genitalia. It is of utmost importance that the first examining physician be judicious in any statement he may make to a patient as to either prognosis or the exact nature of the injury. In most cases the emergency room physician should explain only in general terms what has happened. The specific prognosis should be given by the surgeon who will provide definitive care. Because first impressions are often the most lasting ones, an inaccurate statement made by a physician at the time of initial treatment may jeopardize the entire future treatment and rehabilitation program.

USE OF ANTIBIOTICS IN HAND INJURIES

The routine use of antimicrobial agents as a prophylaxis against infection is not recommended in hand injuries. Certain open injuries that should receive antibiotics include human and animal bites, contaminated crushing injuries, and joint injuries. All wounds should have cultures taken as part of the initial treatment, and an appropriate antibiotic may be prescribed. The antibiotic need not be continued beyond 96 hours unless infection has ensued or other indications arise.

Antimicrobial agents are complementary to adequate surgical care and are not a substitute for it.

SUMMARY

The following are the steps in providing initial care of the hand:
1. The hand injury should be recognized as a bona fide emergency and not relegated to care at the convenience of emergency room personnel.
2. An accurate history of the mechanism of injury, possible contaminants, and the condition of the hand at the time of injury should be ascertained.
3. After superficial inspection, the wound should be covered with a clean (preferably sterile) dressing.
4. The examination for definitive injury should be carried out distal to the wound.
5. Adequate x-ray examination, rather than physical examination, should be utilized to ascertain bone and joint injury.
6. After an accurate estimate of disability has been made, definitive care of an injury to deeper structures should not be done in the emergency room but *only* after the patient's admission to the hospital.
7. In general, tendon lacerations of the palm and fingers are best treated by delayed repair. Repair of tendons in these areas must be primarily done

under ideal circumstances by highly trained individuals who are available to evaluate and treat the patient.

8. In wounds that will no doubt heal by primary intent, and in wounds that involve lacerations of flexor tendons at the wrist level or above, primary repair may be carried out; this same principle also applies to extensor tendon injury.

9. Injuries of mixed nerves (motor and sensory) should be treated by initial wound closure and delayed nerve repair within 4 to 6 weeks.

10. When the patient is recovering from soft tissue repair and awaiting further repair of deeper structures, he must be followed closely, and joint mobility must be maintained. He should be placed in the hands of the surgeon who will give the follow-up care soon after the injury.

11. The prognosis in severe hand injuries is often guarded as to restoration of normal or nearly normal function, even with treatment by the most skilled surgeons; therefore the initial physician must be extremely careful in offering any opinion to the patient on the final outcome.

12. No emergency room physician can be criticized for his initial care of a hand wound providing that his diagnosis is accurate, his findings are recorded, and his attention is directed toward the wound itself.

13. Bites, human and animal, are a special type of injury. These wounds must be thoroughly cleansed and must not be closed.

14. Because of potential contamination, all hand wounds must be considered as a possible source of tetanus and gas gangrene. In animal bites rabies is an additional cause for concern. The use of antirabies serum depends on the state of health of the wounding animal. Antitetanus measures must be instituted in all injuries. Prophylactic use of gas gangrene antitoxin has not proved to be effective.

QUESTIONS

1. Explain the importance of obtaining a clear, accurate history of the position of the hand at the time of an injury.

2. What two important differences between the bite of the human and that of other animals must be considered in treating the lacerated hand?

3. Quantitate the psychologic reaction to a hand injury and discuss the rationale involved.

4. "With regard particularly to hand injuries—if not in general—there may be a tendency to say too much and do too much during immediate care." Defend or argue with this statement.

5. Define "delayed repair" and comment on its desirability as routine practice.

6. Name three criteria of excellence used to characterize emergency room care of the hand injury.

7. Which particular types of hand injury preclude closure as a part of immediate care? Why?

8. Discuss the use of gas gangrene antitoxin in emergency care of the hand injury.

9. Explain the statement that a detailed examination is carried out distal to the site of the hand injury.

10. In assessment of sensation in the injured hand, describe the particular anatomic areas of investigation.

SUGGESTED READINGS

Glass, T. G.: Early debridement in pit viper bites, J.A.M.A. **235:**2513-2516, 1976.

Weeks, P. M., and Wray, R. C.: Management of acute hand injuries, St. Louis, 1973, The C. V. Mosby Co.

CHAPTER 24

Fractures and dislocations

MARSHALL B. CONRAD

The application of an emergency splint should not be a complicated or difficult maneuver. Any ambulance that purports to provide emergency service should be equipped so that emergency splints can be applied with facility. However, other materials that are usually readily available can be adequately utilized. These include triangular bandages or folded towels or sheets to be used for slings and swaths, cardboard or magazines to make excellent short splints, a pillow or blanket to be wrapped around an injured extremity, or material to be used as padding when securing an injured lower extremity to the uninjured leg.

It is important to remember that fractures of the spine and pelvis are difficult to detect; the only indication may be the complaint of pain in the affected area. If the victim is unconscious or cannot communicate, the possibility of such an injury must be kept in mind, and the victim must be handled accordingly.

FRACTURES OF THE SHOULDER

Fractures about the shoulder involving the scapula, clavicle, or upper humerus should be suspected if the victim complains of pain or tenderness or both in the area of the shoulder. The involved extremity may be protected by the victim, and the shoulder on the involved side may sag. These injuries can be adequately splinted by means of a sling and swath using two triangular bandages. One is applied as a sling, and the second is used to immobilize the upper arm to the chest wall. Unless other injuries preclude doing so, these victims are usually more comfortable if transported in a semi-sitting position. Fractures of the upper arm between the shoulder and elbow can be splinted in a similar manner. Fractures about the elbow may be splinted by sling and swath when the elbow can be bent without resistance or increased pain. If the elbow cannot be flexed, then the victim is best transported on a stretcher with the extremity splinted at the victim's side with adequate padding between the arm and the body.

FRACTURES OF THE ARM

Fractures of the upper extremity below the elbow should be splinted using adequately padded boards extending from the elbow to the fingertips. The extremity is then placed in a sling. Padded boards are recommended because they are widely

198

available and are considered to be disposable. Inflatable plastic splints are excellent but require special training in their use. Also they are more expensive than boards and sometimes are difficult to retrieve after use. Injuries of the hand must be managed in a similar manner with a dressing over wounds and immobilization on an adequately padded splint. The hand should be supported on soft padding with the fingers and thumb comfortably flexed.

FRACTURES OF THE LEG

Emergency splinting of fractures involving the lower extremities is somewhat more complicated than splinting fractures of the upper extremities, but the same principles apply. This can be quickly accomplished by adequately trained personnel, provided that the necessary equipment is at hand. For fractures at or above the knee the half-ring traction splint is best. This requires that equipment be available and that attendants be trained in its use. Padded board splints are certainly acceptable, provided that the outer board extends from the axilla on the affected side to below the sole of the foot. The inner board extends from the groin to below the foot. Both boards must be well padded. The application of either of these splints requires a two-person team; one person supports and applies gentle traction to the extremity while the second person applies the splint. Plastic inflatable splints are only suitable for fractures below the knee. Other means of splinting injuries below the knee, such as a pillow reinforced by boards on the outside, serve equally well. Well-padded boards extending from midthigh to below the foot can be used and are easily obtained. Any open wounds should be covered with a clean (or sterile) dressing, of course, prior to applying the splint. It is frequently necessary to realign the extremity before the leg can be splinted if gross deformity is present. This can easily be done by cautiously applying gentle traction. Fractures about the hip are best managed by applying a half-ring traction splint but are equally well handled by supporting the injured extremity on a pillow with the hip and knee flexed slightly and the extremity stabilized by gently strapping it to the stretcher or to the uninjured leg. Fractures of the pelvis usually require no special splinting, but the patient should be transported with care on a firm surface. Frequently the patient is less uncomfortable if the legs are strapped together with adequate padding between them.

DISLOCATIONS

Dislocations of major joints may present special problems. The term *dislocation* is defined as the complete and persistent displacement of the articular surfaces of a joint. Except for certain major joints, these injuries can be splinted in the same manner as a fracture. Dislocations of the shoulder and the hip, however, usually result in gross deformity that makes splinting difficult. Force in attempting to realign these injuries should never be used, and the involved extremity should be supported in the least painful position.

Most dislocations of joints of the lower extremity can be easily splinted provided that voluminous padding is used. As previously mentioned, however, a dislocated hip presents a special problem. Dislocations of this joint usually occur as a result of a powerful force applied in the long axis of the femur with the thigh adducted. This results in a posterior dislocation with or without a fracture of the acetabulum and causes a characteristic deformity. The hip is flexed and adducted and cannot be brought down into normal alignment until the dislocation is reduced. Anterior dislocations occur more rarely, and in this injury the deformity, of course, is in the opposite direction and results in the affected thigh being flexed slightly and externally rotated. A patient with such an injury must therefore be transported with the limb supported and immobilized in the position of deformity. This can best be accomplished by supporting the extremity on multiple pillows or blankets and gently strapping it to the stretcher.

DIAGNOSIS

The following *symptoms and physical signs* indicate that a fracture has probably occurred:
1. Complaint of pain in the area of injury, provided that the victim is conscious and can talk
2. Tenderness elicited by gentle pressure at the site of injury
3. Deformity of the extremity
4. False or unnatural motion at the fracture site
5. Swelling and discoloration

If any of these findings is present, the patient should be handled as if a fracture were present. The possibility of nerve or vascular injury must always be kept in mind and should be noted at the time of the initial examination at the scene. Such information is useful in evaluating the patient's condition and in planning definitive treatment. It is most helpful to the treating physician to know whether there was evidence of vascular or nerve injury at the scene of the accident or whether competent observation indicated that these structures were intact and that evidence of vascular or nerve injury appeared by the time the victim arrived at the medical facility.

As a general rule a fracture, even an open fracture, is not a life-threatening injury. Familiarity with the proper immediate care of fractures is important, however, because of their frequency. Proper emergency splinting does much to prevent or control shock. It follows, then, that after the life-threatening conditions have been dealt with, fractures should be splinted before transportation is attempted. Assuming that a quick but thorough survey indicates that no life-threatening conditions are present, then the victim should be checked for soft tissue wounds and for fractures.

The term *fracture* means a break in the continuity of a bone. This results, except in special cases, from the application of considerable force either directly or indirectly. It is important to note the general area of injury and whether the fracture is open or closed. Closed fractures are those in which the skin over the fracture site is intact. These may be either displaced or undisplaced and may or may not be comminuted. Open fractures are those in which the skin is open so that there is communication between the fracture site and the exterior. These are more serious injuries but, from the standpoint of immediate care, demand only the application of a clean (preferably sterile) dressing before a splint is applied. Other injuries may include abrasions, contusions, sprains, lacerations, and dislocations. It may be difficult even in ideal circumstances to determine whether there is a fracture associated with these other injuries. It is good practice therefore to handle such an injury as if there is a fracture; that is, an appropriate splint should be applied in addition to a dressing if indicated. Major bleeding can usually be controlled with a properly applied pressure dressing. A tourniquet is practically never indicated unless a traumatic amputation has occurred or unless a limb is so badly damaged that it cannot be saved.

QUESTIONS

1. Discuss the importance of the fracture in the total evaluation of first aid priorities.
2. What is the current practice with regard to use of tourniquets in immediate management of injuries to the extremities?
3. Explain the rationale for a classification of fracture types as presented in this chapter.
4. Explore the relative advantages of inflatable plastic as compared with other splinting materials.

CHAPTER 25

Head and spinal injuries

JOHN T. BONNER

When the traumatized patient has sustained central nervous system injury, two primary modalities become particularly important: maintaining the airway and maintaining adequate blood volume.

MAINTAINING THE AIRWAY

As with other organ system injuries, the initial concern is the maintenance of an airway. This is not only necessary for survival of the individual in overall terms but is also especially critical to the central nervous system, which requires adequate oxygenation for survival. An inadequate airway may actually aggravate the neurologic injury and not allow neural tissue to survive because of the lack of oxygen availability. Airway obstruction may not only decrease available oxygen but may also increase expiratory pressure, resulting in increased venous pressure and worsening any cerebral edema that may exist. Also airway inadequacy may allow an increase in carbon dioxide content that may aggravate cerebral edema. Obtaining arterial blood gas levels can be informative and helpful. Physical obstruction, such as vomitus and blood, may often be easily removed by adequate suctioning, but usually a more dependable airway mechanism is needed in the comatose patient to allow assurance of an airway and to permit attention to the care of other injuries. Recently the technique of placing endotracheal tubes has been mastered by most physicians, and it is an expeditious and satisfactory means of maintaining the airway. Tracheostomy is the other method of choice. It should be familiar to all physicians and may become necessary in such situations, especially when extensive oral or facial injuries may not allow adequate placement of an endotracheal tube. Possibility of a neck fracture in traumatized patients specifically precludes excessive movement of the neck in placing an endotracheal tube. In most situations this can be done safely, but occasionally tracheostomy may be the procedure of choice.

As previously mentioned, the possibility of cervical fractures must be given paramount consideration in the patient who is comatose from a head injury to avoid aggravating any neurologic injury to the spinal cord or causing one to occur. This consideration is especially important in extracting injured individuals from damaged automobiles and may require great care. One is rarely justified in dragging an injured person through apertures, such as windows. Such procedures often require twisting and manipulation of the body on its axis and increase the possibility of spinal cord or root damage in the presence of spinal fractures.

Adequate care involves removing the person on a seat or on special extraction boards that are carried by most ambulances, thus allowing the head and neck to stay in alignment with the axis of the body, probably the most important principle involved in such situations. In transporting an individual with a possible spinal fracture, especially fracture of the cervical spine, it is sometimes useful to assign one individual the task of assuring that the head and neck are properly positioned. Cervical halter traction is quite useful in this situation, especially if mandibular injury is not present. Even in the presence of such injuries, care in manually controlling the head to protect the spinal cord is time and energy well spent.

Unless endotracheal tubes or oral airways are satisfactorily placed at the site of injury and adequate suctioning is available, one is rarely justified in transporting the injured, comatose person in the supine position. Transportation on the side in the so-called decubitus position or in the prone position is better because these positions assure a better airway and also there is less likelihood of aspiration if vomiting does occur. Again I emphasize the importance of keeping the head and neck in proper traction and alignment and preventing neck flexion, which can also be satisfactorily done in these positions.

MAINTAINING ADEQUATE BLOOD VOLUME

Shock and low blood pressure cannot, for practical purposes, be attributed to head injuries. Only in the infant, who has a relatively small circulating blood volume and an expandable intracranial cavity because of the lack of suture closure, can an intracranial hemorrhage be sufficient to occasionally cause shock. In the adult intracranial pressure from hemorrhage or other cerebral injuries usually results in hypertension. Thus when shock is present in the traumatized patient, one must look for blood loss in other areas, such as pelvic fracture and intra-abdominal or thoracic hemorrhage. Shock with neurogenic loss of vasomotor tone occurs only in the terminal phase of brainstem decompensation. Coma may be secondary to hypotension itself. It is not an uncommon experience in the emergency room to see a patient awaken on replacement of an adequate circulating blood volume, demonstrating that he may have only a minor head injury or perhaps none at all.

Adequate replacement of circulating volume, especially blood, is important in minimizing cerebral injury and allowing adequate oxygenation of the brain. In replenishing circulating volume one must remember that in the presence of significant head injury, especially one involving the possibility of cerebral edema, excessive fluid replacement should not occur nor should excessive amounts of sodium be given. Aggravation of the cerebral edema may occur and thus worsen the intracranial pathology. In the absence of loss of significant circulating volume, fluids should be restricted and any saline given should not usually be greater than one-half normal in concentration. During a 24-hour period 2,000 ml of fluid with a limited amount of exogenous sodium is usually more than ample for an adult with a head injury and avoids worsening cerebral edema. Steroids, such as dexamethasone (Decadron), 10 mg intramuscularly or intravenously given as a loading dose followed by 4 mg every 6 hours, or methylprednisolone (Medrol), 40 mg given intravenously as a loading dose and 40 mg every 4 hours, are often beneficial initially for cerebral edema in a contused brain.

Steroids do not seem to be as efficacious in this situation as they are in treating the edema surrounding brain tumors; therefore they should not be given as a routine measure but only when clinically indicated. Hypertonic fluids, such as mannitol intravenously, should be given only for specific indications, such as to decrease cerebral edema to allow one time to evaluate the patient for possible operative intervention in lesions such as acute epidural, subdural, or intracerebral hematomas. I favor 1 gm per kilogram of weight of mannitol intravenously administered as a bolus, although many favor 0.5 gm per kilogram.

A Foley catheter should be placed to handle the hoped-for diuresis. Because of the possible rebound phenomenon of initially reducing cerebral edema but then aggravating it, these agents can act as a two-edged sword. Also by reducing cerebral edema, they may allow a hematoma to enlarge proportionally; thus if rebound does occur, it may compromise the situation. Therefore hypertonic fluids do have indications in buying time for evaluation, including diagnostic procedures when operative intervention is a distinct possibility, but because of the rebound side effects, they should be used only for strict clinical indications and certainly not as a routine procedure. When necessary, mannitol seems to be more desirable than urea, since experience indicates that there is less rebound with it.

Anyone who has handled extensive scalp lacerations knows that the scalp is extremely vascular, and a very significant blood loss may occur. Hemorrhage usually can be controlled easily by using digital compression along the scalp edge, placing mosquitoes or other hemostatic instruments on the galea, and turning the instruments back, thus tamponading the bleeding vessels. It is usually a worthless, time- and blood-wasting exercise to attempt to clamp individual bleeders or to tie off individual bleeding scalp arteries. The most important aspect of scalp closure is to close the galea tightly, either as a separate deep layer or with the skin by a mattress suture.

INITIAL TREATMENT

In head and spinal injuries evaluation and treatment are designed to be appropriate for each patient. There are no *routine* procedures as such. This is especially true in the consideration of lumbar puncture, which is certainly not a routine item in the evaluation of the nervous system. There are very few situations in which lumbar puncture is needed or indicated in the acute evaluation of trauma, and in many situations it is extremely deleterious and dangerous to the patient. In the presence of a mass, lumbar puncture may hasten herniation once it has started by upsetting the dynamic balance of pressures that exist. The information that is gained in the acute evaluation of trauma may not be worth the risks involved. Obviously such manipulation is contraindicated.

Control of seizures

Fortunately, seizures are infrequently seen in acute trauma, but if seizures should occur, adequate control by intravenous drugs is necessary. Phenytoin (Dilantin) has little effect in stopping acute seizures, but its use is appropriate for long-term seizure control. Initially, intravenous barbiturates, such as amobarbital (Amytal), can be given to control seizures for an adequate time without long depression, which may mask any progressive consciousness deterioration. Administration of intravenous diazepam (Valium) is also useful, especially with a focal seizure pattern. Intravenous paraldehyde is also used for seizure control, especially if appropriate amounts of other medications have not been successful. One must remember that pulmonary hemorrhages may be a complication of using intravenous paraldehyde, but this is infrequent. Paraldehyde is also well absorbed rectally; thus it is especially useful in infants when there is difficulty in obtaining intravenous routes.

The important feature in obtaining seizure control is in using adequate medication. No exact dosage amounts or limits can be given, since this varies according to the clinical situation, which is determined by the relative refractoriness of the seizure. One must be prepared to support respiration if much anticonvulsant is needed to control the seizures; however, if the initial intravenous medication is carried past a safety margin after seizure has stopped, unnecessary respiratory depression may result. One must not forget the initiation of long-acting anticonvulsants such as phenytoin (Dilantin) for continued control.

Open skull fracture

If an open skull fracture is present with dura exposed or dural lacerations and brain exposed, one should remove and irrigate away the grossly evident foreign material and cover the exposed brain area lightly with sterile sponges. This is the one situation in which induction of general anesthesia may be justified immediately after admission in the emergency room. The patient must be prevented from fighting, bucking, or coughing; the strain caused by such activity progressively herniates more cerebral tissue from the skull defect and results in an excessive loss of brain substance.

THE EXAMINATION

When one has attended to the immediate lifesaving procedures, more detailed attention should then be given to the patient as a whole. A general physical examination is necessary including an adequate neurologic examination, which need not be complicated but should be accurate. The important aspects are the level of consciousness, orientation in the verbally responsive patient, and especially whether the patient's condition is improving or deteriorating. If scalp lacerations are present, careful visual exploration and palpation with a sterile gloved finger can determine whether skull fractures are present in this region. This procedure often reveals fractures that would not be visible on x-ray films. One must take care that subgaleal or subperiosteal hemorrhages are not mistaken for fractures. They are commonly misinterpreted as depressed skull fractures.

Examination of the eyes

The pupillary size and response to light should be noted, as well as the ability of the eyes to move and in the comatose patient the vestibulo-ocular reflexes (doll's eyes) to limited head rotation. Such examination can occur without putting the neck in jeopardy. The corneal response is seldom checked in the emergency room but should be, since it often gives valuable information as to the level of the patient's neurologic injury and often gives hints of possible lateralization. Funduscopic examination should not be neglected, but the presence of papilledema is seldom seen at an early stage of increased intracranial pressure; thus the funduscopic examination is often normal. There are situations in which increased intracranial pressure may be present and retinal vein pulsations are preserved although this is not the usual situation. Examination of the head in neurologic injuries includes noting the condition of the nose and ears and other signs.

Examination of the nose and ears

The presence of hemorrhage from the external auditory canal in the absence of an obvious superficial ear laceration is presumptive evidence of basal skull fracture. Additional support would be given by escape of cerebrospinal fluid. When there is blood in the external auditory canal, most physicians believe that appropriate antibiotic coverage should be given as partial treatment for the basal skull fracture. Irrigation of the blood from the external ear canal for further examination is not indicated, since it could introduce retrograde infection that may not otherwise occur. Allowing bloody fluid from either the ear or nose to drop on a sponge or pillowcase may often verify the presence of cerebrospinal fluid, since the double ring sign is formed by the quick migration of cerebrospinal fluid circumferentially from the drop around the central blood spot. In the absence of hemorrhage from the external auditory canal, the tympanic membranes and the pharynx should be carefully visualized because the presence of blood or fluid behind them is also evidence of basal skull fracture. The clear fluid can be further verified as cerebrospinal fluid by obtaining a positive result with a glucose stick. Nasal secretions, except in a patient with an upper respiratory infection, usually test glucose-negative; however, blood in the fluid negates the validity.

There are other external manifestations of basal skull fracture, such as the well-known "Battle sign." This is ecchymosis above the mastoid region reflecting the dissection of cerebrospinal fluid and blood into the mastoid air cells and overlying tissue. Bilateral periorbital ecchymoses (or the initial development of such by discoloration medially around each eye in the absence of direct injury to the eye) is also indicative of basal skull fracture. Dissection of blood and cerebrospinal fluid through the ethmoid air cells and into the loose areolar tissue around the eyes produces the colloquially identified "coon's eyes" because of similarity to the periorbital markings of the raccoon.

Examination of the neck

In the comatose, disoriented, or irrational individual or one presumed to be under the influence of drugs such as alcohol, attention must be given to prevention of aggravation of a neck injury by maintaining the axial orientation, which has been mentioned before, by adding either halter traction or sandbags around the sides of the head to prevent head turning. The ability of the awake and rational patient to voluntarily move the neck with little or no discomfort is reassuring. Significant neck injuries usually elicit enough paravertebral muscle spasm to make neck motion uncomfortable and thus are self-protective. An awake or rational individual who is able to and wants to move his head around does not need such protective measures and is unlikely to have a significant neck injury.

Examination of range of motion and reflexes

Other important features in the neurologic evaluation are the ability of the person to move his extremities and whether he moves them equally and symmetrically. This may be ascertained in the comatose patient by his response to noxious stimuli, such as pressure over the supraorbital nerve or squeezing the clavicle to elicit periosteal pain. Any difference in ability to move extremities is an important observation concerning possible lateralization. The difference in tone of the extremities, such as suggestion of spasticity, is also important lateralizing evidence. One must interpret extremity examination in light of possible local injuries or fractures. Change of tone and paresis can often be easily elicited by noting the difference in the rate or direction of fall of extremities when elevated and, especially in lower extremities, by the amount of rebound the leg has after being dropped from a height against the mattress. The side with more paresis has less tendency to bounce on rebound and thus gives important lateralizing information. The deep tendon reflexes should be carefully evaluated for possible asymmetries, ankle and knee clonus, presence of Babinski responses, and symmetry and lateralization of responses. The ability of the individual to respond to noxious stimulation of the extremities should also be noted. Paresis is often uncovered by difference in withdrawal ability, remembering that differences in sensation reception also aid in laterality and modify response. The superficial reflexes, abdominal and cremasteric reflexes in males, and abdominal reflex in females should also be examined and asymmetry should be noted to obtain important possible lateralizing information. Although often neglected, the examination of superficial reflexes is one that often offers valuable information. The activity of the superficial reflexes can be considered to some extent the "neurologic sedimentation rate" because it gives some indication of the severity of injury.

Notation of change of state

In evaluating the patient with a head injury it is important to note whether his condition is static or whether he is changing in level of consciousness or in other parameters of neurologic function. If his condition is improving, it is unlikely that he has a significant mass that would need acute treatment. One who shows progressive improvement is highly unlikely to have a mass at all. Even with the improving patient, close observation is important, since it is possible that he may start to deteriorate as a result of a progressive extrinsic or intrinsic lesion or progressive cerebral edema, usually secondary to contusions. Therefore as a patient's condition improves, generally it is inappropriate to manipulate him by performing diagnostic procedures such as arteriography.

The deteriorating patient is of great concern, especially if his condition is showing lateralization. This is the person who needs accurate and appropriate diagnostic measures or exploratory burr hole or twist drill placement to treat a mass before brainstem compression has progressed to the point where the patient cannot be saved.

Recording an adequate history

It should be clear that detailed examination and observation of the neurologic function are important, are easily and quickly accomplished, and are not overly complicated. One of the more important details is to accurately record significant findings at the time of initial examination and also during subsequent examinations so that judgment as to whether the patient is changing clinically should not be left to memory. During stressful situations, especially when multiple-system trauma is present or when many injured persons arrive at the same time, clinical confusion is quite common. Right-left disorientation is especially common among observers. Jotting down significant details is not time wasted and may be the factor allowing appropriate judgment to be made on patients, saving much time and morbidity in the long run. Therefore the dearth of records on traumatized persons and the subsequent confusion and lack of clinical information, even in the better emergency rooms, is completely inexcusable.

Roentgenographic evaluation

The most important factors in initially evaluating trauma, as in other aspects of medicine, are the combined product of history and physical examination with clinical appraisal being the paramount source of information. Although other examinations, such as x-ray studies, often add further significant information, they are in a true sense ancillary to clinical appraisal. Roentgenograms *should not* be obtained until the patient has been sufficiently stabilized for movement, and most modern hospital emergency rooms have x-ray facilities present or available on a portable basis that are of good quality and adequate for initial evaluation. Computerized axial tomography, when available, can be a rapid, low-risk method of great aid in evaluating the possibility of intracranial masses. Echo techniques have not proved dependable enough in most hands to be very useful. Because of the high incidence of neck injuries associated with head injuries, at least a single lateral cervical spine film should be obtained with the skull films of such patients.

SPINAL INJURIES

The handling of spinal injuries is an especially critical consideration in the initial care of acute trauma. It must be reiterated that such injuries often accompany head injuries. Evaluation for spinal injuries is essential in both the history and the physical aspects to prevent aggravation of these injuries (with neurologic consequences) during transportation and care of other systemic injuries. Spinal fractures do not of necessity involve nervous system injury, but there are many tragic situations in which the initial trauma does not cause neural damage but subsequent evaluation and handling result in such damage. The fact that the head and neck should be kept in the same axis as the remainder of the body has been previously emphasized. Torsion of the thoracic or lumbosacral areas must be avoided by utilizing the log-rolling technique in comatose individuals to protect against neural damage. In positioning these patients a degree of hyperextension of any of the involved areas is certainly much more desirable than any flexion, and, at times, it is more desirable than the neutral position.

Initial care

Initially, use of conservative therapy versus the value of open operative decompression in the various injuries is a long and complex topic that need not be discussed in detail. This subject may be summarized by stating that the general experience is that the patient who is improving should be allowed to improve on his own and not be considered at that time for an operative decompression. The conservative treatment involves traction and attempted closed reduction of the fracture, especially in the cervical region, by such methods as cervical halter traction on arrival while initial evaluation is occurring. Then as early as possible, one places more permanent skeletal traction, such as the well-known Crutchfield tongs or other appliances such as Barton or Gardner tongs. Patients with spinal cord injury should have a Foley catheter placed as soon as possible after admission to allow bladder decompression or preferably initiation of sterile intermittent catheterization to prevent overdistension that may, in itself, add months to the rehabilitation process. After the initial evaluation of patients with paraplegia and quadraplegia and the placement of tongs in patients with cervical fractures, the patient should be placed on equipment such as a Foster frame or circle bed during the initial care period to prevent compromise over skin pressure points and the development of decubiti. Foster and Stryker frames are generally preferable to circle beds, which while turning tend to put excessive weight on the axis of the body and thus the fracture. This may cause fracture movement or dislocation.

As with head injuries, a complete review of the various types of pathology in spinal injuries is beyond the scope of this discussion; however, one of the more common injuries is the musculoligamentous injury of the neck and low back, the initial care of which is often poor in the emergency room situation. Musculoligamentous (myofascial strain) injury of the neck is often termed *whiplash injury*, a term of dubious medical background and out-of-proportion medical-legal litigation overtones. After determination that cervical fracture is not present, appropriate care usually involves using adequate analgesics. Muscle relaxants are often beneficial to the patient. Cervical collars often provide temporary usefulness for paravertebral muscle spasm for a few days until this phase has passed. After that time they should be removed because continued immobilization often causes spasm to continue and also causes joint degenerative changes in the cervical spine. In addition, these collars become severe psychologic crutches for many patients. Lumbar and cervical disc protrusions are usually initially treated conservatively unless a significant neurologic deficit is present.

Examination

Examination of the back itself, the most obvious maneuver, is often neglected, and there is loss of significant information. Swelling or prominence of frank hematoma over the spinal area is suggestive of local injury that is likely to involve bony fracture. In the conscious patient, local tenderness may often be elicited over the area of injury by mild percussion up and down the spinal axis. The location of paravertebral muscle spasm that is made apparent by local scoliosis or tilt is suggestive of local injury, and it is manifested not only by discomfort of the patient in that area but also by actual palpation of the paravertebral muscle spasm by the examiner. The spinal processes may often be quite prominent as a gibbus at the area of fracture. Often there is a frank fracture dislocation resulting from a flexion or torsion injury or a compression fracture of the vertebral body. Open injuries involving the spinal column, whether they be by sharp or blunt trauma or by gunshot wound, obviously need care to control local hemorrhage and temporary sterile tamponade dressing to avoid retrograde infection prior to operative debridement, especially if spinal fluid communication exists.

Neurologic deficit may be gross and unmistakable or it may be quite subtle; nevertheless it is usually demonstrable even in those patients who are comatose. The ability to voluntarily move extremities may show deficits or asymmetries or both. Observed deficits in reflex response to noxious stimuli are also important observations that may imply neural damage. One must remember that in acute cord injuries, spinal shock may be present for variable lengths of time, minutes to months, and thus flaccid paralysis may be present, although varying degrees of spastic paralysis are frequently seen in acute trauma. There may be the usual spasticity to passive movement of the extremities, hyperactive deep tendon reflexes combined with ankle clonus and up-going toes, and absence of superficial reflexes. The presence of priapism is always suggestive of spinal cord injury above the sacral area. In the awake, cooperative patient, identification of the injury level is usually accurately done by examining the extremities for specific root deficits and in the case of the trunk with a pinwheel or usual safety pin, bilaterally eliciting the sensory level. In the awake patient this sensory examination should be done with care because both an upper and lower sensory level may frequently be elicited; the upper level occasionally exhibits dysalgesia as well as hypalgesia and, at times, hyperesthesia. The upper sensory level, which is the one most suggestive of the level of pathology, is called the primary sensory level and the lower is the secondary. When the level is up to the region of the clavicles, one then examines the upper extremity in detail for root distribution sensory loss, as well as doing specific muscle testing and reflex eliciting to determine site of lesion. A discussion of the neurologic findings representative of the various lesion levels is beyond the scope of this book and can be found in most good neurology and neurosurgery texts and correlated with a knowledge of the anatomy.

Information may also be gained by examining the patient for sweat level, which is another useful but neglected technique. Such a level may be determined by sweeping one's hand lightly up the trunk of the patient and noting the position where additional "drag" occurs, identifying the region where moisture represented by perspiration begins, or one may use starch. Occasionally the discrepancy of moisture that exists above and below this level may be observed by using an ophthalmoscope with a bright light and actually visualizing beads of sweat above the level and noting a relative or absolute absence below the level. Cord injury in the thoracic area (or above) often results in a sympathectomy with relative hypotension that is quite sensitive to postural change. Again, completeness of examination is important but is only useful for evaluation if properly recorded, even if in an abbreviated, shorthand fashion. Repeat evaluations are necessary and, as in the situation with head injuries, the patient's condition when initially seen is of paramount importance. The patient who is improving is of less immediate concern than the patient who is deteriorating in neurologic function.

PERIPHERAL NERVE INJURIES

Plexus and peripheral nerve injuries are also frequently seen in acute injuries, more often in a wartime environment. Brachial plexus injuries often result from a stretch mechanism and not infrequently include avulsion of the brachial roots themselves from the spinal cord. With direct injury to the brachial plexus area, neighborhood injuries are also often present, such as subclavian artery lacerations or aneurysms. Tenderness or fullness on palpation high in the axilla is often present, as is tenderness on palpation in the supraclavicular area and bruits on auscultation of the proper areas in associated subclavian artery injuries. Such injuries and associated neighborhood injuries are less common in the lumbosacral plexus region. Peripheral nerve injuries are common in orthopedic injuries of the extremities and are discovered only if proper neurologic examination of such extremities is done. There are obvious medicolegal connotations.

It is usually agreed that laceration of peripheral nerves is best repaired after a waiting period of 3 to 6 weeks, but many good and valid arguments can be proposed for the acute repair of such injuries. I believe that delayed repair is usually preferable so that the limits of the central neuroma and central scar may be apparent; thus there is somewhat more assurance of a successful repair at the first procedure. In acute situations the nerve ends should be identified and approximated so that they do not retract and may be more easily anastomosed in the future. Small wire sutures are valuable tagging devices for the nerve ends in the acute situation, since they not only have the tensile strength to keep the ends in approximation but they also serve as satisfactory radiographic and palpable surgical aids in the future procedure. Delayed repair of peripheral nerve injuries is also more easily done because the epineurium is thicker and thus stronger for suturing. Furthermore in the cleaner, secondary wound under elective circumstances, the surgeon is less likely to make the well-known error of suturing a nerve to a tendon.

• • •

The initial care of injuries is only partially considered unless one reflects on some of the mechanisms of trauma and their prevention. It has been widely publicized and it is apparent in most hospital emergency rooms that alcohol is a major contributor to severe and fatal automobile crashes. Alcohol and other drugs do alter and influence the clinical picture. It must be remembered that a portion of the depression in a head injury may be secondary to the alcohol level in an intoxicated individual. It is all too easy, however, to write off such presentations as intoxication. This is a diagnosis of exclusion only. For medicolegal reasons one should be hesitant to make a firm diagnosis of alcohol intoxication unless one is prepared to support it by such means as verifying blood alcohol levels. This is often impractical. The best course is to enter an impression of "possible alcohol intoxication" and to be certain not to underestimate the degree of head or spinal injury present.

Many vehicular injuries and deaths would be prevented by the proper use of restraints such as seat belts, shoulder straps, and infant seats. The large risk factors of motorcycles, used either on or off the road, must also be considered.

QUESTIONS

1. How do (a) airway obstruction, (b) hypotension, (c) coughing, and (d) vomiting compromise neural tissue?
2. What blood pressure and pulse changes are usually associated with increased intracranial pressure, and what is responsible for these changes?
3. What are the possible complications of use of steroids in head injuries, and what means should be utilized to minimize such risks?
4. Why is it important to tightly close the galea

aponeurotica in scalp lacerations? What complications might occur if it is not properly closed?

5. What are the risks of basal skull fracture, and what are the various methods and philosophies of treatment?

6. What is the incidence of posttraumatic seizures, and what factors participate in their production or avoidance?

7. What are the various mechanisms of spinal cord and root trauma, and what are the therapeutic implications?

8. What are the neurologic implications in patients with major nonspinal orthopedic injuries?

9. What are the factors considered in deciding whether to hospitalize or treat as an outpatient an individual with a concussion?

10. What concerns are added when wounds of the central nervous system are caused by gunshot?

11. What advice would you give to a football player who has just received a concussion or a neck injury without spinal cord or root symptoms and who has normal x-ray films?

SUGGESTED READINGS

Caveness, W. F., and Walker, A. E.: Head injury conference proceedings, Philadelphia, 1966, J. B. Lippincott Co.

Comarr, A. E., and Kaufman, A. A.: A survey of the results of 858 spinal cord injuries, J. Neurosurg. **13:**95-106, 1956.

Evans, J. P.: Acute head injury, Springfield, Ill., 1950, Charles C Thomas, Publisher.

Foltz, E. L.: Head injuries, Northwest Med., pp. 705-715, 1963.

Haymaker, W., and Woodhall, B.: Peripheral nerve injuries, Philadelphia, 1953, W. B. Saunders Co.

Heaton, L. D., Coates, J. B., and Meirowsky, A. M.: Neurological surgery of trauma, Washington, D.C., 1965, Office of the Surgeon General, Department of the Army.

Kahn, E. A., Crosby, E. C., Schneider, R. C., and Taren, J. A.: Correlative neurosurgery, Springfield, Ill., 1969, Charles C Thomas, Publisher.

Plum, F., and Posner, J. B.: Diagnosis of stupor and coma in contemporary neurology series, Philadelphia, 1972, F. A. Davis Co.

Seletz, E.: Injuries of peripheral nerves—principles of treatment, Pac. Med. Surg. **74:**161-164, 1966.

Ward, A. A.: The physiology of concussions, Clin. Neurosurg. **12:**95-111, 1966.

Youmans, J. R.: Neurological surgery, Philadelphia, 1973, W. B. Saunders Co.

CHAPTER 26

Eye injuries

RICHARD O. COE, Jr., and JOHN A. FABRE

GENERAL CONSIDERATIONS

There are but a few true ocular emergencies that require the proper treatment within 30 minutes to several hours after onset. These include orbital cellulitis, gonococcal conjunctivitis, *Pseudomonas* corneal ulceration, acute iridocyclitis, acute closed-angle (congestive) glaucoma, retinal detachment (prior to macular involvement), central retinal artery occlusion, and various types of trauma to and about the eye. These cases are serious; however, it is equally important to manage other types of eye conditions that the patient terms an *emergency*. These patients are usually prompted to seek help at all hours whether they experience a simple redness of the eye or more profound ocular discomfort. Mismanagement of a so-called emergency may create a serious ocular problem later.

In the management of an unconscious patient, even without ocular problems, two things must be done: searching for the possibility of contact lenses, and ensuring that the eyes are protected from exposure by closing the eyelids, patching the eyes closed, or applying ophthalmic ointment.

Topical anesthetics delay epithelial regeneration. Except in the actual removal of a superficially embedded corneal foreign body, topical anesthesia should not be used in the treatment of acute ocular pain. In a patient with welder's keratoconjunctivitis or sunlamp keratoconjunctivitis, one is tempted to make use of these agents; however, it should be remembered that this delays corneal epithelialization. Icepacks with sedation constitute a superior form of treatment. For the physician who occasionally deals with acute ocular disease, the antibiotic-steroid ophthalmic preparations should be avoided. Herpetic and fungal keratitis have been increasing as a result of the widespread promiscuous use of these preparations. Often the patient develops a sensitivity with the first administration of an antibiotic preparation. Later when antibiotics are prescribed during a true infection, the patient develops an allergic blepharoconjunctivitis.

Occasionally a patient with a mildly infected eye with tearing comes in for treatment. This condition is mistaken for a simple conjunctivitis, when in actuality it is the beginning of a viral (usually herpes simplex) keratitis, which progresses rapidly in the presence of steroids. If one is in doubt and if the patient demands treatment, one should dispense or prescribe one of the nonspecific zinc eyedrops (Zincfrin).

If the case is diagnosed as mild mucopurulent conjunctivitis after culture and sensitivity testing has been taken, one of the 10% to 15% sulfacetamide preparations should be prescribed. The ever-popular antibiotic eyedrops should be saved for a true emergency.

History

A precise history, brief but to the point, must be recorded for every patient who is seen on an emergency basis.

Visual acuity

An initial, best visual acuity must be taken on each eye. If the glasses are not available or if a refraction problem is suspected, a simple pinhole punched in a card or piece of plastic will suffice for the patient to view the chart. If a standard visual acuity chart is not available, the examiner may hold any print (for example, a newspaper) at a distance and record the size of the print and the *maximum* distance at which that particular type could be recognized by the patient.

Technique of examination

Gentleness should be stressed. A thumb placed on either the upper or the lower orbital rim can retract a lid with a rolling maneuver. Absolutely no pressure should be applied on a globe suspected of having a perforating injury. The examiner should not wrestle with any child suspected of a serious perforating ocular injury. It is best to examine this type of patient under general anesthesia in the operating room, and the examination should preferably be made by a qualified ophthalmologist.

A strong, focal bright light is essential for satisfactory gross examination. Shining it from one side and varying the angle will create less of an ordeal for the patient and provide a better technique for the examiner, particularly in identifying corneal abrasions or lacerations and in estimating the all-important anterior chamber depth because the transparent cornea domes forward from the flat iris diaphragm.

Binocular magnification of some sort is extremely desirable.

Ophthalmoscopy is essential. Ten percent phenylephrine (Neo-Synephrine) or tropicamide (Mydriacyl) is a rapid mydriatic that should be used on every ocular injury in which intraocular penetration is suspected and not frankly evident.

Orbital x-ray films should be made of any and every eye injury caused by a foreign body, particularly a missile-like injury (for example, history of a sudden sharp pain while operating a lathe, hammering a nail, or running a lawn mower).

TRAUMA
Orbital injuries

The real danger in orbital injuries lies in failure to recognize their presence. Because paranasal sinuses virtually encompass the orbits, meningitis or orbital cellulitis may result from trauma about the face. X-ray studies should include not only the facial bones but also the orbital foramen. When penetrating injuries are discovered, the possibility of retained foreign bodies within the orbit should also be considered.

Although there are many signs of orbital fracture, some of the more important findings are described here:

1. Diplopia may occur, particularly when the orbital contents sag into the maxillary sinus. These orbital floor fractures may be produced by a baseball or fist type of blow. The absence of diplopia in a "fresh" contusion about the face should not cause one to dismiss the possibility of orbital fracture with displacement. As the associated swelling diminishes, the patient's diplopia may appear as much as 1 week later.

2. Anesthesia is another important finding. Fractures of the orbital roof may create pressure on the supraorbital nerve, resulting in anesthesia above the eyebrow. Fragmentation in the area of the infraorbital foramen produces anesthesia over the cheek and the ala of the nose and upper lid.

3. Rhinorrhea may be the hallmark of a torn dura in the anterior fossa, associated with fractures of the prominent supraorbital rim and frontal sinus. The sharp crista galli may penetrate the dura mater and arachnoid in medial orbital wall fractures.

4. Diminished vision must create suspicion of a fracture of the posterior orbital roof where the bony optic foramen encases the optic nerve.

Lid injuries

Ecchymosis. Blood seepage under the loose areolar tissues of the eye is commonly termed a *black eye*. This in itself is no real emergency; use of an icecap suffices. The physician finds it his responsibility to proceed in an orderly manner and to rule out orbital fracture and contusions to the globe.

Burns. Aside from general supportive treatment to the patient as a whole, only cleansing is necessary for first- or second-degree burns. Third-degree burns are another matter and should be referred immediately to an ophthalmologist. No debridement should be done by the physician initially attending the emergency; this should be left to the discretion of a specialist.

Lacerations. Although it is important to initiate prompt repair before lid swelling occurs, adherence should be made to the general principles of surgery, such as antitetanic measures, irrigation, and hemostasis. In extensive lid lacerations without corneal involvement the cornea should be protected from exposure by instilling a sterile antibiotic ophthalmic preparation prior to the referral. An apparently simple puncture type of injury to either lid may, in actuality, also involve the intraocular structures.

Simple suturing is usually adequate when less than one fourth of the eyelid is missing. Margin involvement and severance of one or both canaliculi must be considered. Lid margin repair by direct suturing should be the procedure of choice for the occasional operator when referral to an ophthalmologist is an impossibility. The technique should strive to attain good apposition of lid margin to avoid notching after healing.

Injuries to the globe

Contusions. Blunt trauma to the globe is almost a study within itself. No intraocular structure is "safe." Tears and ruptures can occur in almost any of the eye's component parts. It may not be noticeable objectively, yet severe edema may develop in the macular area, resulting in a visual acuity of 20/200 or less. Most ruptures occur in the upper nasal quadrant, concentric with and adjacent to the limbus. Hyphema may be immediate, delayed, or both. Hemorrhage can occur as late as 10 days after the injury. Eyes have been lost between the time of thoughtless discharge from treatment for a so-called tiny clot in the anterior chamber (or just a smoky appearance in the anterior segment) and the patient's next visit 7 days later. Any blood in the anterior chamber may be the hallmark of more severe hemorrhage. Observation in a hospital and binocular patching are essential. It is best for the general physician to refrain from the instillation of any miotic or mydriatic eyedrops, leaving this to the discretion of a specialist. The so-called secondary hemorrhage is usually more severe than the initial one, thus making it quite necessary for the patient to be under an ophthalmologist's care at the time.

Foreign bodies. Most small, penetrating intraocular foreign bodies remain undetected because insufficient time was taken to elicit a history or because the scope of the ocular examination was narrow. The only sign of such an injury may be a tiny area of corneal edema, a "spot of subconjunctival hemorrhage," or a slightly eccentric pupil. Injuries sustained from air guns, sand blasting, hammering of nails, metal chips from lathes, or chipping of stone are all subject to this suspicion.

It is unfortunate that greater pain results from the presence of a foreign body near the limbus of the cornea than from one nearer the center because central corneal lesions heal more slowly and produce more serious permanent visual disability. Also administration of tetanus toxoid (or TAT) should not be neglected following an injury that is exclusively corneal. Tetanus has been recorded 10 days following a simple corneal injury.

Corneal injuries resulting from a fleck of sand, metal, or splinter embedded in the superficial cornea should be irrigated initially. If this does not dislodge the foreign body, a drop of 0.5% tetracaine or 5% proparacaine hydrochloride (Ophthaine) should be instilled, and the patient should be made comfortable in a supine position. A sterile 20-gauge needle on a syringe (used as a handle) can be brought in from the side and the foreign body can be gently lifted from the cornea. Binocular magnification is necessary, along with good oblique focal illumination. It should be remembered that the degree of corneal injury is proportional not only to the depth of the foreign body and the time elapsed until its removal but also to the amount of trauma inflicted in attempts to remove the foreign body. It is desirable to place even these simple problems in the initial care of an ophthalmologist. Corneal penetration deeper than Bowman's membrane should always be referred immediately to an ophthalmologist.

Lacerations. Nonperforating lacerations of the cornea should be thoroughly irrigated, preferably with sterile physiologic saline. This treatment should be followed by the instillation of some broad-spectrum antibiotic drops or ophthalmic ointment. Referral is urgent. Penetrating corneal lacerations with various degrees of anterior segment involvement should be treated by binocular patching with a shield placed over the injured eye. No attempt should be made to remove any visible foreign bodies or blood clots. At times the iris may resemble a blood clot, and the attempted removal by forceps would produce more dangerous results than gentle irrigation with sterile saline.

Abrasions. "Clean" abrasions of the cornea should be gently irrigated, followed by frequent instillation of antibiotic drops (or 10% to 15% sulfacetamide). Small abrasions can be left unpatched. Larger ones are extremely painful and should be carefully patched using two or three eye pads in thickness and enough tape to keep the lid from opening. Patients with such injuries should be seen again within at most 24 hours and preferably 12 hours later. If the abrasion is obvious, staining with fluorescein is not only unnecessary but hazardous because fluorescein itself is an excellent culture medium for *Pseudomonas aeruginosa*.

Irradiation burns. Snowblindness, sunlamp conjunctivitis, and the more severe welder's keratoconjunctivitis are all caused by injurious exposure to ultraviolet light. The initial symptoms usually begin 12 hours following exposure. No other condition is more frequently mismanaged, usually by the unwise multiple instillation of topical anesthetics. If any instillation is indicated, it is usually only at the time of initial examination. The severity may range from a chemosis of the bulbar conjunctiva to a diffuse corneal epithelial desquamation. Ice compresses, head elevation, analgesics, and sedatives are the accepted forms of treatment.

Chemical burns. The emergency treatment of chemical burns of the eye (whether acidic, alkaline, or refrigerant) consists of immediate, profuse, and prolonged irrigation with water (sterile physiologic saline, ideally). Acidic burns are not quite as serious as the others because of stoppage by an action in which the acid combines with and coagulates the superficial tissues. Alkaline burns soften and penetrate in a relentless fashion; in these cases, irrigation for at least 30 minutes should be performed and followed by instillation of 1% atropine drops to prevent the iris from adhering to the lens or cornea (secondary iritis). Some potentially dangerous refrigerants are oil soluble; therefore instillation of olive or mineral oil should be used in irrigating them from the eye. If the conjunctiva is involved, an ophthalmic ointment should be instilled to help deter symblepharon formation.

Thermal burns. Thermal burns from an open flame are usually not very serious. Boric acid ophthalmic ointment instilled several times daily and 2% homatropine usually suffice.

MEDICAL CONSIDERATIONS
Acute conjunctivitis (purulent)

Neisseria gonococcus can produce the only real emergency situation of the conjunctival diseases. The condition in the adult is usually unilateral with a copious discharge of pus almost literally pouring from a beefy red, tremendously swollen conjunctiva. Corneal perforation is always a hazard. Scrapings must be taken from the raw conjunctiva for immediate fixing and staining, in addition to culture and sensitivity studies for later information. *Neisseria catarrhalis* and *Meningococcus* are also gram-negative, intracellular diplococci; however, they present a much less severe clinical picture.

The cornea should be carefully examined, preferably after irrigation. Any loss in inherent luster (and in uptake of fluorescein dye) is the first evidence of corneal involvement. If a penicillin ophthalmic ointment is not immediately available, one of the chlortetracycline (Aureomycin) ointments should be immediately sought.

Treatment of ophthalmia neonatorum is essentially the same.

Corneal ulcer

Any corneal ulcer is an urgent case; however, when the causative organism is *Pseudomonas aeruginosa*, it is an ocular emergency in the truest sense. An eye can be lost because of this organism within 48 hours. Presumptive evidence is the appearance of a blue-green cast. Any corneal infiltrate should undergo immediate culture and sensitivity studies; the edge should be delicately scraped for pathogenic material. The appearance of a clear center in an ulcer is usually not a sign of healing but more than likely eventually it is identified as the herniation of Descemet's membrane through the necrotic stroma. Some of these patients can have an eye saved by a lamellar keratoplasty, if referred to the ophthalmologist in time.

The red eye

Table 26-1 shows the salient points in differentiation of acute conjunctivitis, acute glaucoma, and acute iridocyclitis. It is important for the attending physician to recognize and know the significance of a deep ciliary injection. It is the hallmark of serious intraocular disease. Referral should be immediate. Both acute iridocyclitis and acute glaucoma have this sign. This radial spoke-like sunburst type of injection is most intense where clear cornea joins white sclera and fades in intensity peripherally from the limbus. Some describe a purplish hue; however, the pattern is the important feature. A crosslike pattern, created by engorgement of the penetrating anterior ciliary vessels at the insertion of the four rectus muscles, may also be present. In acute iridocyclitis the pupil is miotic as a result of spasm and irritability of the iris sphincter, and may be slightly irregular if portions of its margin adhere to the lens. The pupil is large in acute glaucoma because the iris is paralyzed by the extremely high intraocular pressure.

Acute iridocyclitis should be treated with cycloplegics. If early posterior synechiae are present, they may be broken with 10% phenylephrine (Neo-Synephrine). The crucial danger point is attempting to dilate an "irritable" eye when acute glaucoma is already present. This is more likely to happen by mistake if the patient arrives for emergency treatment during the time a self-limited remission of an acute attack is taking place. The treatment for acute (angle-closure) glaucoma is primarily surgical and the patient should be placed immediately in the care of an

Table 26-1. Differentiation of acute conjunctivitis, acute glaucoma, and acute iridiocyclitis

	Acute conjunctivitis	Acute iritis	Acute glaucoma
Incidence	Very common	Common	Uncommon
Discharge	Watery or purulent	Watery	Watery
Visual acuity	Normal	Slight reduction	Marked reduction, halos
Pain	Minimal	Moderate	Severe
Conjunctival injection	Diffuse	Ciliary flush	Ciliary flush
Cornea	Clear	Clear	Steamy
Pupil	Normal	Miotic	Semidilated
Pupillary light response	Normal	Poor	Nonreactive
Intraocular pressure	Normal	Normal or decreased	Marked elevation

ophthalmologist, if possible. Otherwise 2% to 4% pilocarpine drops should be instilled every 15 minutes. There are cases in which these measures fail. Osmotic agents must then be instilled—Osmitral is a good example.

Central retinal artery occlusion

Sudden blindness in any eye should instinctively make the physician reach for an ophthalmoscope. In cases of central retinal artery occlusion, the posterior pole of the eye appears blanched and the macula stands out as a "cherry-red spot." The arterioles are threadlike and no amount of digital pressure creates a venous pulsation that can be seen with an ophthalmoscope. Paracentesis of the anterior chamber or retrobulbar injection (accepted treatment by an ophthalmologist) is not to be attempted by anyone else. Inhalation of amyl nitrite, nitroglycerine administered sublingually, and inhalation of carbon dioxide alternating with oxygen and ocular massage can all be resorted to by the general physician. The prognosis in most cases is extremely poor, even if detected within the first 30 minutes; however, the accepted methods of treatment should be faithfully executed. Patients older than 55 years with a tentative diagnosis of central retinal artery occlusion should have sedimentation rate determination to rule out the diagnosis of temporal arteritis. Treatment in this case consists of large-dose systemic steroid administration. These patients have bilateral disease with the second eye being potentially involved within hours of the first.

Retinal detachment

Any patient who complains of a curtain blocking his field of vision, coupled with light flashes or black spot, should be carefully examined (with dilated ophthalmoscopy) for a detached retina. The red reflex may be absent in one or more quadrants, and ophthalmoscopy, particularly for the occasional observer, may be puzzling. A large, grayish, wrinkled curtain may be evident. All efforts should be directed toward evaluating macular involvement. If the macula is intact, the case is definitely an emergency. Prior to calling the ophthalmologist, bed rest (flat on the back) is advised and binocular patching should be performed. It ceases to be a true emergency if the macula is detached, although the case remains urgent. Surgical treatment has improved in the past 10 years, and no case should be slighted. Even a slight haze in the media (early vitreous hemorrhage) may actually be caused by an undisclosed retinal break. Cases of so-called iritis have later been identified as unsuspected retinal separation.

QUESTIONS

1. In patients with periorbital trauma careful inspection should be done to rule out what other injuries?
2. What is the primary objective in repairing a marginal lid laceration?
3. What is the major complication necessitating close followup of patients with superficial corneal abrasions?
4. In all patients seen with a corneal or conjunctival foreign body, history and examination should seek to rule out what?

5. In all patients seen with obviously penetrating injuries what should be the only treatment before immediate referral?
6. Identify the initial mode of treatment for patients with chemical injuries.
7. Outline history, examination, and possible treatment for patients seen with a complaint of red eye.
8. Discuss history, physical findings, diagnosis, and emergency treatment of central retinal artery occlusion. Remember the possibility of temporal arteritis.

9. What history and examination findings are suggestive of retinal detachment?
10. What types of injuries suggest the need to obtain x-ray studies?
11. Specify the appropriate culture media and stains used when evaluating a conjunctivitis in patients of different ages from neonates to adults.

SUGGESTED READINGS

Fox, S. A.: Ophthalmic plastic surgery, New York, 1970, Grune & Stratton, Inc.

McKinlay, R. T., and Cohen, D. N.: Ophthalmic injuries: handbook of initial evaluation and management, Trans. Am. Acad. Ophthalmol. Otolaryngol. **79**:880, 1975.

Newell, F. W., and Ernest, J. J.,: Ophthalmology: principles and concepts, ed. 3, St. Louis, 1974, The C. V. Mosby Co.

New Orleans Academy of Ophthalmology: Symposium on industrial and traumatic ophthalmology, ed. 3, St. Louis, 1964, The C. V. Mosby Co.

Oksala, A.: Treatment of traumatic hyphema, Br. J. Ophthalmol. **51**:315, 1967.

Paton, D., and Goldberg, M. F.: Injuries of the eye, the lids, and the orbit, Philadelphia, 1968, W. B. Saunders Co.

Paton, D., and Goldberg, M. F.: Management of ocular injuries, Philadelphia, 1976, W. B. Saunders Co.

Read, J. E., and Goldberg, M. F.: Comparison of medical treatment of traumatic hyphema, Trans. Am. Acad. Ophthmol. Otolaryngol. **78**: 799, 1974.

Scheie, H. G., and Albert, D. M.: Adler's textbook of ophthalmology, Philadelphia, 1969, W. B. Saunders Co.

Vaughn, D., and Asbury, T.: General ophthalmology, Los Altos, Calif., 1974, Lange Medical Publications.

CHAPTER 27

Athletic emergencies*

FRED A. WAPPEL

To properly understand athletic injuries, the trainer and the physician should know precisely how the injury was sustained, so that they may be able to visualize the areas receiving the greatest stress, the direction from which the stress came, and the damage that occurred to the joints and other areas of the body. Bilateral comparison in examination is helpful in detecting irregularity, bone displacement, swelling, and other symptoms that aid in diagnosing the injury.

Immediate examination on the field of play by the trainer has proved to be beneficial to the physician who sees the athlete. Marked pain, swelling, and stiffness are not always immediately present; thus the athlete may not be apprehensive during examination. A goal of immediate care on the field is to lessen swelling and decrease pain. It is important to calm the athlete and to offer reassurance.

INTERNAL INJURIES
Concussion

With a mild concussion generally the athlete is incoherent and dazed, and occasionally he sees spots before him. There may be loss of memory and headache. There may be a period of unconsciousness during which the athlete should not be touched or moved. Return of consciousness may not bring coherency. Amnesia may be present. He should be encouraged not to try to remember preceding events because this frustrates him and causes additional apprehension. The neck as well as the head may be injured. Neurologic tests of pinching and pinpricking should be administered before the athlete is moved. Direct questioning should be avoided because it may cause fear, emotion, and shock. Observation should be made of any pupillary dilation.

If these tests are negative, the athlete should be hospitalized for observation, particularly if he was unconscious for a lengthy period. The athlete who was never

---

*Athletic injuries are seldom discussed in the medical curriculum. In fact, few physicians feel confident to manage their immediate diagnosis and treatment unless they have had special exposure to and experience with this specialized group of injuries. One reason is that these injuries occur in eager, young, and active individuals in the best physical condition. An improper decision may result in serious or permanent damage. Mr. Fred Wappel, a veteran intercollegiate trainer, presents a brief summary of immediate measures needed in the care of some frequently encountered athletic injuries.

unconscious but who was incoherent or dazed, with a temporary loss of memory, should never be left alone. He must be accompanied by a friend, coach, or trainer and must be placed immediately in the care of his family or roommate. He must *not* be left alone because he may have a relapse, suffer amnesia, and wander off alone, not knowing who he is or where he lives.

Occasionally the athlete may become violent. Anticipating this problem, the physician or trainer should kneel and straddle the athlete at the waistline and re-assure him when he regains consciousness.

Finally, the athlete may "swallow his tongue." In this case, the jaws lock and the athlete may suffocate if prompt treatment is not initiated. An oral screw is used to pry open the jaws; the tongue should be placed in its normal position, using the tongue-seizing forceps. Usually, however, simply positioning the head as outlined in Chapter 12 opens the airway satisfactorily. Mouth-to-mouth resuscitation should be administered if necessary.

Whenever an oral screw is not available, tongue depressors may be used by staggering them one on top of the other and taping them together. The bottom blade is placed between the jaws and they are wedged in as rapidly as possible until one of the fingers can remove the tongue from the airway. Needless to say, this procedure must be accomplished within 4 minutes.

Ruptured spleen

The athlete who receives a blow to the left upper abdominal quadrant may suffer a ruptured spleen. The symptoms and signs of a ruptured spleen may be pain in the left upper abdominal quadrant and shoulder, weakness, rapid pulse, paleness, apprehension, thirst, and sweating.

Pain may be present in the left shoulder (supraclavicular fossa) because of an irritation of the diaphragm. The phrenic nerve innervates the diaphragm, and the pain in the shoulder is referred pain. An athlete who has any of these symptoms should be seen by a physician immediately or placed in a hospital for observation and examination.

Ribs in the left upper quadrant should be examined carefully before a hasty generalization is made.

Kidney injuries

With any trauma to the posterior lower aspect of the rib cage, a kidney injury should be suspected, and proper examination should be made before the athlete returns to the contest. Generally there is pain in the back over the area of the kidney. A urine sample should be taken immediately to determine whether there is any hematuria. If blood is present, the urine sample should be retained and the athlete should be seen by a doctor immediately.

Needless to say, this athlete should not compete in athletics if marked kidney damage is present. An athlete who has only one kidney should never be permitted to participate in contact sports.

Bladder

Bladder injuries are rare in athletics. One reason is that the athlete generally keeps his bladder empty because of nervous tension.

Hematuria has been discovered after running. This is usually of no consequence. Examination should be made by the physician, however, as a precautionary measure.

Rib cage injuries

Injuries to the rib cage are classified into two categories: injury to the ribs and injury to the costal cartilages.

The rib cage injury usually involves symptoms of pain, point tenderness, bony irregularity, inability to breathe deeply, and inability to lie down without discomfort.

Palpation determines whether there is any bone irregularity. Usually injury to the costal cartilage produces a detectable separation. By no means should the athlete be picked up by the belt to restore respiration. The ribs may be fractured and the lung punctured.

An elastic rib belt should be applied for comfort until x-ray studies determine the extent of the injury. The rib belt should be worn day and night, if necessary, for comfort and support. The 6-inch elastic bandage is adequate to wrap around the rib cage for comfort if a rib belt is not available.* Ice should be applied immediately and continued for a minimum of 12 hours.

Hyperventilation

Hyperventilation is defined as a greater respiratory rate and/or depth than is necessary for physiologic needs of the body. Hyperventilation is a result of fright and apprehension following injury. Direct questions such as: "Do you have any feeling in your arms and legs?" may alarm the athlete further and should be avoided until the condition has been relieved. The athlete has a conscious feeling of needing more air, begins rapid breathing, and exhales too much carbon dioxide.

A paper bag is held in place over the mouth and nose to permit rebreathing of the expelled air, which is increasingly rich in carbon dioxide. The athlete is instructed to breathe slowly, which is not easily accomplished in this condition.

The bag should remain in place until respiration returns to normal. The athlete may lose consciousness, but he regains it within a short period of time. Occasionally heavy breathing begins again, and the same procedure is once more followed.

HEAD, NECK, AND BACK INJURIES
Sunstroke or heat stroke

These matters are treated in Chapter 14.

Nosebleed

Nosebleed is discussed in Chapter 31.

Cervical spine injury

When an athlete is lying motionless on the field, whether conscious or unconscious, he should not be moved until a doctor is summoned. Anything should be suspected at this point. The athlete should be observed to determine if he remains motionless and to rule out spinal injury. If he regains consciousness and moves his

---

*Elastic rib belts are manufactured by Du Puy, Warsaw, Ind.; Richards Mann, Memphis, Tenn.; Zimmer U.S.A., Warsaw, Ind.; and Baka Manufacturing Co., Inc., Plainville, Mass.

body, more precise examination may begin. The symptoms of cervical vertebral involvement are pain, stiffness in the neck, limited range of motion, muscle spasm, referred pain in the arms, and general lack of peripheral sensitivity. A physician should be summoned immediately. The athlete should not be moved, and no equipment should be removed, particularly the helmet, until there is voluntary head movement. The subject is discussed in further detail in Chapter 25.

An athlete who is suspected of having a neck injury should not be permitted to return to a contest, particularly in a contact sport, until x-ray films have been taken and he is cleared for competition. An x-ray study is made of all cervical vertebral injuries, no matter how minor they may seem. This is a hard and fast rule that must not be ignored.

Many athletes who do not report neck injuries immediately feel the matter to be of no significance. After an athletic event, an athlete may sit slouched over in front of the locker with marked pain, stiffness, and limited range of motion and in a partial state of shock. This athlete should be handled in the same way as the athlete on the field who is suspected of having a cervical vertebral injury.

SHOULDER INJURIES
Acromioclavicular separation

Acromioclavicular separation occurs as a result of falling directly on the shoulder or from a blow directly on the shoulder as in tackling as well as falling on the elbow. The athlete should be made comfortable and the arm must be placed in a sling with the elbow supported until the diagnosis can be made by the physician. Normally the complete or severe separation is easiest to detect. Elevation of the clavicle is distinctly prominent. The moderate separation will show partial elevation, and the mild separation will show slight elevation. Bilateral comparison of x-ray films is important. Some athletes deomonstrate normal elevation of both joints.

If the separation is severe, surgery may be indicated; however, this procedure is debatable. If the separation is mild, the arm should be placed in a sling and ice should be applied to the shoulder for a minimum of 6 hours. The sling should be worn until pain disappears. If the separation is moderate, it should be approximated with an acromioclavicular splint.*

The acromioclavicular splint should be worn for 14 to 21 days depending on the point tenderness, continued relaxation of the joint, and further x-ray studies to determine the amount of reduction. The arm should be placed in a sling, and ice should be applied for a minimum of 24 hours.

Dislocation

Shoulder dislocation in athletics generally occurs when the arm is in abduction and external rotation. The joint capsule usually tears anteriorly and inferiorly. On rare occasions, usually in wrestling, the posterior aspect of the joint capsule tears.

The dislocation of the shoulder is easily recognized by noting a hollow pit at the superior portion of the deltoid muscle. The condition is generally accompanied by fixation of the arm. The athlete is apprehensive at moving the arm from its fixed

---

*Acromioclavicular splint manufacturers are Du Puy, Warsaw, Ind.; Richards Mann, Memphis, Tenn.; Zimmer U.S.A., Warsaw, Ind.; and others.

position. Immediate muscle spasm makes reduction without administration of relaxants difficult to accomplish unless one is particularly skilled in this manipulation. When manipulation is being attempted without analgesics, one must be cautious not to apply a force so great that more extensive tearing will result. It is important, however, that reduction be accomplished immediately if at all possible, to minimize muscle spasm.

When the athlete is moved, the arm should be placed in a comfortable position and stress should be taken off the shoulder joint. This may be accomplished by placing towels, a pillow, or a similar bulky object under the elbow and upper arm so that the shoulder joint will be as relaxed as possible under the circumstances. The arm should then be placed in a sling, or a sling may be improvised by taping posteriorly from the shoulder girdle, under the elbow, and back to the shoulder girdle.

An x-ray study should be made immediately to eliminate the possibility of fracture. An effective method of reduction by the physician consists of placing the athlete on the affected side with the arm hanging off the end of the table and his head resting on another table. A 10-pound plate with a tape extension is applied to the athlete's wrist and a reduction is accomplished by the hanging weight. Ice should be applied to the area immediately after reduction to minimize hemorrhage.

After reduction, the athlete should be placed in a universal shoulder immobilizer for at least 4 weeks, to permit the joint capsule to scar down and lessen the possibility of recurrence.

ELBOW INJURIES
Dislocation

Elbow dislocations generally occur when the arm is extended with the hand stabilized on the ground or floor, so that the elbow is forced into hyperextension. Symptoms are displacement of the elbow joint, pain, fixation, swelling, and greatly diminished range of motion. A physician should be summoned immediately. However, if the athlete is to be taken to the hospital, the elbow should be cradled in a pillow for comfort and held against his body. An x-ray study should be made to determine whether a fracture is present.

After reduction, the elbow should be wrapped with an elastic bandage from the hand to the axilla. The elbow should be elevated, and it should be encased in ice for a minimum of 24 hours.

Hyperextended elbow

When the arm is extended with the hand fixed on the ground or floor, the elbow may be forced into hyperextension so that it does not dislocate but the ligaments, muscles, and joint capsule are stretched and distended. Symptoms include swelling of the medial condyle, limited range of motion, pain, and tenderness.

The elbow should be examined for swelling and to determine passive range of motion for flexion, extension, supination, and pronation. Palpation is helpful in determining any bony irregularity or chips.

The elbow should be elevated, wrapped with an elastic bandage, and encased in ice for 1 hour. It should then be wrapped with an elastic roller bandage and cushioned by foam rubber. The wrap should extend from the hand to the axilla. The arm should be placed in a sling, and the athlete should be referred for examination and x-ray study. Even when initial swelling and other symptoms are absent, the elbow should be iced and wrapped because it usually swells and becomes symptomatic several hours later.

HAND AND WRIST INJURIES
Navicular fractures

The carpal navicular is more subject to injury than are any of the other carpal bones. It may be fractured in a fall, which forces the wrist into hyperextension, or by other violent action to the wrist. Pain, particularly in the snuff box area, limited range of motion, and swelling characterize the injury. Range of motion tests should be accomplished to determine the amount of immobility. Immediately after injury, pain, swelling, and limited range of motion are frequently absent, but these symptoms may begin several hours later.

Ice should be placed on the wrist immediately and should be maintained until x-ray study and examination are instituted. If the wrist is painful, a longitudinally halved type-carton or wooden split padded with cotton or any soft material should be placed under the wrist; an elastic bandage should be used over this splint or an air splint should be applied. An x-ray study should follow.

Many physicians cast this injury at once because a fracture is not always detected immediately. If a fracture is not detected on a recheck x-ray film after 10 to 14 days, the cast is removed and the athlete may resume activity. Otherwise the cast is retained, and the athlete is removed from participation in athletics until the fracture unites. Healing is slow because of the poor blood supply, and in many instances this fracture does not unite.

Fracture of metacarpals

The reader is referred to Chapter 23 for a discussion of hand injuries.

Forearm injuries

Fracture of the radius or ulna is identified by displacement of bone, bone irregularity, swelling, pain, limited pronation and supination, and inability to grip with the hand. Any bony irregularity or displacement should be noted before active motion is accomplished. Pressing the radius and ulna together with the hand elicits sharp pain if either bone is fractured, although pain may also be present with a contusion. After determining that pronation and supination can be accomplished, the athlete should be asked to grip the hand of the examiner firmly so that muscular strength may be evaluated. An x-ray study should follow.

Whenever there is a question of fracture, the forearm should be wrapped with a 3-inch elastic bandage from the hand to the elbow and the arm should be placed in a sling. If a fracture is present, the forearm should be wrapped with an elastic bandage and placed on a pillow, blanket, air splint, or any available splinting material until a physician can give further treatment.

INJURIES TO THE CREST OF ILEUM AND THE GROIN
Groin

Although groin injuries have never presented a serious problem in athletics, muscle strains are frequently detected in this area. Symptoms include pain with hip flexion, abduction, hyperextension, and rotation. There is a limited range of motion, and the characteristic walk favors the involved hip. Treatment of groin strain consists of ice for a minimum of 12 hours and rest. Moist heat helps restore muscle function in a few days. When the athlete is able to walk normally without pain, a spica wrap is applied to the upper thigh and lower abdominal area with 2- to 4-inch elastic roller bandage. This spica wrap supports the hip muscles and aids hip flexion, enabling participation in athletics even though there is slight pain. The injury is rarely disabling.

Crest of the ileum contusion

The crest of the ileum is subjected to trauma when the athlete fails to properly wear hip pads designed to protect this area. Pads are frequently worn too low, exposing the crest to trauma. Occasionally, a shoulder or helmet hits this point with terrific force and the injury cannot be avoided. Symptoms include marked pain and limited range of motion, particularly trunk rotation. There is swelling, and coughing or sneezing cause acute pain. Swelling is noted on visual examination. Fortunately fracture of the crest of the ileum is rare, and treatment for contusion is the same as that prescribed for other contusions.

KNEE INJURIES

Although considered to be a hinge joint, the knee is not a true hinge. In flexion it has the ability to go into a medial or lateral rotation. The knee does not have a true joint capsule for stabilization, unlike other joints; therefore it is particularly subject to a variety of injuries. The cartilages that lie on the condyles of the tibia are injured if forced rotation takes place. The collateral ligaments are injured if the stabilized knee is hit from a medial or lateral plane. The cruciate ligaments are injured if the body is hit from either the front or the back while the leg is in complete extension and the foot is stabilized. Multiple damage (to the medial collateral ligament, to the medial cartilage, and to the anterior cruciate ligament) occurs when the cleats of a football player are stabilized in the ground during forced medial rotation. This injury, classified as the "unholy triad," has been occurring frequently in athletics during recent years.

When examining a knee injury, it is important to know how the injury occurred. The knowledge of this fact enables one to understand the structural derangement that takes place and the exact anatomic location of injury. Palpation is an excellent means of determining any irregularity around the joint, and point tenderness is an important indicator of ligamentous tissue damage or derangement. (Point tenderness over the joint margin, medially or laterally, may indicate either cartilage or meniscus damage.)

Medial collateral ligament involvement

The ligament may be torn or severed when the athlete is subjected to a forceful blow from the side while the foot is stabilized. The medial collateral ligament is longer than the lateral collateral ligament and has a deep branch that attaches at one point on the outer rim of the medial cartilage border. Generally when the medial ligament is stretched, torn, or severed, the medial cartilage is also torn. There is inability to bear weight and point tenderness over the ligamentous area. Swelling is highly variable with time and with the degree of injury. There is pain, and the joint may be unstable.

A visual examination should be accomplished before the individual is moved, to determine any displacement of bone. The athlete should be calmed and the leg should be completely extended before an abduction test is performed. One hand is placed on the lateral aspect of the knee and the other hand is placed medially on the ankle. Pressure is exerted on the knee joint to determine whether there is any relaxation of the medial ligament. Then the knee is placed in partial flexion and the same procedure is repeated. Comparison with the opposite knee determines the amount of relaxation of the ligament if there is any question of tearing.

If the medial ligament is stretched or slightly torn (which may only involve a few fibers), ice and pressure should be applied for a minimum of 1 hour, and application of ice during the entire evening is recommended. The knee will not become stiff and sore for several hours after activity. Foam rubber should be placed under a 4- or 6-inch elastic roller bandage. Crutches are generally unnecessary with this type of sprain.

If the medial ligament is partially torn and relaxation is present, the athlete cannot bear weight well. In this case the knee should be wrapped with an elastic bandage before the athlete is carried from the playing area. Ice and pressure should be applied immediately. The ice should be placed in large plastic bags encasing the knee to control hemorrhage and swelling. Ice should remain for at least 24 hours. The extent of relaxation and gapping of the joint should be determined by x-ray films during forced abduction. Avoidance of weight bearing and bed rest with elevation are important during the first 24 hours. When the medial ligament is completely severed, orthopedic consultation must naturally be requested.

Lateral collateral ligament involvement

The ligament is torn or severed when the knee is subjected to a forceful blow from the medial side while the foot is stabilized. The symptoms are generally the same as those encountered in medial involvement except that the athlete generally bears weight well with this type of tear or sprain. The lateral ligament is much shorter than the medial one and neither pain nor immobility is marked.

The examination procedure is reversed from that of the medial ligament, with one hand placed on the medial aspect of the knee and the other hand placed laterally on the ankle. Procedures to determine the extent of injury and the nature of treatment are the same as those for the medial collateral ligament.

Anterior and posterior cruciate ligament involvement

The anterior cruciate ligament is generally torn or severed by forced hyperextension at the knee. The posterior cruciate ligament is torn or severed if the tibia is forced backward while the knee is in complete extension. Both ligaments have been known to rupture when the athlete is struck below the partially flexed knee while the cleats of the football shoe are locked in the ground, thereby forcing medial rotation of the knee. Concomitant tearing at the medial collateral ligament and the medial cartilage may also occur. The extended knee generally lacks stability. Pain may be present, although little swelling is detected until several hours after injury.

During examination the knee is flexed at 90 degrees and the drawer sign is used in the following manner to determine the extent of tearing or possible severing. The hands are placed below the knee with a firm grip around the leg; the leg is pulled forward and pushed backward. The distance that the leg glides forward and backward determines the severity of injury. Slight displacement anteriorly or posteriorly indicates only mild damage; however, if the ligament is completely ruptured, the knee glides forward or backward with no resistance.

In mild and moderate tearing of ligaments, the knee should be immediately encased in ice to limit hemorrhage and swelling. The ice should be continued for a minimum of 24 hours and in some cases up to 48 hours. The leg should be wrapped from the foot to well above the knee with an elastic bandage, and it should be elevated. The physician may wrap the knee heavily with cotton wadding and place it in half or full cylindrical cast. Crutches are issued. If the cruciate ligament is ruptured, the physician handling the case decides whether surgical intervention is needed.

Medial and lateral semilunar cartilage involvement

The medial cartilage is injured more frequently than the lateral cartilage. Its injury is caused primarily by the forced medial rotation of the knee from partial flexion while the cleats of the shoe are locked in the ground, thus tearing the cartilage. The cleated shoe is the largest cause of all cartilage injuries. The cartilage is also torn if the knee is hit from either the medial or the lateral side while partially flexed and while the shoe is stabilized. Forced medial or lateral rotation tears the cartilage. The primary symptom of any torn cartilage is locking of the joint in partial flexion. In walking the knee may collapse or give way. The knee may also present a clicking sensation when walking or squatting. Pain and point tenderness are present at the joint margin, although these may be delayed symptoms. If an athlete says he "cuts up field and feels the knee give way," this is a positive indication of a cartilage tear. Walking is possible, but comfort depends on the degree of tearing. Fluid is not always immediately present, but if the cartilage is torn, fluid will increase or decrease, depending on the activity of the athlete.

If the medial ligament is sprained or ruptured, generally the medial cartilage is torn. When the abduction test is applied, the cartilage will "pluck." The presence of the McMurray sign (the knee presents a "click" when going into extension) is a good indication of posterior tears of the cartilage. The athlete is placed on a table with the knee flexed at 90 degrees. The heel is grasped and rotated in external rotation and the knee extended by circling the leg. A "click" or pain from this action indicates tearing.

The immediate treatment of a torn cartilage consists of ice, pressure, and immobility with crutches. Ice and immobilization should be continued for at least 24 hours. Crutches may be indicated for a longer period of time. A pressure bandage with foam rubber should be worn at all times to support the knee and to control synovial fluid increase. Treatment is generally conservative until point tenderness and pain subside; however, if the knee cannot be unlocked with manipulation or traction, surgery is, of course, advised. Traction has been used to unlock the cartilage, and, with conservative treatment, some athletes have been able to complete a season with the knee taped without ill effects. It must be remembered that pain and the knee "giving way" should not be tolerated when the athlete is participating in an event.

During his convalescence the athlete must maintain quadriceps tone by such methods as isometric contraction and progressive resistive exercise.

ANKLE INJURIES
Sprain

A sprain is fibrous tearing of ligaments, either partially or completely. The identifying features of a sprained ankle may differ markedly, depending on the severity of the sprain. The manner in which the athlete walks gives an indication of the severity of his sprain. The symptoms are inability to bear weight, swelling resulting from internal bleeding (hemorrhage may or may not appear immediately; swelling, in many instances, does not begin for 5 or 6 hours), pain, and point tenderness over ligamentous tissue. Bony irregularity is an indication of fracture. Derangement of the ankle joint is an indication of severe ankle injury, which, although not often seen in athletics, is not beyond possibility.

On the field, the athlete should be calmed before any examination begins. An attempt should be made to determine how the injury occured. Only after careful observation of the position of the ankle and foot should the shoelaces be cut, and the shoe should be removed with care. Pressing the tibia and fibula together helps to determine the possibility of a fracture, which is indicated by marked pain with this action. Palpation of the ligaments surrounding the joint reveals tenderness, swelling, or bony irregularity. If possible, determination of range of motion will enable evaluation of the degree of injury. If range of motion is limited, the athlete should be carried off the field to receive a more complete examination.

If range of motion is good and pain is not severe, bearing weight on the ankle will determine whether there is any limitation while standing. In the absence of pain and if the attending physician consents, the athlete may return to the game. It must be emphasized, however, that the injury may not present any immediate symptoms. If, with continued activity, the athlete begins favoring the ankle, he should be removed from the game immediately for treatment.

Treatment should be initiated with elevation, ice, and pressure. Ice should be packed entirely around the ankle and lower limb. Heavy ice-filled plastic bags have proved to be the most effective means for controlling hemorrhage. A regular icebag does not offer adequate hypothermia and does not control hemorrhage to any marked degree. Ice, pressure, and elevation should be continued for a minimum of 24 hours and in some cases as long as 48 hours or until a physician examines the injury.

Ice should be applied when the athlete returns home and should be continued throughout the night.

The use of foam rubber under the elastic pressure bandage, when swelling is present, is a general practice at the University of Missouri. The bandaging is removed when the athlete goes to bed and is reapplied when he awakens. He continues this procedure until swelling subsides.

The elastic wrap is applied with mild pressure, beginning at the toes, enclosing the ankle, and ending below the calf. If the toes swell, the wrap is too tight and should be reapplied. Elevation of the foot reduces the temporary swelling.

QUESTIONS

1. Why do athletic injuries (which obviously overlap greatly with other areas of this text) deserve special consideration here?
2. Before any special treatment of athletic emergencies per se, what general principles of first aid must apply?
3. Discuss the particular importance of accurate history and careful initial examination of the athletically injured patient.
4. Why is the knee joint of particular concern in the context of this chapter?
5. What is the importance of accurately determining and recording body positioning at the time of a knee injury?
6. Of what special implication is loss of consciousness in treating the patient who sustains injury during athletics?
7. What are the implications of hyperventilation in the handling of athletic emergencies?

SUGGESTED READINGS

Klafs, C. E., and Arnheim, D. D.: Modern principles of athletic training, ed. 4, St. Louis, 1977, The C. V. Mosby Co.

Litton, L. O., and Peltier, L. F.: Athletic injuries, Boston, 1963, Little, Brown & Co.

Moseley, H. F., Shoulder lesions, ed. 3, New York, 1953, Paul B. Hoeber, Inc.

O'Donoghue, D. H.: Treatment of injuries to athletes, ed. 2, Philadelphia, 1970, W. B. Saunders Co.

CHAPTER 28

Abdominal trauma

Despite the use of antibiotics, despite blood replacement techniques and the availability of blood substitutes, and despite other refinements in treatment, the morbidity and mortality from major abdominal trauma are still excessively high. The crux of the problem—the hope for increased survival rates—rests on the early management of patients with abdominal trauma. Early management is basically a matter of prompt diagnosis to institute immediate and effective treatment.

PROMPTNESS: THE SINE QUA NON

Delays in diagnosis of abdominal trauma are attributable to several factors. Patients arrive in the emergency room with multiple injuries, injuries of more *apparent* urgency than whatever trauma has been provoked within the abdomen. A shocklike state may mask the signs of intra-abdominal trauma to the extent that the clinical picture may be considerably altered. The patient with alcoholic intoxication is difficult to diagnose accurately at an early stage; some drug addiction problems present a similar picture. The unconscious patient can give no history, and his abdominal examination may be difficult to interpret. The onset of peritonitis from sharp or blunt perforation may be insidious and may escape early detection. If the patient arrives in the emergency room within a few minutes after receiving the trauma, there may be no intra-abdominal signs to indicate perforation of a hollow viscus.

The general priorities previously emphasized apply equally to the patient with suspected abdominal trauma. Patients with abdominal injury often have associated fractures of extremities, head injuries, and thoracic injuries. A proper assessment of the overall importance of these injuries must be made.

The pathology may include a multitude of possibilities and countless combinations of injuries. In evaluating any blunt or penetrating injury of the abdomen, one should keep in mind the possibility of a lacerated liver, a ruptured spleen, trauma to the pancreas, torn mesentery, diaphragmatic rupture, urinary bladder rupture, laceration of the vena cava or aorta, retroperitoneal hematoma or renal injury, ruptured duodenum or jejunum, gastric or colonic perforation, or injury to the gallbladder, portal vein, or abdominal portion of the esophagus.

As always, the need for adequate ventilation is obvious. Nasogastric suction should be started. An intravenous infusion using a large-bore needle should be done. In some instances a subclavian catheter should be inserted to obtain central venous pressure monitoring. Regardless of the complaints of the patient, analgesics or narcotics should not be administered until a diagnosis is made. At the time of venipuncture, blood should be obtained for typing and cross-matching as well as for measuring serum electrolytes and serum amylase levels.

The history of the injury may provide important clues. The location and nature of any blunt trauma should be noted. Initial complaint of radiation of pain to the left supraclavicular fossa may be noted after a splenic tear, for example.

By observing the patient, the respiratory excursions can be noted. With intra-abdominal hemorrhage or peritoneal contamination, splinting of the abdominal muscles is observed and respiratory activity is generally of a thoracic nature. If abdominal contents are exposed, prompt covering with the most sterile dressing available is indicated.

Undue apprehension and thirst should lead one to suspect abdominal hemorrhage. These are often complained of before a significant fall in blood pressure is noted. Palpation of the abdomen for areas of maximal discomfort, muscle guarding, or rebound tenderness should be carefully done. If the patient is in shock, the findings may be partially obscured. Evidence of rebound tenderness indicative of peritonitis usually takes a matter of several hours to develop.

Percussion is significant if the usual area of liver dullness is absent as a result of the accumulation of free air in the peritoneal cavity over and above the liver. On auscultation the absence of bowel sounds is significant, particularly if one has listened carefully for a period of 2 to 3 minutes in each quadrant.

Despite suggestive findings on inspection, palpation, percussion, and auscultation, early diagnosis of an intra-abdominal catastrophe may be delayed unless one exhausts one's armamentarium while the patient is still in the emergency room.

ABDOMINAL PARACENTESIS AND/OR PERITONEAL LAVAGE

Abdominal paracentesis is of the greatest help in determining the presence and nature of any free intra-abdominal fluid. One can diagnose a ruptured spleen or intra-abdominal hemorrhage within a few minutes of the patient's arrival in the emergency room and thereby facilitate prompt removal to the operating room. High amylase readings in the aspirated fluid may indicate trauma to the pancreas. Aspirated fluid with high leukocyte counts points to early peritonitis; occasionally bile may be aspirated. We have never aspirated urine but such a possibility may occur. A urinary catheter is generally inserted at the time of the patient's admission, however, to rule out a urinary tract injury. Fluid removed from the abdomen can be checked for peritoneal ammonia. Levels above 3 mg per milliliter suggest a perforated bowel or urinary extravasation.

Although different techniques are described for the abdominal paracentesis, including the four-quadrant tap, the single midline abdominal paracentesis is preferred. A small subcutaneous wheal is made with procaine hydrochloride (Novocain) or lidocaine (Xylocaine). After a scapel has been used to incise the skin for several millimeters, a No. 14 needle is inserted into the anterior abdominal wall through which an intracath or appropriate polyethylene catheter is inserted. As the needle is slowly advanced, so also is the catheter advanced within the needle. At the moment the needle moves beyond the posterior rectus sheath and the peritoneum into the intra-abdominal cavity, the catheter advances freely beyond the needle. At this point the needle is withdrawn and the catheter is inserted to the desired depth and to some degree in the desired direction.

Of particular aid is proper positioning of the patient to aspirate a representative quantity of intra-abdominal fluid content. The knee-chest position has proved to be of particular value for small quantities of fluid that gravitate in such a manner that aspiration is possible. If aspiration fails to reveal any blood or fluid, then the catheter should still be maintained in place and observed at several-minute intervals because a positive tap can often be obtained simply by capillary action of the fluid within the polyethylene catheter. By insertion of the catheter with proper positioning of the patient, a positive tap is almost always obtained if there is any free abdominal fluid. The same tubing used for the paracentesis may also be used for a peritoneal dialysis. This test has become increasingly popular as an adjunct in determining intra-abdominal complications.

Diagnostic peritoneal lavage may be performed with 1,000 ml of Ringer's lactate solution in an adult or 300 to 500 ml in children. The connected infusion bottle is then lowered to floor level, creating a siphon to return the peritoneal fluid. As little as 75 ml of free blood in the peritoneal cavity colors the perfusate salmon pink, an indication for laparotomy. In addition to amylase determinations, microscopic examination for fecal material or bacteria should be done.

DIATRIZOATE TEST FOR INTESTINAL PERFORATION

In the case of perforation of the stomach, the small intestine, or (occasionally) the colon, we have found the urine precipitation test for diatrizoate salts after the ingestion of Gastrografin to be a valuable diagnostic aid. Gastrografin is not normally absorbed in any appreciable amount within the gastrointestinal tract. If, however, it escapes into the peritoneal cavity, it is rapidly absorbed and subsequently excreted by the kidneys. Its early detection in the urine can be made by adding *concentrated* hydrochloric acid a drop at a time to a test-tube specimen of the patient's urine. If a white, chalky precipitate is seen, the diagnosis of a perforation can be made, providing that the patient has not been taking penicillin. Penicillin salts precipitate in a similar fashion. The latter problem can be circumvented, however, by first checking a control sample of the patient's urine for a precipitate. In this case the specific gravity of the patient's urine can be measured at 15-minute intervals to note whether diatrizoate is present, as indicated by the gradual rise in urine specific gravity. In several instances we have seen the specific gravity rise rapidly within 30 minutes to 1.050. The diatrizoate salts can be administered via the nasogastric tube. With adults 50 to 60 ml is an appropriate dose. In babies the hypertonicity of the Gastrografin may contraindicate its usage.

As mentioned, it is important to avoid a false-positive test by first doing a control or by utilizing specific gravity determinations. A false-negative reaction may be obtained if dilute rather than concentrated hydrochloric acid is used.

X-RAY DIAGNOSIS

Should abdominal x-ray films be used? Although abdominal x-ray films may provide useful information, the urgency of the information is lessened by the previously mentioned examination and test. In the case of a foreign body such as a bullet, the path of the bullet and the nature of the injuries may be more nearly ascertained or suspected by the location of the bullet or foreign body. A rupture of the diaphragm may be suspected early by use of the chest film. In many instances, however, the patient is not able to stand in an upright position for an accurate determination of free air beneath the diaphragm because of the semishock state. For an accurate determination of the intra-abdominal air, the patient should be in an upright position for at least 3 to 5 minutes. A film in the lateral decubitus position can be obtained in lieu of a film in the upright position and, while its accuracy is somewhat less, its value is still a real one.

STAB WOUNDS

Controversy continues over the early management of stab wounds of the abdomen. The advocates of mandatory laparotomy point to the risk of undiagnosed perforation of a hollow viscus or laceration of the liver, spleen, or a major vascular component. Those urging selective management with a conservative approach in a sizable number of cases stress the reliability of current diagnostic observations.

A stab wound with questionable peritoneal penetration can be investigated through an incision, longitudinally placed by preference, approximately 3 cm to the side of the stab wound and carried down to the peritoneum by muscle-splitting action. This is not best performed in the emergency room, of course, but should be done in the operating room where the exploration, if positive for intra-abdominal penetration, can be further extended into a laparotomy. Avoiding a laparotomy is particularly advantageous in the alcoholic patient or in an individual with upper respiratory infection or active pulmonary disease. The patient may have just eaten, and the possibility of vomitus aspiration increases the risk.

Renal and major venous injuries in penetrating abdominal trauma can be anticipated preoperatively by use of a venogram.

Although pancreatic injury should be suspected in any trauma to the upper abdomen, particularly as in an automobile accident, the preoperative diagnosis is difficult to make. A rise in serum amylase level is, however, usually noted within a few hours of injury.

SUMMARY

The immediate care of the patient with abdominal trauma must, in addition to emphasizing the possibilities of other injuries elsewhere in the body, center on the urgency of an early diagnosis. With the present diagnostic armamentarium in addition to a careful evaluation of the circumstances of the injury and the physical findings, *prompt* diagnosis should usually be established.

QUESTIONS

1. Why is promptness preeminent in dealing with abdominal trauma?
2. Compare use of the diatrizoate test with abdominal x-ray films in specific situations.
3. Which particular problems may best be evaluated by use of abdominal paracentesis?
4. Define *free abdominal fluid* with particular regard to its diagnostic significance.
5. Characterize several symptoms of abdominal hemorrhage.
6. Comment on the controversial nature of managing stab wounds of the abdomen.
7. Explain the significance of free air beneath the diaphragm in the diagnosis of abdominal injury.
8. What are the particular advantages of the Gastrografin test? What are its disadvantages for emergency-care application?
9. Relate diagnostic competence to early administration of analgesia, particularly in cases of abdominal trauma.
10. What is the main hope for increased survival in patients with abdominal trauma?

CHAPTER 29

Chest trauma

The initial management of the victim of thoracic trauma may often require the application of immediate lifesaving measures. Gunshot wounds, stab wounds, and blunt trauma to the chest provoke most of the serious injuries that require urgent attention. Of the large number of deaths from automobile accidents each year in the United States, it is estimated that more than half of these deaths result from injuries to the contents of the chest. The immediate and effective initial supportive measures followed by careful observation may suffice in almost three fourths of all cases of chest trauma. A relative few will require immediate operation.

This text is concerned with those emergency measures required in the immediate care of the patient; therefore most of the subsequent remarks in this chapter are not concerned with decisions made after x-ray studies, electrocardiogram, blood gas level determinations, and aortography. It is necessary for the immediate care to be rendered with a particular view toward recognizing those emergencies that require early surgery and whose early recognition therefore is imperative. Immediate operation in patients sustaining thoracic trauma is most commonly required by hemorrhage and shock, cardiac tamponade, injury to the great vessels, and rupture of the diaphragm.

As cautioned in other chapters, extensive multiple-system injuries and bleeding sites are especially common in patients who have received blunt trauma.

Although intrathoracic hemorrhage frequently originates from an intercostal or internal mammary vessel, it may also result from a lacerated lung or torn mediastinal structures. Thoracic injuries are different in certain ways from injuries in other anatomic areas. Of particular concern is the intrathoracic pressure. When the normally negative intrathoracic pressure relationship is disturbed, the cardiopulmonary dynamics are altered. Therefore the immediate goal in the management of the patient with a thoracic injury is restoration of cardiopulmonary function as nearly to the normal state as possible. This even supersedes the control of hemorrhage. Ventilation takes precedence.

Of first priority is a necessity to inflate the lung. If ventilation does not occur properly, there exists an immediate need to locate the cause for an unexpanded lung or portion of lung. As previously emphasized, the patient should be completely disrobed to adequately view the chest wall for any evidence of paradoxic motion, open wounds of the chest, signs of rib fractures, or stab wounds.

RECOGNIZING A CHEST INJURY

In many instances the presence of chest trauma is obvious, but in instances of multiple injuries including unconsciousness from a head injury, the intrathoracic injuries may not be so apparent. Of particular importance is the observation that the patient is experiencing dyspnea, is complaining of chest pain, has hemoptysis, or is coughing. A rapid respiratory rate, mucous membrane or nail beds indicative of inadequate oxygenation, or the presence of blood-tinged sputum should certainly indicate that all is not well within the chest. Other significant clinical observations include a chest wall that is moving in a paradoxic fashion, the obvious presence of a sucking wound of the chest, distended neck veins in the presence of shock, deviation of the trachea in the suprasternal notch, absent or distant breath sounds or heart tones, stridor or a crowing type of respiration, and marked restlessness. Most of these findings, if allowed to persist by failure to correct the underlying pathophysiology, rapidly lead to respiratory failure and shock.

The frequently emphasized point throughout this book is pertinent here and must be repeated: To adequately examine and diagnose the problem, one must disrobe the patient and observe the chest wall, palpate, and auscultate. Unless this is done, the presence of paradoxic motion, an open wound, or crepitus may be overlooked. (Crepitus in this case refers to the presence of air within the superficial layers of the chest wall.)

Without adequate ventilation and perfusion the patient may rapidly become confused and agitated. The resulting depressed state of consciousness suggests that a head injury is present. The patient's cerebration may be rapidly restored if adequate respiration once again takes place.

PNEUMOTHORAX

If lung ventilation is impossible on one side of the chest, a tension pneumothorax may be present. This situation involves a rapid buildup of intrapleural tension that causes a collapse of the lung on the involved side with displacement of the mediastinal structures to the opposite side. In displacing the mediastinal structures, the heart and great vessels including the large veins are compromised and cardiac filling is disturbed. This progressive buildup of pressure must be relieved by venting the intrapleural air to the outside. A large-bore needle may be the only means available, and if a needle is not available, even a stab wound may be lifesaving. Although a large-bore tube ideally should be inserted or attached to an undersealed drain, these approaches may be mandatory on an immediate basis.

The open sucking wound of the chest produces a marked shift toward the contralateral lung with subsequent compression. When the air is expired, the mediastinum shifts backwards producing the so-called mediastinal flutter with its associated hypoxic effect.

Ideally a large petrolatum gauze dressing is best for immediate application over the sucking wound with an adequate amount of overlying gauze to support the pressure. Obviously more definitive management of the wound is indicated after the patient arrives in the emergency room or the operating room.

A pneumothorax without a great deal of tension is seldom an indication for emergency care prior to arrival in the emergency room. Usually a tube thoracotomy is employed after admission, if the pneumothorax is greater than 20%.

CARDIAC ARREST

Cardiac arrest in association with chest injuries is not uncommon. Closed-chest cardiac massage and proper management of the airway and artificial ventilation as discussed in Chapter 12 usually suffice. Nevertheless open and direct cardiac massage may be the only effective means of resuscitating some of these victims. For example, cardiac tamponade requires opening of the pericardium and direct cardiac compression unless adequate decompression of the pericardial sac is quickly achieved with needle aspiration. Other indications for direct cardiac massage are discussed in Chapter 12.

CARDIAC TAMPONADE

Once one is assured that ventilation is occurring, the next procedure of immediate priority relates to the possibility of the pericardial tamponade. Since rapid filling of the pericardial sac with blood markedly compresses the vena cava and the chambers of the heart, the venous return to the heart is seriously impaired. Adequate diastole (filling of the ventricular components of the heart) is prevented, thereby limiting the amount of cardiac output with a resultant fall in coronary artery filling and decreased blood pressure. Because of the nature of steering wheel injuries and many other cases of blunt trauma to the chest, a cardiac tamponade effect can occur, involving a laceration or puncture wound of the heart or intrapericardial portion of the aorta. One can suspect acute hemopericardium of sufficient nature to cause a cardiac tamponade by clinically observing distended neck veins, a low peripheral arterial pressure, and a high systemic venous pressure.

Immediate decompression of the pericardial sac is indicated and can be done through a needle aspiration of the left parasternal fifth or sixth interspace. This effort at decompression often enables the patient to be transported to the hospital for a thoracotomy, pericardiotomy, and correction of the underlying pathology. Nevertheless problems may occur in patients with multiple injuries. The usual signs of cardiac tamponade may not be evident in association with hypovolemia, hypotension, and respiratory distress.

BLUNT CARDIAC TRAUMA

The possibility of cardiac injury during blunt trauma should be strongly suspected in all accident victims who may have a thoracic or upper abdominal injury. Of the more than 5,000,000 automobile injuries that occurred in 1973, it has been estimated that as many as 900,000 were varying degrees of cardiac trauma and almost 3,000 resulted in death. Not only can a deceleration injury occur, but other possible mechanisms include a direct blow to the myocardium or direct chest compression of the myocardium between the sternum and the thoracic vertebrae. Jackson and Murphy, as noted in the suggested readings at the end of this chapter, present a complete summary of the various types of nonpenetrating injuries to the heart in an automobile accident. The injuries to the myocardium may range from severe contusions, lacerations, and rupture to septal perforation as well as hemopericardium and tamponade. There is always the possibility that myocardial contusion may provoke a sudden episode of ventricular fibrillation.

Although the immediate management of cardiac injury during blunt trauma is somewhat limited, it is important to be aware of many possibilities of injury to or rupture of the aortic, mitral, or tricuspid valves, pericardium, cardiac septa, and coronary arteries. A number of these injuries are managed successfully by prompt surgery. As mentioned, early recognition of pericardial trauma and immediate peri-cardiocentesis may be lifesaving.

RUPTURE OF THE HEART

Frequently the rupture involves the right or left atrial appendage because these are the weakest and thinnest portions of the heart. A major intracardiac rupture can be confirmed by observing cyanosis in the upper part of the patient's body in association with shock and a high central venous pressure. A high central venous pressure almost certainly indicates cardiac tamponade unless there has been sufficient bleeding from the great vessels to compress the superior vena cava.

MASSIVE BLOOD LOSS

Massive blood loss within the chest may occasionally pose an insurmountable problem. In many instances the bleeding is from low-pressure vessels. If the blood volume interferes markedly with lung volume, a repeated thoracocentesis may stabilize the patient. When possible the insertion of a thoracotomy tube is indicated. In spite of severe exsanguination, many patients with stab wounds of the heart or injury to the great vessels can be saved.

If it is apparent that the patient has suffered a deceleration type of injury, a rupture of the aorta just distal to the left subclavian artery resulting from the shearing effect should be suspected. A tracheal deviation (possibly resulting from a large hematoma) or a systolic murmur is further evidence that an aortic injury may have taken place. Asymmetry of the radial pulses, paralysis of the vocal cords, or a superior vena caval syndrome type of compression all should prompt one to go quickly to the emergency room. A posteroanterior film of the chest can determine the presence of a widened mediastinum.

Although the majority of patients with a hemothorax do not require a thoracotomy, they require observation and monitoring in the emergency room. Recurrent hypotension and recurrent bleeding often prompt emergency thoracotomy after arrival in the hospital.

FLAIL CHEST

The markedly reduced ventilation occurring as the result of paradoxic motion with a flail chest can be improved by a number of rather simple techniques. Inserting a cuffed endotracheal tube and inflating the lungs under positive pressure ventilation may stabilize the flail chest. Simply turning the patient onto the injured side or maintaining pressure against the involved side may prevent some degree of paradoxic motion over the flailing portion of the chest. Further efforts to stabilize the chest by mechanical means can be taken in the emergency room and a tracheostomy can also be performed.

RUPTURE OF DIAPHRAGM

Although it is relatively uncommon, there may be sufficient trauma of either a penetrating or blunt nature to rupture the diaphragm. Rupture of the diaphragm with herniation of the abdominal contents into the thoracic cavity occurs most commonly on the left side. This complication calls for early surgery and its diagnosis is usually confirmed by roentgenograms. Of an immediate nature is the need to give intermittent positive pressure respiration if the patient is in marked cardiorespiratory distress from compression of pulmonary tissue by the abdominal viscera that have been drawn up into the thoracic cavity.

EMERGENCY TRACHEOSTOMY

Even under optimum conditions, a tracheostomy may be a difficult technical procedure. There are few times when an emergency tracheostomy should be performed immediately because an endotracheal tube can be used to establish an effective airway in a more rapid manner. The cricothyroid membrane puncture as described in Chapter 10 may serve well if there is obstruction of the airway and no endotracheal tube is available.

PHYSIOLOGIC CONSIDERATIONS

Although one is exposed to a great deal of instruction concerned with the physiology of respiration, a brief review of pulmonary function is appropriate. A proper working understanding of the pathophysiology of urgent lifethreatening thoracic injuries is the crux of understanding proper therapy.

If one considers the respiratory process as simply an adequate exchange of gases between the patient and his environment, one can separate pulmonary function into the phase or process of ventilation and that of gas exchange.

Ventilation simply refers to the ability or technique of getting oxygen into the lungs. Once it has reached the lungs, the mechanism by which oxygen gets into the circulating blood while carbon dioxide exits from circulation is referred to as gas exchange. Adequate gas exchange or the diffusion of oxygen and carbon dioxide across the alveolocapillary membrane, of course, depends on the adequate circulation of blood through the lungs.

Where can things go wrong? Interference with the mechanism of either the ventilatory phase or the gas exchange phase can lead to serious disruption.

To begin with, the arrival of oxygen in the lungs can be interfered with in a number of ways. If the lung volume is reduced by a pneumothorax, the air within the pleural cavity collapses the lung on the involved side and often interferes with the expansion on the opposite side. Blood in the thoracic cavity (hemothorax) likewise reduces lung volume and thereby diminishes ventilation. If the integrity of the diaphragm has been interfered with as in a traumatic rupture, the abdominal viscera may herniate into the thoracic cavity to the extent that lung volume becomes markedly reduced.

With ventilation there is an important time relation in which lung volume has to be expanded and collapsed over a time period. The term *tidal volume* refers to the volume of air that enters or leaves the respiratory tract with each breath. This aspect of ventilation may be interfered with if there is an obstruction of the airway by vomitus, blood, or foreign objects. When a massive crushing injury to the chest produces a stoving-in effect or a fracture of multiple ribs, the chest expansion occurs in a paradoxic fashion. One may observe an inspiration expansion of the uninvolved side of the chest and a collapse of the flail portion, whereas with expiration the involved side shows expansion. The air in the normal side may be expired not only into the trachea but to the abnormal side as well. A somewhat similar effect is produced with an open pneumothorax or a so-called sucking wound. In an injury that results in an open wound to the chest, air is sucked through the wound into the thoracic cavity on inspiration, thus collapsing the lung on the side of the injury and moving the mediastinum to the opposite side. This decreases ventilation on the uninvolved side and also decreases cardiac output. Pulmonary ventilation is dependent on other factors, such as central nervous system control of respiratory rates and depths, normal functioning of the respiratory muscles used in respiration, and an effective elasticity of the lungs. This last factor is called lung compliance. None of these last factors is considered to be of major importance in the immediate care of lung or thoracic injuries.

In addition to adequate pulmonary ventilation, effective and adequate pulmonary gas exchange must be present; otherwise respiratory failure and shock quickly occur. The relationship of ventilation and gas exchange is fundamental. If ventilation perfusion inadequacies are of significant magnitude, obvious signs of hypoxemia or hypoventilation are present. Examples of chest trauma that may produce a marked derangement of the ventilation perfusion rate are hemothorax, pneumothorax, and bronchial obstruction. *Immediate* care of the patient suffering thoracic trauma is followed as soon as possible by the more definitive measures available in the emergency room and operating suite of the hospital. As in other seriously injured patients, an intravenous route should be rapidly established to replace any blood loss and to combat hypovolemia. Measures as outlined in Chapter 4 are employed. Occasionally a patient benefits by being moved directly to the operating room to receive more effective resuscitative measures. For example, a patient with a penetrating wound of the heart can be taken first to the operating room where further observation, probably pericardial paracentesis, and ideal monitoring can be accomplished.

Again, it should be emphasized that the *immediate* measures employed for patients with serious chest trauma are of the utmost importance and, if properly employed, are extremely rewarding. Generally speaking these measures are relatively simple. Some of these measures have been outlined in this chapter. One should refer also to Chapters 4, 10, and 12 because of an obvious overlapping of information.

SUMMARY

The morbidity and mortality of chest injuries are directly proportional to the effectiveness of early therapy. The need for ventilatory support as soon as possible is usually evident. As previously emphasized, there is a high percentage of multiple organ system involvement: Head injuries, visceral lacerations, and ruptured spleens, as well as fractures, occur with great frequency. Immediate care requires a high degree of alertness, knowledgeability, and often decisive action.

QUESTIONS

1. Discuss the role of *immediate* surgery in treatment of the victim of chest trauma.
2. Describe the clinical features of diagnosing chest trauma in the accident victim.
3. What is pneumothorax? How is it diagnosed and treated in the first-aid routine?
4. What is cardiac tamponade? What is its importance in the management of chest trauma?
5. In what important sense is blunt chest trauma a "hidden killer"?
6. Discuss rupture of the aorta and its significance in the total picture of chest trauma.

7. Define hemothorax and relate the condition to the total picture of thoracic trauma.
8. What is a flail chest, and what is its emergency treatment?
9. What are the two main phases of pulmonary function, and how may each be most often interrupted in emergency situations?
10. What is the primary emergency treatment of pneumothorax?

SUGGESTED READINGS

Bassett, J. S., et al.: Blunt injuries to the chest, J. Trauma 8:418, 1968.

Beall, A. C., Jr., et al.: Considerations in the management of penetrating thoracic trauma, J. Trauma 8:408, 1968.

Jackson, D. H., and Murphy, G. W.: Nonpenetrating cardiac trauma, Mod. Concepts Cardiovasc. Dis. 45:123-128, 1976.

Kish G., et al.: Indications for early thoracotomy in the management of chest trauma, Ann. Thorac. Surg. 22:23-28, 1976.

PART EIGHT

Special considerations

CHAPTER 30

Pediatric emergencies

GERARD J. VAN LEEUWEN

Most parents and many physicians regard all acute illnesses in children as being emergencies. It is impractical to present all of these occurrences in a brief chapter. The management of pediatric emergencies is documented adequately in standard pediatric textbooks. This presentation is designed to help one to recognize and partially manage some of the more frequently encountered emergencies with special emphasis on those that are least likely to be discussed in other areas.

FEVER

What is fever? The exact mechanism of the febrile reaction is not clearly understood. A subnormal body temperature, especially in an infant, is greater cause for alarm than is fever. This indicates that a moderate degree of fever is not detrimental but suggests resistance on the part of the afflicted individual.

Hyperpyrexia, or a rectal temperature of greater than 104° F, has more serious implications. Persistent fever of this degree may either be a result of or lead to dehydration, and it may result in a febrile convulsion and possible brain damage.

There are many approaches to the therapy of pyrexia when such therapy is deemed advisable. It must be remembered that even though salicylate (aspirin) is primarily considered an antipyretic in children, it is also an effective analgesic. There is little physiologic reason for prescribing aspirin for fever when the hyperpyretic stage has not been reached; however, all clinicians and parents vouch for its efficacy in making the child more comfortable, and aspirin is the most widely used antipyretic. The maximum total amount of aspirin that can be tolerated safely within a 24-hour period is 2.0 grains per kilogram of body weight. A safe and usually adequate antipyretic dose is 1 grain per year of age, given every 4 hours. Thus a 5-year-old child may be given 5 grains of aspirin every 4 hours as an antipyretic. Liquid medications containing salicylates are commercially available and easily administered. It is my clinical impression, however, that they are less effective than tablet forms and are more easily used to excess. Aspirin can be given to even the smallest infant by crushing the tablet between spoons and adding any desired kind of liquid vehicle.

Overdosage of salicylate may result in (among other things) renal damage. Salicylates should therefore be avoided in any condition in which improper or decreased renal function may be present, especially in newborn and premature infants, the vomiting patient, and the dehydrated patient.

Many pediatricians today prefer using acetaminophen (Tylenol) in place of aspirin. This is acceptable. Dosage is different than aspirin: up to 1 year—60 mg; 1 to 3 years—60 to 120 mg; and 6 to 12 years—240 mg. Preparations of this type come as drops, elixir, and tablets.

Bathing the child for 15 to 30 minutes in lukewarm water may be effective as a substitute or adjunctive measure. Properly executed alcohol sponging is very effective in reducing fever. The naked child should lie on a towel and an alcohol-soaked towel should be placed on his body for a few seconds. The towel should be removed, and the skin should be allowed to dry before the child is turned over; the process may be repeated for as long as deemed necessary. Cold water enemas are cruel, generally ineffective, and potentially dangerous.

UNCONSCIOUSNESS

Perhaps it is appropriate to list a broad etiologic classification of the conditions that might render a pediatric patient unconscious. Primary intracranial disorders include convulsive disorders, infections, tumors, vascular conditions, and trauma. Systemic conditions affecting the central nervous system are metabolic disorders such as diabetes mellitus, hemorrhagic and cardiovascular conditions, infections, and intoxication. This discussion is limited to the emergency management of a convulsion and a discussion of intoxication caused by the ingestion of poisonous material.

All major seizures are recognized and managed (at least acutely) in essentially an identical manner, irrespective of whether the etiology is fever, poisoning, or unknown. The seizure is usually preceded by some sort of warning or aura; many older children are aware of it and can describe it as peculiar visual disturbances, auditory hallucinations, or simply a sort of "premonition." The seizure then begins with spasm of the larynx followed quickly by generalized muscle tonicity and subsequent clonic movements. Fecal or urinary incontinence usually follows and, finally, sleep.

Once a convulsion has started, it can in no way be halted. If the seizure is prolonged beyond the usual 3 to 5 minutes, termination may be assisted by giving diazepam (Valium), 0.5 mg, every 2 or 3 minutes, directly into a smoothly running intravenous tube. Because the process cannot be abruptly halted, management is aimed at prevention of bodily injury, particularly holding the patient so that he does not fall or bump his head. The time-honored method of inserting something between the teeth serves no purpose once the seizure has begun and may possibly harm the patient and the operator. The postseizure sleep state is often misinterpreted as coma. Distinguishing between the two states requires an experienced clinician.

If the seizure does not respond to diazepam or other drug therapy and is prolonged beyond 20 to 30 minutes, the diagnosis of status epilepticus is made. Then additional management may include special attention to prolonged anoxia, dehydration, and aspiration pneumonia. Adequate oxygenation and administration of intravenous fluids are usually necessary, and antibiotics may be required to combat pneumonia.

In this prolonged state of seizure, drug therapy is of utmost importance. Probably the best drug is diazepam titrate, 0.5 mg every 2 to 3 minutes, as previously outlined. The patient must be observed closely for respiratory depression during this therapy.

Some authorities advocate the use of phenobarbital intramuscularly, 4 to 7 mg per kilogram of body weight. One half of this dosage is given each 30 minutes until most of the manifestations of the seizure are terminated. Other physicians prefer intravenous administration of short-acting barbiturates given continuously and slowly until the seizure stops.

POISONING

Despite complete coverage of poisoning in Chapter 21, certain pediatric aspects of the subject are discussed briefly here.

Children who have ingested hydrocarbons or corrosive agents should not be induced to vomit because of two factors: the danger of aspiration and the re-exposure of the epithelial surfaces to corrosive action. For other poisons (and contrary to common practice) spontaneous or induced vomiting is a more effective procedure in emptying the stomach than is gastric lavage.

Drugs may be used to induce vomiting. Syrup of ipecac has withstood the test of time, although the results are not consistently predictable. Two teaspoons given orally is usually followed by vomiting in 15 to 20 minutes. Extreme caution must be exercised to avoid the use of other forms of ipecac since this agent may in itself be damaging to the central nervous system. More recently the administration of intramuscular apomorphine, 0.06 mg per kilogram of body weight, has been advocated. This results predictably in violent vomiting a few minutes after injection.

If lavage is required, the following points should be kept in mind. A large-caliber rubber tube should be passed into the stomach (usually through the mouth of a pediatric patient). Water is always a safe lavaging agent, although if the specific neutralizing agent is known and available, it should be used. The patient's head should always be kept down to prevent aspiration. At the conclusion of the procedure a neutralizing agent or a cathartic, such as mineral oil, may be instilled. The universal antidote—which contains activated charcoal, tannic acid, and magnesium oxide—may be used if specific agents are not available.

Accidental overdosage of aspirin is probably the most common poisoning in pediatric patients. Again, the maximum amount that can be tolerated within a 24-hour period is about 2 grains per kilogram of body weight; therefore 1 grain per kilogram can usually be tolerated in one ingestion. Fortunately most instances of aspirin poisoning are relatively mild and consequently require very little therapy. If an excessive amount has been ingested, the stomach should be emptied promptly. Alkalinizing fluids should be given because an alkaline urine facilitates the excretion of salicylate. In mild situations carbonated beverages or baking soda may be given orally. For most severe instances bicarbonate must be given intravenously. Intramuscular vitamin K is usually given to prevent hypoprothrombinemia. Very severe cases may require exchange transfusion or dialysis.

The major hydrocarbons accidentally ingested by children today are power mower gasoline and cigarette lighter fluid. The ingestion of hydrocarbons even in small amounts is often followed by a chemical pneumonitis; central nervous system depression may follow ingestion of large amounts. Emptying the stomach is crucial only when apparently more than 4 ounces was taken. Vomiting should be avoided because of the likelihood that aspiration may increase the severity of the pneumonitis. The patient must be observed very closely for pneumonitis and should have a chest x-ray film taken a few hours after ingestion.

RESPIRATORY OBSTRUCTION

Although respiratory obstruction may occur with many infections, it may be complete or nearly complete in three particular situations: severe laryngotracheobronchitis (LTB), acute epiglottitis, and foreign body aspiration. Lateral soft tissue x-ray films of the neck differentiate between the first two. LTB usually responds to cool mist with oxygen if cyanosis is present. The condition is self-limited and subsides within a few days.

Epiglottitis usually occurs in the 3- to 7-year age group. The onset is abrupt, unlike LTB, which is usually gradual. The patient exhibits severe air hunger, drools, and is concentrating on only one thing, his next breath. Lateral soft tissue x-ray films of the neck in extension demonstrate the enlarged epiglottis. The striking difference in severity and outcome of LTB and acute epiglottitis cannot be overemphasized. Most deaths from epiglottitis can be prevented if it is always suspected, or at least considered, in upper airway obstruction.

In epiglottitis if the obstruction is nearly complete, a tracheostomy must be done. In the absence of a skilled operator insertion of several 13- to 15-gauge needles into the trachea may be lifesaving. Insertion is made into the trachea above the suprasternal notch, posteriorly in a caudad direction. There is current interest in attempting nasotracheal intubation before doing a tracheostomy.

Epiglottitis may be caused by a virus but more commonly by *Haemophilus influenzae*. Therefore careful culturing and prompt administration of ampicillin or chloramphenicol is indicated.

Children may aspirate any type of foreign body. If the child is younger than 15 months, the object is usually a safety pin; if the child is older than 15 months, it is usually a vegetable particle, especially a peanut. Less than 2% of these objects are ejected spontaneously; this may occur immediately after aspiration. If the object is visible in the larynx or throat, one may try to retrieve it while the patient is placed in an inverted position to lessen the likelihood that the object may enter the lower respiratory tract.

Objects that pass the larynx usually pass through the trachea and enter a bronchus. Such movement of the particle decreases the urgency but also makes diagnosis more difficult. Inspiration and expiration films and fluoroscopy are usually diagnostic. Diagnostic and removal bronchoscopy should be performed early.

ALLERGIC ASTHMA

The only promptly effective method of therapy for an acute asthmatic attack is prevention. This, of course, is not possible with the first attack. By the same token anxiety generated in parents who observe their child's acute respiratory embarrassment, coughing, and wheezing makes them especially cooperative in attempting to prevent further attacks.

The recognition of an acute asthmatic attack is aided by knowing that the patient has a positive allergic history, especially a family history, and by noting that in the absence of obvious infection he suddenly begins to wheeze. Attacks are often precipitated by fatigue, apprehension, or (obviously) exposure to allergens. In many patients the attack is preceded by a type of aura that the parents and the patient quickly learn to recognize from such symptoms as sneezing, slight coughing, or throat clearing.

Once an attack seems imminent or the warning signs have appeared, the patient is put to bed in a room that is as free as possible of common allergens such as house dust, feathers, wool, or animals. The room should also be free of odors such as paint and tobacco smoke. The child is then given three medications on a 4-hour basis: nose drops or spray, an antihistamine cough preparation, and a specific bronchodilator. Every physician develops his favorite set of drugs; mine vary from time to time. When Tedral is used as a bronchodilator, parents must be warned about the potentiating effects of ephedrine and theophylline, which occasionally results in agitation and central nervous system stimulation of the patient.

If these procedures do not abort or modify the attack, the physician should be contacted. Epinephrine may then be given by injection. Epinephrine in an aqueous solution of 1:1,000, 0.01 to 0.025 ml per kilogram is injected subcutaneously (maximum dose, 0.50 ml). If there is marked improvement in 20 minutes, epinephrine in an aqueous solution of 1:200 (Sus-Phrine) may be administered; one half of the first injection may be given subcutaneously and the patient should be sent home. If there is little improvement after two injections of the 1:1,000 solution of epinephrine at 20-minute intervals, the child should be hospitalized. Some parents can be taught to administer epinephrine when indicated, but they often overdose the patient. Isoproterenol is the most acceptable inhalator and is most effectively used with a nebulizing apparatus.

If the patient does not respond after administration of epinephrine, he is said to be in status asthmaticus, and he must then be hospitalized. As in all situations involving pulmonary disorders, asthmatic or otherwise, the importance of adequate hydration cannot be overemphasized. Water may be given orally if possible, otherwise intravenously. Other nonspecific measures include administration of oxygen, steam, iodides, and usually antibiotics. Specific therapy usually consists of corticosteroids and aminophylline. It is rarely necessary, and usually not advisable, to prescribe corticosteroids in asthma of childhood except in status asthmaticus.

MENINGITIS

A patient with meningitis always produces anxiety not only in his immediate family but also in the school and community. The method of transmission from one individual to another is not clearly understood. With our present knowledge it seems advisable to prophylactically treat all persons who have been in contact with cases of meningitis caused by *Neisseria meningitidis*. Such therapy should consist of rifampin, 10 to 20 mg per kilogram per day, one dose daily for 7 days.

In the infant the symptoms of meningitis appear quite different than those seen in the older child or adult. Not observed in the infant are the high fever, headache, and stiff neck commonly seen in the patient who has reached a degree of neurologic maturity (closure of fontanels and sutures). It is deceptively common for infants to be hypothermic rather than febrile. Classic signs include bulging of the fontanel and projectile vomiting (manifested by headache in the adult and caused by increased intracranial pressure). Both of these findings may be difficult to assess by an untrained person.

Anyone remotely suspected of having meningitis should immediately seek expert attention. No illness of a medical nature is a greater emergency than meningitis. When the physician is able to identify the organism, specific antimicrobial agents are prescribed. In the absence of specific diagnosis, "therapy of unknown organisms" is directed toward simultaneously treating all of the usually incriminated organisms. This consists of ampicillin, 300 to 400 mg per kilogram per day, in divided doses every 4 hours, and chloramphenicol, 100 mg per kilogram per day, divided into 4-hour doses, until the culture reports are available. The chloramphenicol is recommended because of recent reports of some resistant strains of *Haemophilus influenzae*.

VOMITING AND DIARRHEA

Infants and small children are very prone to develop gastroenteritis, and they dehydrate very easily. Vomiting is especially common with any febrile illness and is, in fact, often the first symptom of such illness. Both vomiting and diarrhea are often caused by acute viral enteritis and occasionally by food poisoning.

An adequate history often reveals the cause of vomiting or diarrhea. A very ill child with bloody and mucoid stools usually has a bacterial enteritis. A child who has eaten spoiled food is rarely the only one who partook. If primary bacterial enteritis or that secondary to food poisoning can be excluded, the situation is generally less alarming.

How can dehydration be recognized? Several physical findings appear and are related more to the patient's age than to the degree of dehydration. Failure to tear with crying, dry mucous membranes, decreased or absent urinary output, depressed fontanel, and dry skin with loss of turgor all indicate dehydration.

Vomiting can often be controlled by a short (1- to 2-hour) period of complete abstinence followed by small frequent sips of clear liquids, such as tea, water, or 7-Up. Bland solid foods may be given after 8 hours (banana, cereal, toast, and the like) followed by dilute, boiled skimmed milk after 24 hours. Diarrhea also usually responds to these procedures. There is very little benefit from the use of kaolin, pectin, or opium medications for their intestinal coating action, and they may cause recurrence of vomiting. Very few children fail to respond to this regimen. If they do fail, medical attention should be sought promptly.

A large number of pediatric emergencies have been omitted from this discussion, partially because they are discussed elsewhere in this volume (cardiovascular and metabolic emergencies and care of the premature infant), and partially because these types of emergencies are not often encountered.

QUESTIONS

1. What is the correct dosage of aspirin for pyrexia in a child up to age 10 years?
2. Why should salicylates be avoided in a dehydrated patient?
3. In a 5-year-old child, what is currently the most accepted manner of arresting a grand mal seizure of longer than 5 minutes' duration?
4. After ingestion of small but significant amounts

of which agents should vomiting be avoided if possible?

5. Name two drugs that may be used to induce vomiting after ingestion of an overdose of a drug.

6. What clinical features differentiate croup and epiglottitis?

7. What is the most common foreign body aspirated in a 6-month-old child?

8. What is the definition of status asthmaticus?

9. When is rifampin used in relation to meningitis?

10. Which antibiotic(s) should be used in a 3-year-old child with proved meningitis until culture and sensitivity reports are available?

CHAPTER 31

Otolaryngologic emergencies

JAMES M. LANDEEN

HEMORRHAGE
Lacerations

Severe lacerations to the face, oral cavity, or neck may injure sizable arteries or veins and may cause exsanguination. A 7-year-old girl stepped from a car with soft drink bottles in her arms, headed for a grocery store. She fell on the curb, breaking the bottles. In resuscitation attempts at the hospital, the last of her intravascular fluid was pumped out a laceration of the left common carotid artery by closed cardiac massage. If pressure had been applied immediately to her neck, it may have saved her life.

Oral cavity lacerations may cause bleeding so severe that only bulky packing with gauze may apply the necessary tamponade. This packing may, however, cause airway obstruction. One must be prepared to place a nasal pharyngeal airway or to provide an airway through a cricothyrotomy or tracheostomy.

Unnecessary damage to nerves and intact blood vessels occurs by wildly stabbing into facial lacerations with hemostats trying to stop bleeding. One should use pressure first, then controlled ligation. Large veins that have been opened in head and neck lacerations may be a source of an air embolus. Pressure over these areas can help prevent embolization and blood loss. As long as the wound is cleansed and kept moist with saline compresses, primary suture may be delayed for hours.

Laceration of the ear is dangerous because of the possibilities of perichondritis, stenosis of the external ear canal, and tissue loss. If the injured party brings a portion of his ear along with him, it should not be thrown away. Later if it cannot be primarily sutured in place, it can be buried in surrounding tissue to keep it alive for future reconstruction. Hematomas of the external ear associated with lacerations and trauma need sterile drainage. This may be done with a needle or small surgical incision that does not cut into the cartilage. A hematoma here (as well as a septal hematoma of the nose) may elevate the perichondrium away from the cartilage, thus robbing the cartilage of its nourishment and leading to necrosis and structural collapse. Blood in the external ear canal is best left alone. Its source may be an ear canal laceration or the middle ear. Placement of a sterile cotton pad in the concha of the external ear is all that is necessary.

Epistaxis

One of the problems of being a rhinologist is that one acquires the title *nosebleed doctor*. The nosebleed problem is created by blood flowing from a "hole," nonvisualization of this "hole," the blood being spewed onto you as it traverses the lips, an excited patient and family, and a disagreeable hour of the night.

Children bleed spontaneously from the nose. They also have epistaxis from blood dyscrasias or trauma. Generally this is easily managed because it is anterior in nature: external pressure by pinching the nares together, cold compresses to the bridge, or light intranasal packing of Vaseline gauze or Gelfoam. Severe nosebleeds in young males demand an investigation to rule out juvenile angiofibroma, a benign but extremely vascular tumor. Control of severe epistaxis is difficult because the measures used in usual hemorrhage control, such as tamponade, suturing, cauterizing, and direct visualization, are not easily applied. The adult patient may be diabetic or hypertensive, but one must not forget that multiple myelomas may initially present as a nosebleed.

Besides anterior packing, posterior packs may be necessary. Posterior packing may seem mystical because of the strings and catheters. Even more mystical is the patient's endurance when these packs are placed by an inexperienced physician. It can resemble a medieval torture routine to an observer. The key here is sedation and topical anesthetization. The classic posterior pack is made up of gauze or preferably lamb's wool, which has strings attached to it. Small No. 8 red rubber catheters are placed into the oropharynx via the nose and retrieved through the mouth. One set of strings is attached to the catheters, which are again pulled out the nose, placing the pack securely into the posterior aspect of the nose. These strings are then carefully tied over the columella so as not to cause necrosis. The other set of strings is brought out the mouth with no tension on the soft palate and taped to the cheek. Therefore one string holds the pack and the other retrieves it at the time of removal. When posterior packs are placed, anterior packing is also necessary. Vaseline gauze, ½ inch wide, is carefully layered in. Another means of packing the nose is by inflating a 30-ml Foley catheter balloon while it is in the nasopharynx and pulling it anteriorly until snug. Stevens' nasal balloons are contoured for the turbinates (both left and right) and inflated for pressure. A word of caution here: The pressure from inflation may be so severe as to cause necrosis and subsequent stenosis in the period following removal. Cases have been reported in which inability to control epistaxis by means of nasal packing has necessitated the bilateral ligation of the external carotid arteries in the neck. Though not an emergency room procedure, transmaxillary sinus antrum ligation of the internal maxillary artery has replaced the external carotid artery ligation. The arterial ligation of the internal carotid supply is performed by a curvilinear incision above the medial canthal ligament of the eye, giving access to the anterior and posterior ethmoid arteries.

Postoperative bleeding

Postoperative head and neck cancer patients occasionally develop flap necrosis with carotid artery exposure. This exposure to drying combined with preoperative irradiation makes this artery subject to spontaneous rupture. In large head and neck services family members are asked to stay with these patients while the artery is vulnerable. This constant observation for a rupture provides someone who can apply finger pressure while calling for help. The ligation of the artery can take place later in the operating room.

Postoperative tonsillectomy or adenoidectomy patients who are bleeding need to be returned to the operating room immediately. A primary concern is recognition of this potential catastrophe because more than one child has been found the next morning dead in his bed with a gastrointestinal tract full of blood after swallowing it all night.

The exasperating patient is one who is bleeding at 1 AM from a dental extraction. Having the patient apply pressure by biting a sterile gauze pad or Gelfoam packing is usually all that is necessary to stop the bleeding.

HEAT AND COLD
Frostbite

Frostbite occurs in the nose, ears, and extremities. Our primary concern is with the nose and ears. Warming should be accomplished rapidly. The nose and ears should not be traumatized. Brisk rubbing and excessive manipulation are mentioned only to condemn them. Frostbite is the effect of the cold on the blood vessels. Vasoconstriction is followed by hyperemia and edema caused by permeability of the capillaries. Regional capillaries filled with clumped red cells cause ischemia; therefore the prevention of intravascular clotting is the key factor in determining the final tissue loss. Infected gangrenous tissue should be surgically excised.

Burns

Burns of the head and neck, either thermal or electrical, demand and deserve special management by a burn specialist such as a plastic surgeon. Burn therapy is a specialty all its own. In ingested chemical burns of the deglutition tract the agent must be identified, neutralizing fluids should be started, and the oral cavity must be inspected. A pleasant surprise is to look into the mouth of a child who is suspected of having drunk lye only to see normal mucosa. Later this patient, if indeed burned, may need complete endoscopy to determine the condition of the pharynx, esophagus, and larynx.

TRAUMA
Barotrauma

Otitic barotrauma occurs with sudden changes in atmospheric pressure. These pressure changes are not equalized in the middle ear cleft because of eustachian tube malfunction, causing severe otalgia. This is most commonly produced on descent in aircraft or by skin diving. Relief can be gained by pushing air into the eustachian tube by catheterization, Valsalva maneuver, or politzerization. If these are all unsuccessful, a paracentesis of the drum head under strictly sterile technique is necessary. Barotrauma of the sinuses gives acute pain. Cannulation of the sinus ostia is avoided. One should give antihistamines, analgesics, systemic steroids such as 40 mg of triamcinolone injected intramuscularly, and a nasal spray to shrink the edema around the ostia.

Cosmetic trauma

Medicolegal problems associated with cosmetic surgery are commonplace. If a recent postoperative rhinoplasty patient sustains trauma to his nose, extremely conservative treatment should be used. The surgeon who operated should be notified, and he should handle the case. By all means no attempt should be made to shift the nose back to where one thinks it belongs.

Maxillofacial trauma

Patients with severe maxillofacial trauma also sustain cervical spine injuries in a high percentage of cases. This fact should not be overlooked in immediate care and transport. Hemorrhage can be controlled with pressure and packings. The mandible and the maxilla can be temporarily immobilized with Barton's dressing. This dressing relieves pain and prevents sharp fragments from lacerating vessels. The airway is in danger from the tongue, dislodged teeth, broken dentures, blood, mucus, and associated laryngeal fractures. Laryngeal fractures are diagnosed by the presence of subcutaneous emphysema in the neck, ecchymosis over the anterior neck, and loss of prominence of the thyroid cartilage (the Adam's apple). Definitive care of these wounds may take place hours to weeks later. Intermaxillary fixation is readily accomplished with a healthy set of teeth. If the patient is edentulous, his dentures are used in place of his natural teeth for intermaxillary fixation. If the dentures are broken, they can easily be repaired and utilized. A search at the scene of the accident may prove its worth later. When teeth are missing, they must be accounted for. If they cannot be found either outside or inside the mouth, x-ray films of the abdomen and chest are necessary.

The most common maxillofacial fracture involves the nose. This fracture should not be underestimated. A simple push to realign and a pack for epistaxis are not enough. Too many people end up unhappy with their crooked noses because time and effort were not made to properly align the fractured nasal bones and nasal septum. Emergency care is usually concerned with the epistaxis, which has already been discussed.

An interesting problem is the dislocated mandible. The condyle of the mandible has slipped out of the glenoid fossa anteriorly. The patient may have yawned widely, screamed as in childbirth, or attempted to get his mouth around too much food. The thumbs should be wrapped with something to protect against a bite, the mandible should be grasped bilaterally, and pressure should be applied manually with the thumbs over the molar teeth, pushing downward and posteriorly. If the patient can shut his mouth, you have been successful in relocating the mandible. A patient with chronic dislocation needs the jaw wrapped shut and a preventive medicine lecture should be given.

Skull trauma

Temporal bone fractures can produce sensorineural hearing loss, vestibular loss, and cerebrospinal fluid otorrhea. Conductive hearing loss is caused by (1) hemotympanum, (2) laceration of the tympanic membrane, or (3) disruption of the ossicular chain. Suction should not be applied to the external ear canal; it should not be wiped out with Q-Tips, and no antibiotic drops or ointment should be instilled in the ear canal. A sterile gauze or cotton ball dressing should be placed in the concha of the external ear. Bed rest, sedation, antibiotics, and antivertiginous medications can be started systemically. One of the most important observations and accurate recordings is the fast component of the nystagmus, when present. Cerebrospinal fluid drainage from the ear canal can be determined by the clear drainage or the "halo" effect when mixed with blood.

INFECTION
Ear

Otitis externa pain is produced by elevation of the pinna. It is distinguished from temporomandibular joint pain, which is anterior to the tragus of the ear. The pain of the mastoiditis is posterior to the auricle over the mastoid portion of the temporal bone. Topical application of antibiotic drops with steroid and placement of a gauze wick in the canal to keep the medication against the canal wall gives relief. Systemic antibiotics and analgesics are sometimes necessary. Once the edema begins to subside, healing is well on its way.

Acute otitis media may rupture the tympanic membrane by fluid pressure in the middle ear. If rupture appears imminent, a myringotomy is performed to relieve the pressure. A poorly visualized, moving tympanic membrane of an irritable child may prove disastrous if a myringotomy is attempted. A dislocated stapes, which allows the infectious material of the middle ear to enter the perilymph, may produce permanent loss of hearing and labyrinthine function as well as meningitis. The child should be sedated and wrapped securely in sheets, and the incision should be performed in the posterior inferior quadrant of the tympanic membrane. Do not hesitate to place children under general anesthesia for the sake of the patient, parents, and the doctor. This procedure must be done accurately and safely.

Acute mastoiditis is still a problem. Some clinicians mistakenly think mastoid problems departed with the entry of antibiotics. The ear is characteristically pushed outward and downward away from the head. It should not be drained. This patient must be referred to an otologist for surgical drainage by a simple mastoidectomy. Chronic drainage from the ears is not a surgical emergency. It should be referred to an otologist.

Nose

The furuncle of the nose is potentially dangerous since it may communicate via venous channels to cause a cavernous sinus thrombosis. This "pimple" must not be underestimated. It should be treated with systemic antibiotics and moist heat and drained only when "ripe."

Pharynx

Peritonsillar abscesses demand incision and drainage. Symptoms consist of trismus, drooling, pain, voice change, and shift of the soft palate. Local infiltration by lidocaine (Xylocaine) is ineffective to control pain. Adults under sedation can be drained in a sitting position by placing a hemostat in the proper place and spreading. In this position and awake, the adult can handle the gush of pus and slight bleeding. Children need to be taken to the operating room and placed under general anesthesia. The need for a tonsillectomy in approximately 4 weeks is emphasized.

An enlarged epiglottis can cause airway obstruction, necessitating a tracheostomy. The epiglottis can reach an amazing size when infected. The "hot potato" voice characterizes this problem.

If diphtheria is clinically evident (positive for the bacterial agent on Gram stain) a tracheostomy is indicated. Diphtheria is like mastoiditis—it is still around.

FOREIGN BODIES
Pharynx

Friday night fish fries are notorious for creating the midnight rendezvous to remove a fish bone. The search should begin at the inferior pole of the tonsil, the base of the tongue, and then the piriform sinus of the hypopharynx. In my experience less than 50% of these patients have a bone recovered. A common physical finding is a small area of erythema and edema where the bone may have been lodged at one time. If the initial examination with a mirror is negative, inform the patient that a direct view with a laryngoscope and esophagoscope may be necessary in the operating room, if the symptoms persist several hours later.

Nose

Foul, unilateral nasal discharge in children represents a foreign body until proved otherwise. The objects are rocks, toys, coins, vegetable matter, flowers, or practically anything. If the time interval since placement is short, the objects may generally be removed easily by anterior grasping with a nasal forceps. The foreign body should not be dislodged posteriorly where the child can aspirate the object. The excited, uncooperative child should be sedated or general anesthesia may be scheduled for safe removal. It is always a good idea to inspect the ears of these patients. They are fond of all their orifices but play favorites. It is amazing how a child can become a chronic offender despite disagreeable experiences at removal.

Ear

Ear canal foreign bodies can be insects, vegetable matter, toy parts, paper, and beads. Removal should not be attempted with suction, curettage, or forceps if the child is fighting. If sedation is unsuccessful, general anesthesia should be scheduled. A tympanic membrane rupture, ossicular chain injury, or otitis media is a high price to pay for carelessness. The tympanic membrane must be intact before an irrigation is attempted to remove insects or other foreign bodies. A large insect needs ether to kill it before removal. A small insect washes out with water.

Esophagus

The conventioneer who consumes too much alcohol and steak may lodge a large bolus of meat in the cricopharyngeus, cardiac junction, or midportion of the esophagus where the aorta crosses. Visualization requires esophagoscopy in the operating room. Meat tenderizers should not be given because this may cause esophageal rupture leading to mediastinitis and a possible fatality. Swallowed coins may lodge at the cricopharyngeus only to pass into the stomach with relaxation under general anesthesia.

QUESTIONS

1. A young man in a motor vehicle accident is bleeding extensively from severe head lacerations and maxillofacial fractures. The pulse pressure is narrowing, the pulse rate is increasing, and the blood pressure is dropping. His teeth are missing, and the airway is questionable. What is the most appropriate course of management?

2. A postoperative tonsillectomy-adenoidectomy patient vomits 300 ml of blood. "Watchful waiting" is suggested. Is that correct?

3. A young lady is slapped in barroom tussle. She complains of "roaring" in the right ear and hearing loss. What is the problem? Is irrigation needed?

4. If hoarseness in acute head trauma demands laryngoscopy, what about oral burns in a 3-year-old child who has been discovered with a can of lye?

5. Sky King comes from the airport with an earache, headache, and hearing loss. He has been flying with a recent cold. Is this problem tension and noise induced?

6. Unilateral purulent nasal discharge in a child is most likely caused by what?

7. Certain manipulative procedures in conditions of the ear, nose, and throat should not be attempted in uncooperative patients without general anesthesia. Give some examples.

8. Outline progressive management of epistaxis. What is the difference if it occurs in the postoperative rhinoplasty patient.

9. Brisk manipulation may be dandy in romance, but how should frostbite cases be handled?

10. Can otalgia be distinguished by the character and location of the pain?

CHAPTER 32

Obstetric and gynecologic emergencies

RUSSELL E. HANLON† and DAVID G. HALL III

The vast majority of births in the United States today occur in hospitals and under medical supervision. However, an occasional expectant mother is faced with delivery in suboptimal conditions outside a medical facility without the benefit of attendance by trained medical personnel. In addition, recent societal trends have resulted in couples electing to conduct their own labors and deliveries at home under normal conditions. Certain unpredictable problems affecting both mother and infant may and do occur with any pregnancy, labor, delivery, and the immediate puerperium. Heavy blood loss during late pregnancy, labor, delivery, or the first few hours following delivery may portend a serious, life-threatening dilemma for both mother and infant that may require immediate corrective action within a medical institution. In addition, some newborn infants do not initiate spontaneous or effective respiration and require proper resuscitative techniques to prevent irreversible brain damage or death.

With these thoughts in mind this chapter stresses the basic principles of diagnosis and immediate management of obstetric and gynecologic difficulties in adverse conditions. In all cases the best medical personnel and facilities available should be obtained as quickly as possible.

SIGNS AND SYMPTOMS OF LABOR

The onset of true labor may be preceded by a "bloody show" occurring within 24 to 48 hours of the onset of labor. Frequently the "show" is not seen until labor is established. This small amount of thick blood-streaked mucus is the result of expulsion of the plug of mucus occluding the cervix during pregnancy. In some patients labor is preceded by rupture of the membranes (amnion and chorion) signified by a gush of clear fluid (amniotic fluid) from the vagina. The amniotic fluid may be recognized by its characteristic musty odor and colorless, sometimes slightly turbid appearance, which differentiates it from urine, which sometimes escapes from the bladder involuntarily during late pregnancy. Rupture of the membranes most commonly occurs in advanced labor but occasionally occurs as much as 24 hours prior to

---

† Deceased.

the onset of labor in the term patient. Rarely, rupture of the membranes may occur days or even weeks prior to the onset of labor.

MANAGEMENT OF LABOR AND DELIVERY

When a patient is encountered in labor, the first question concerns the location of medical facilities and the availability of trained medical personnel. In most circumstances this simply means telephoning the physician and transporting the patient to the hospital where she has been previously scheduled for delivery. If the patient has no physician and has received no prenatal care, a police officer can usually give directions to a hospital where care can be provided, any many times he provides transportation. Moreover in some areas policemen have received training in emergency delivery. Unless delivery is imminent, as signified by signs of the second stage in a multipara or actual "crowning" (presentation of the head) in a primigravida, it is probably best to transport the patient to a hospital if one is reasonably available. If this is not feasible, her physician (if she has one) or any physician (if she does not) should be notified immediately. Any patient in advanced labor should be transported in a reclining position either in an ambulance or (lacking this) the rear seat of an automobile. The patient should remove any underclothing that might obstruct delivery during the trip. Under no circumstances should any attempt be made (either mechanically or medically) to delay delivery.

On rare occasions, precipitate delivery may occur in public places, commercial aircraft, or crowds. When this occurs, it is best to place the patient in a reclining position in an area of maximum privacy and cleanliness. No attempt should be made to provide analgesia or anesthesia unless one is experienced in the management of labor. Pain relief is rarely essential to successful labor and, indeed, may prove harmful if injudiciously administered.

Occasionally in isolated areas, in an emergency, or by the decision of the family, labor and birth may occur without benefit of traditional medical support. Notwithstanding the fact that unpredictable calamities can occur, the majority of labors and deliveries are completely normal, and a successful outcome can be anticipated in the absence of trained personnel and modern facilities.

A calm, reassuring attendant is the best sedative possible even under ideal conditions; therefore when labor and delivery are to be conducted by a nonphysician, this may be even more significant. Early in labor, certain preparations should be made. The mother should lie on a clean, flat surface. If a bed is available, it should be protected with waterproof sheeting. If this is lacking, six to eight layers of newspapers placed beneath the sheet provide some protection. In addition, clean folded sheets or mattress pads may be placed beneath the buttocks. They can be changed intermittently when they invariably become soiled with amniotic fluid, mucus, and fecal material. Materials to be utilized during the actual delivery should be prepared. A knife, scissors, or other sharp instrument that has been thoroughly cleansed and two strips of fabric measuring approximately 10 inches in length to be utilized as a cord ligature should be boiled in water for 20 to 30 minutes. If ordinary kitchen forceps are available, they should be sterilized in the boiling water with a string attached to the handle to recover other articles from the water. The water and instruments contained therein should be allowed to cool before use. Although presterilized and packaged cord ties and clamps are available, they are unlikely luxuries in the emergency situation. Suitable substitutes may be found in gauze bandages 1 to 1½ inches in width, narrow strips of clean, white cloth, or even shoe laces. Narrow caliber ties should be avoided because they tend to cut into the soft, gelatinous cord.

A second large vessel of water containing several washcloths should be boiled for 20 to 30 minutes and allowed to cool for use in cleansing the perineum. All attendants should scrub their hands and forearms thoroughly with soap and water if possible. They should utilize a rich lather and a liberal, thorough rinse before handling the perineum or the infant. Prior to the initial scrub, the fingernails of the attendants should be thoroughly cleansed with a nail file if available. If the patient is not in advanced labor and the decision has been made to conduct delivery outside a medical institution, a plain water enema is desirable to evaluate the lower bowel and to decrease the risk of fecal contamination during labor and delivery.

After the attendant has thoroughly scrubbed his hands, a sterile cotton pledget, if available, is placed in the introitus to prevent contaminated substances from entering it. It is essential during this and other cleansing procedures of the vulva that nothing enter the vaginal orifice, including the hand of the attendant. A rich lather is made in the hairy area of the vulva with soap and water. After the washing procedure, the sterile pledget in the vaginal introitus is removed and replaced with a fresh one. The entire vulva and inner thighs are cleansed with water, working from above downward and from the introitus outward to the inner thighs.

It is advisable that the patient receive no solid foods during her labor. She may, however, be encouraged to drink small amounts of water. The patient should also be encouraged to empty her bladder frequently during labor; however, she should not use the toilet if delivery seems imminent. Ambulation is permissible during the first stage of labor provided that the membranes have not ruptured. Following rupture of the membranes or during the second stage, the patient should remain in a supine position. Signs of the second stage are strong contractions, 2 to 3 minutes apart, accompanied by a bearing down sensation (as though the patient needed to have a bowel movement), increased bloody show, and bulging of the perineum. At this time the top of the infant's head may be visualized at the maternal introitus. Preparations for delivery should now be accelerated.

The patient should try to avoid bearing down as much as possible. She should assume a supine position in bed with her knees elevated. The attendant should again thoroughly scrub his hands with soap and water for 10 minutes if time permits. If they are available, he should wear sterile rubber gloves. The perineum should again be cleansed as previously described, and a clean pad should be placed beneath the buttocks. Once the head is crowning (95% of infants are born head first), a hand should be placed lightly against the presenting head during contractions to prevent sudden expulsion, which could result in severe maternal lacerations. No other assistance is necessary, and, indeed, the attendant should let the infant be born by itself. Under no circumstances should the attendant's hand enter the vagina nor should any attempt be made to pull the infant from the vagina. Birth need not occur in a hurry.

Usually after the head is delivered, the shoulders follow with the next few contractions. If the membranes cover the head after it is delivered, the sac should be torn with the fingers to allow the amniotic fluid to escape and to permit the infant to breathe. A check should be made to be certain that the umbilical cord is not wrapped around the infant's neck. If the cord is wrapped tightly around the neck, it may impede the progress of delivery and result in airway obstruction after the head has emerged but before completion of the delivery, or it may result in fetal blood loss as a result of tearing the umbilical cord. If the cord is found around the neck, a gentle attempt should be made to slip the loop over the fetal head. If this fails, then one should attempt to slip the cord back over the shoulders as the baby delivers and await the completion of the delivery. After the shoulders are delivered, the remainder of the body slips from the vagina without difficulty. The sole manipulation by the attendant should be to support the infant as it emerges from the introitus. The attendant should avoid touching the mother's rectum, if possible, during delivery.

After the head has emerged, milking the trachea with a gentle, stroking action of the fingers from the base of the neck to the chin aids in clearing the trachea of secretions.

The newborn infant is slippery and difficult to hold. As the shoulders emerge, by placing the right hand behind the neck of the infant with the thumb and index finger around the sides of the neck, the attendant is able to achieve control of the baby without a tight or possibly injurious grip. The body, as it emerges, should be supported with the left hand to avoid contact with the bed, which should be regarded as contaminated.

INITIAL CARE OF THE NEWBORN INFANT

After the baby is born, he should be held head down. This is best accomplished by holding him up by the ankles, utilizing a firm grip with the index finger inserted between the ankles, and supporting the shoulders with the other hand. The infant should be held just above the bed or any soft, flat, clean surface to avoid injury if he is inadvertently dropped.

The baby should not be spanked, although sometimes gently rubbing the infant's back or slapping the soles of the feet may aid in stimulating respirations. Tension on the umbilical cord should always be avoided when it is still attached to the placenta within the uterus. When the infant begins to cry, he should be placed on the bed near the mother with a clean blanket or sheet beneath him. He should be placed on his abdomen with the head turned to either side. The nose and pharynx may be gently suctioned with a small, rubber bulb ear syringe, if available, to clear the respiratory passages of mucus and debris.

Infant resuscitation

A newborn infant normally cries and breathes within 1 minute of birth. Although normally pink in color after respirations are well established (except possibly the hands and feet), an infant who does not breathe may become cyanotic (dusky bluish in color), or if anoxia has been present or continues long enough, the infant may be pale and limp. If respirations have not been established within 3 minutes, resuscitative measures should be instituted, particularly if cyanosis is progressing. The most available and efficient method is mouth-to-mouth resuscitation. The infant should be placed on his back with the head extended. This may be facilitated by placing a folded sheet or blanket beneath the shoulders. The airway should be cleared as much as possible by gentle rubber bulb suction or wiping the mouth out with a cloth. The mouth of the attendant should then be placed to the nose or nose and mouth of the infant, and the attendant should then inhale and partially exhale into the external nares of the infant. In general the mouth-to-nose technique is more satisfactory in newborn infants than the usual mouth-to-mouth technique utilized in adults. If only the nose is included within the lips of the attendant, the mouth should be firmly closed by finger compression to prevent escape of air. It is possible to severely damage the infant's lungs by this method, but the risk can be minimized by using a "puffing" technique, utilizing the cheek musculature of the attendant rather than forcibly exhaling. The effect can be gauged by placing a hand on the chest of the infant and observing chest expansion. A short puff about every 5 seconds is sufficient. This effort should be continued until spontaneous respirations are established, or until efforts are obviously futile as signified by absence of a palpable or available heartbeat, absence of corneal reflexes, and complete lack of muscle tone. It is advisable, however, to attempt to initiate respiration for 5 to 15 minutes in the absence of these signs because occasionally an infant who appears lost may be revived.

DELIVERY OF PLACENTA

Following the delivery of the infant, uterine contractions usually cease for several minutes as the uterus accommodates to its markedly diminished intracavitary volume. The placenta normally separates from its implantation site as a result of decreased area of the site. Soon rhythmic contractions resume and the placenta is expelled. This usually occurs within 20 minutes but may last longer than an hour. Bleeding may be anticipated. An increase in bleeding as well as a rise in the height of the uterine fundus above the symphysis pubis and advance of the cord from the introitus are signs of placental separation. When any of these signs appear, it is well to gently massage the uterine fundus suprapubically to aid in contraction. If bleeding seems excessive, putting the infant to the breast reflexly stimulates uterine contractions. Under no circumstances should traction be put on the umbilical cord in an effort to deliver the placenta.

Following completion of the third stage if an experienced nurse is in attendance, ergonovine, 0.2 mg, or an oxytocic drug (Pitocin, Syntocinon), 10 units, may be administered intramuscularly to aid in contraction of the uterus, thereby minimizing blood loss. Ergonovine may also be administered intravenously in the same dosage. Following delivery, the perineum should be inspected for tears or lacerations; if they are present with bleeding, pressure should be applied with a sterile gauze pad or sterile cloth for 20 to 30 minutes. This usually controls the bleeding. If bleeding does not occur, no further emergency treatment is necessary, although surgical repair is desirable if facilities are available.

TYING THE CORD

Attention should now be directed to the umbilical cord, which still attaches the infant to the recently delivered placenta. There is no need to rush this procedure; time should be taken, if needed, to ensure sterility of the cutting instrument and cord ties. Contamination during this procedure may be an important source of infection to the newborn infant. The cord should be tied firmly and carefully, about 6 inches from the umbilicus, using a square knot. A second ligature should then be placed approximately ½ inch from the first tie. The cord is cut on the placental side of the two ties approximately ½ inch from the second tie, using the previously sterilized sharp instrument. Special care should be taken in tying the knots to avoid tension on the cord at its entrance to the umbilicus. The cord can easily be torn loose at this point, resulting in blood loss by the infant. If sterile ties and instruments are not available, or if medical attention can be anticipated in a relatively short time, it is best to wrap the placenta with the infant, as fetal blood does not flow back through the placenta after delivery. No special treatment of the cord stump is necessary, and, indeed, no medication of any kind should be applied to the stump.

ECTOPIC PREGNANCY

An ectopic pregnancy is a pregnancy existing within the maternal body but outside the uterine cavity. The majority of such pregnancies are located within the fallopian tubes and are known as tubal pregnancies. The wall of the tube eventually becomes weakened by invasion of the developing placental tissue and subsequently ruptures and bleeds. This is usually accompanied by intraperitoneal bleeding that may lead to blood loss shock and death if appropriate corrective actions are not taken. The signs and symptoms include (1) missing of one or two menstrual periods, (2) vaginal bleeding, small in amount, (3) sharp, unilateral lower abdominal pain followed by progressively more generalized lower abdominal pain, and (4) signs of hypovolemic shock. This is a serious surgical emergency, and the treatment is surgical. Transportation to a hospital facility is mandatory.

ABRUPTIO PLACENTAE

One of the most serious complications of pregnancy is abruptio placentae, which is defined as the separation of the placenta from its site of implantation in the uterus at any time during the last 20 weeks of pregnancy. The prognosis for both fetus and the mother varies with the degree of separation. Most mothers who develop abruptio placentae also have toxemia of pregnancy characterized by hypertension, proteinuria, excessive weight gain, and edema. In placental abruptions only a small portion of the placenta may be involved or indeed the entire placenta may become dislodged. Abruptio placentae is rarely associated with abdominal trauma. Separation of the placenta leaves the vessels at its base open and bleeding. Because the uterus is still distended by the fetus, the organ is unable to contract and retract to effect hemostasis. As the clot behind the placenta enlarges, the placenta tends to become further separated. Blood may dissect beneath the membranes and present through the cervix into the vagina or it may actually infiltrate the myometrium and other pelvic structures. The signs and symptoms of this disorder include (1) lower abdominal pain, (2) vaginal bleeding, (3) tender, rigid, sometimes boardlike uterus, and (4) shock out of proportion to visible blood loss. Further complications may include loss of the ability of blood to clot, failure of the uterus to contract after delivery (uterine atony) with postpartum hemorrhage, and, rarely, renal failure in the postpartum period.

The keystone of emergency management is recognition of the condition, vigorous shock therapy, and immediate transport to a medical facility.

• • •

The keynote of the modern practice of obstetrics, as well as first aid management in all areas, is expressed in the dictum *primum non nocere* (first, do no harm). In the vast majority of obstetric situations a minimum of aid is necessary for the health of both mother and infant.

GYNECOLOGIC EMERGENCIES

There are a few gynecologic conditions in which emergency management may be considered crucial.

Both the internal and external female genitalia are well protected by their anatomic location against all but the most severe trauma. Occasionally, however, lacerations of the external genitalia may occur, accompanied by heavy bleeding. This may usually be controlled by simple pressure applied at the site of bleeding until more definitive medical care can be obtained.

In the past, attempts have been made to treat nearly all types of bleeding from the internal genitalia with the use of a tight pack of gauze or cloth introduced into the vagina. In most cases this is not only futile but dangerous. There are basically two situations that justify using this procedure. The first of these is in patients who develop massive, life-threatening vaginal bleeding with carcinoma of the uterine cervix. Vaginal packing in this instance is a temporary measure while the patient is being prepared for surgery and ligation of the hypogastric arteries bilaterally. Occasionally serious bleeding may result from vaginal lacerations caused by rape or sexual perversion. A pack should be used only if bleeding is life threatening and if more definitive therapy is not available. The preferred packing material is sterile 2-inch gauze. A tight pack inserted under direct vision with good lighting may result in control of hemorrhage under the circumstances described. The pack, however, should be removed as soon as possible when definitive therapy is available.

QUESTIONS

1. Discuss the medical importance of using planned medical supervision during childbirth.
2. List and explain the signs of the various stages of labor.
3. Describe the best handling of precipitate delivery in public places.
4. List several advance provisions that should optimally be made by a nonphysician who must conduct delivery.
5. List the various steps in preparing the patient herself for emergency delivery.
6. What is the best means of holding the newborn, and why is it best?
7. Discuss the steps for initiation of respirations in the newborn and their expected effectiveness.
8. Describe the means of proper attention to tying and severing the umbilical cord.
9. What antisepsis, if any, should be applied to the cord stump? Explain.
10. Explain the meaning of abruptio placentae and its importance in the obstetric-gynecologic first aid picture.
11. Define ectopic pregnancy, and discuss its implications in emergency care.
12. Describe the current medical opinion of the vaginal pack in control of hemorrhage.
13. What is the best sedative possible even in ideal birth conditions?
14. Describe briefly the procedure of the management of labor and delivery.

CHAPTER 33

Genitourinary emergencies

GILBERT J. ROSS, Jr.

Most of the acute illnesses and injuries involving the genitourinary system are associated with one or more relatively repetitive features that include severe colicky pain, hematuria, chills and fever, acute urinary retention, abdominal mass, and certain obvious disturbances of the external genitalia.

Basic principles, particularly the importance of a searching history and careful examination of the urine, must be constantly kept in mind. Special cognizance needs to be taken of the location and distribution of pain in this area, because it is often as ambiguous as it is severe. The nature of any bleeding, general state of prior health, and the use of various drugs must be critically evaluated.

ACUTE URINARY RETENTION

Acute urinary retention is most commonly seen in conjunction with prostatic obstruction. It is particularly prone to occur in men with incipient prostatism following various surgical procedures or following the use of medication with anticholinergic properties. Other factors that may precipitate acute retention are other forms of urethral obstruction, neurologic disturbances, and bleeding with clot retention. The objectives are clear: to relieve the distension by catheterization without injuring the delicate tissue of the urethra.

Generally it is advisable to initiate catheterization in the male with the installation of an antimicrobial ointment into the urethra. A well-lubricated 18 F catheter should then be gently passed using firm pressure at the membranous urethral area if required to overcome spasm. If the catheter cannot be passed and the obstruction appears to lie at the level of the prostatic urethra, an abundant quantity of sterile lubricant should be instilled and an 18 to 20 F coude-tipped catheter may be employed using counterpressure in the rectum if there is difficulty in negotiating the curve of the bulbous urethra.

In the event that the catheter interrupts in the urethra below the level of the prostate, there is a real possibility of a urethral stricture. If small (12 to 14 F) coude-tipped rubber catheters do not pass through the area easily, the stricture has to be dilated with filiform and follower catheters. This highly specialized procedure, although less hazardous than the passage of metal sounds, may easily damage the urethra and should never be attempted by the uninitiated.

In small male infants even the tiniest of the rubber catheters may be too large, but tiny polyethylene feeding tubes in the range of 5 F make admirable urethral catheters for short-term use.

If urethral manipulation for acute urinary retention is unsuccessful or not feasible, and if the bladder is significantly distended well above the pubis, one of the commercially available trocar cystotomy sets (12 to 16 F) may be used to provide suprapubic drainage. After the bladder has been identified by palpation and percussion, a midline skin wheal is raised with 1% lidocaine and the depth and position of the bladder is then more specifically delineated with a No. 22 spinal needle. With this information in hand, the trocar with the investing plastic catheter can be safely advanced into the bladder, the balloon inflated, the trocar removed, and the catheter sutured to the skin.

BLEEDING FROM THE LOWER URINARY TRACT

Bleeding from the prostatic urethra in the male or from the female urethra characteristically occurs at the beginning and end of voiding; whereas bleeding arising from the bladder or upper urinary tract always occurs throughout urination. This localization is most important in dictating the nature of subsequent investigation and management.

Bleeding from the prostatic urethra or bladder is often severe enough to require blood replacement and to produce acute urinary retention because of clots accumulating in the bladder. As a general rule if the bladder can be evacuated and kept decompressed, virtually all prostatic bleeding stops spontaneously and hemorrhage from the bladder is often, though not invariably, decreased or arrested. This is contingent on the nature of the bladder abnormality initiating the hematuria. In any case as long as clots remain in the bladder, bleeding usually persists. The major objective in treatment is to render the bladder clot-free.

Catheterization should be performed with a relatively large catheter (22 to 24 F), the internal diameter of which is adequate to allow clot evacuation as accomplished by copious irrigation with sterile saline. At times it may be advisable to chill the irrigant in an effort to expedite hemostasis.

Not infrequently the decompression of a chronically distended bladder results in profuse bleeding as well as certain undesirable septic sequelae; however, if the bladder is decompressed, the bleeding usually stops.

RENAL COLIC

The patient with acute renal or urethral colic building on a background of acute obstruction is frequently in such severe pain that immediate symptomatic measures are often required, provided that certain criteria are met: red cells in the urine, relative assurance that the problem is not that of an acute surgical abdomen, and some confidence that one is not dealing with an attempt to acquire narcotics for nonmedical purposes.

Narcotics in relatively large dosage are needed for adequate analgesia. There are no admonitions concerning which of these agents may be the most effective or which should be avoided. None of the common narcotics can be clearly shown to have an adverse effect on the smooth muscle of the genitourinary system, and the drug of choice is the one with which the physician is most familiar.

Although the use of antispasmodics is subject to some dispute, it is our impression that they are a valuable adjunct in the management of urethral colic. Anticholinergic agents, such as propantheline bromide, in an initial adult dose of 30 to 45 mg intravenously or intramuscularly, may prove to be of distinct value.

It is imperative to obtain an excretory urogram at the time of the pain in the event that the difficulty is caused by an acute and intermittent hydronephrosis, which returns spontaneously to normal following the episode of pain.

SEPSIS

Infection in the urinary tract encompasses a wide range in the severity of the infection. The most disastrous complication of urinary infection is gram-negative rod septicemia with septic shock. Perhaps the least hazardous is the localized bladder infection commonly seen in young women.

The usual circumstances that prevail prior to the development of septicemia are the combination of a gram-negative rod urinary tract infection with iatrogenic trauma or obstruction with stasis and residual urine. Clinical circumstances are most frequently traumatic catheterization, lower urinary tract instrumentation in the presence of infected residual urine, upper conduit system obstruction with entrapment of infected urine, and, occasionally, a neglected perinephric, scrotal, or prostatic abscess.

The clinical history is often quite clear. When such a patient is seen with actual or impending shock apparently unrelated to myocardial disease or blood loss, immediate affirmative action should be taken while diagnostic studies are under way.

The bladder should be catheterized to monitor the urine output and to assure that any question concerning residual urine is dispelled. Blood and urine cultures should be obtained concomitantly with the introduction of a venous catheter for monitoring central venous pressure (CVP). If the CVP is low, the extracellular space should be volume-expanded while antibiotic therapy is initiated. In the absence of any prior bacteriologic studies, the choice of antibiotics necessarily has to be arbitrary.

Because of the necessity for broad antimicrobial coverage, a combination of gentamicin and cephalothin is a reasonable point of departure, taking cognizance of the necessity for dosage modifications in the event of depression in renal function. The use of vasoactive drugs and steroids can be momentarily deferred while response to the initial treatment is evaluated and additional studies are undertaken to categorically rule out the possibility of upper urinary tract obstruction if this is not already abundantly clear.

In addition to volume expansion and antimicrobial agents, metabolic acidosis may require correction on an emergency basis. The rapid development of profound metabolic acidosis is not uncommon with fulminant sepsis, and blood gas determinations are required to assess the need for sodium bicarbonate and the quantity necessary to control and reverse the acidosis.

Even in the absence of a septicemia, the patient with acute bacterial prostatitis, an acute pyelonephritis, or a scrotal or perinephric abscess may be gravely ill. In addition to the usual antibacterial therapy, supportive management often requires parenteral fluids and the use of a cooling blanket. A known or suspected abscess must be dealt with promptly. Categorical assurance that there is no obstruction with incarceration of infected urine along the course of the urinary conduit system must be obtained, or, if such a situation does exist, it must be promptly rectified.

TRAUMA

Most renal injuries can initially be managed conservatively with strict bed rest and blood replacement as deemed necessary. There is relatively little more that can be done in terms of immediate care other than the acquisition of proper urographic studies. The decision to intervene surgically in renal injuries is usually clinical, and it is imperative to obtain a meticulous baseline assessment of the size of any flank mass. This assures that the repeated physical examination critical to the management of renal trauma can be meaningfully evaluated.

Bladder and urethral injuries with extravasation are true surgical emergencies. The initial management should involve a high index of suspicion following pelvic trauma, treatment of hemorrhagic shock, and examination of the urine (if any is forthcoming) for blood. Catheterization is the preliminary step in obtaining a cystogram to evaluate the nature of the injury.

Frequently a catheter cannot be passed because of partial or total disruption of the deep bulbous urethra. Occasionally a catheter passes into the area of the bladder, but no urine is obtained because the prostatic urethra has been avulsed from the membranous urethral area and the catheter tip is lying free in the retroperitoneal space. In either instance a retrograde urethrogram should be obtained to identify the site and nature of the injury. If the disruption is above the triangular ligament area (urogenital diaphragm) the urethrogram shows amorphous extravasation above the symphysis. Partial or complete urethral tears in the deep bulb below the triangular ligament show extravasation below the symphysis best visualized on oblique films (see discussion of external genitalia).

Contrast media used for cystography and urethrography must always be suitable for intravenous use because there may be rapid absorption from an extravasation into the bloodstream.

EXAMINATION OF THE ACUTELY ILL PATIENT

An order of priorities must be established with attention given first to the most urgent aspects demanded by the clinical situation. Following such fundamentals as assuring patency of the airway and initiating any other resuscitative procedures that may be required, the acutely ill or injured patient should be systematically examined. The scope of the examination should not be unduly conditioned by information obtained through the medical history.

Although the stabbing pain of renal or ureteral colic produced by acute obstruction is most clearly perceived over the renal or abdominal area, lower ureteral obstruction may be quite confusing since such pain typically radiates into the scrotum or labia due to overlapping innervation with the genitofemoral nerve arising from L1 to L2. In contrast acute obstruction of the intramural ureter produces bladder symptoms with straining to void as well as frequency. Testicular pain is equally ambivalent because, although it is classically visceral with localization in the lower abdomen, there is concomitant local involvement often radiating into the groin.

Rectal examination

Rectal examination in the male is imperative not only to establish the status of the prostate and lower rectum but also to allow bimanual examination of the bladder, to assess anal sphincter tone, and to evaluate the effect of suspected pelvic trauma on the genitourinary system.

Following pelvic fractures, there is an understandably high incidence of injury to the lower urinary tract. Rectal examination may be most valuable in localizing any bone fragments and in aiding the assessment of a possible injury to the bladder or prostatic urethra. In the event of a shearing injury of the prostate, only a soft, poorly defined mass can be palpated in the area of the prostate since the urethra has been divided at the triangular ligament and the bladder and prostate have been displaced superiorly.

Only the most infrequent and gentle prostatic examination should be employed in the presence of suspected acute bacterial prostatitis or a prostatic abscess since it is possible that forceful palpation may instigate a bacteremia or septicemia.

SCROTAL MASS

Despite the accessibility of the area to examination, an acutely painful scrotal mass may present a difficult diagnostic problem. Epididymitis, torsion of the testis, incarceration of an inguinal hernia, torsion of the appendix testis, and testicular tumor are among the common conditions that must be considered. Helpful diagnostic maneuvers include auscultation for bowel sounds, transillumination if there appears to be an element of free or loculated fluid, and of, course, palpation. Occasionally aspiration of hydrocele fluid may facilitate subsequent palpation.

The most pressing problem in diagnosis is to distinguish clearly among torsion of the testis, incarceration of a scrotal hernia, and epididymitis in view of the radically different treatment employed. Torsion and the incarcerated hernia require prompt operation if a viable testis is to be saved or if a bowel resection is to be avoided. In contrast the management of epididymitis is essentially medical.

Torsion should be suspected when the testis is noted to be abnormally high in the scrotum, whereas epididymitis usually shows selective involvement of the epididymis early in the course of the disease. Unfortunately in both instances a delay in diagnosis (and treatment) may result in a large, tender, confluent mass without any distinguishing features. Less specific ancillary factors must often be relied on that include the precipitous onset often associated with torsion, the relative rarity of epididymitis in prepubertal children, and the frequent association of lower tract infection with epididymitis. An incarcerated hernia can usually be recognized by hearing bowel sounds over the mass. If there is some dispute concerning whether bowel sounds are present, an x-ray film should show bowel gas within the scrotum.

Unfortunately, physical examination can be notoriously misleading in dealing with scrotal pathology. In recent years the use of one of the small, portable Doppler ultrasonic flowmeters has proved to be invaluable in clarifying the differential diagnosis when confronted with an acutely painful scrotal mass. If auditory characteristics of a well-filled capillary bed are heard with the probe on the testis, there is virtual assurance that one is not dealing with a testicular torsion. It should also be emphasized that a significant delay often occurs in the diagnosis of testicular tumor because an erroneous diagnosis of epididymitis is entertained long after physical findings have become equivocal.

The therapy employed for epididymitis consists of rest, scrotal support, icebags to the scrotum, and antibacterial therapy. If there is a posterior urethritis associated with infected urine, urologic evaluation should be performed after the infection has been asymptomatic for some weeks.

DISORDERS OF EXTERNAL GENITALIA

Trauma to the external genitalia or urethra may be associated with a variety of findings including obvious loss of penile or scrotal skin, blood at the meatus, hematuria, or evidence of extravasation of urine or blood into soft tissues. Power takeoff injuries are particularly prone to denude the penis, and not infrequently they totally avulse the scrotum.

Damage to the bulbous urethra may produce a rupture with blood and extravasated urine following well-defined tissue planes. The same physical findings occur when extravasation develops in conjunction with a urethral stricture and periurethral abscess or urethral carcinoma. If the blood and extravasted urine are confined by Buck's fascia, the extravasation presents as a swollen indurated penis. If Buck's fascia is not intact, the extravasation also fills the scrotum and the superficial perineal pouch and extends up the lower abdomen deep to Scarpa's fascia. Tissue reaction and necrosis may be extensive if drainage of the extravasation has been delayed.

Some seemingly minor disorders of the penis may also be responsible for acute and potentially serious difficulty. For example, meatal stenosis or phimosis may be so severe that it produces acute or, more insidiously, chronic urinary retention. Insect bites are quite common in children and should be suspected in the event of sudden, rather painless penile swelling.

Paraphimosis, the fixation of a retracted prepuce, may produce severe swelling and pain. In certain instances the strangulating preputial ring may be sufficient to compromise the blood supply of the glans. Paraphimosis can usually be manually reduced by exerting steady pressure on the glans penis with the thumb and first two fingers of one hand while attempting to slide the prepuce over the corona with the opposite hand. If attempts at manual reduction fail, emergency dorsal slitting can be performed by incising the constricting ring after infiltration with local anesthesia.

Phimosis rarely produces acute symptoms unless the acute pain and swelling of an associated balanitis make it necessary to perform an emergency dorsal slit or circumcision. More commonly, the reaction subsides with the application of warm soaks and systemic antibiotics. A subsequent, elective circumcision can be performed.

ACUTE GONOCOCCAL INFECTION

Acute gonococcal infections are frequently seen in the emergency room. The diagnosis of acute gonococcal urethritis in the male usually presents no problem, and gram stains are usually strongly positive for gram-negative, intracellular diplococci. In females gram stains are frequently negative or falsely positive, and positive cultures from the endocervical or anal canals are required to establish the diagnosis. Both areas should be cultured by using either Thayer-Martin or Transgrow media depending on whether a prolonged period of transportation to a central laboratory is envisioned.

At the time of this writing, recommendations concerning therapy are for 4,800,000 units of aqueous procaine penicillin G divided into two simultaneous intramuscular injections in conjunction with 1 gm of probenecid given at least one-half hour prior to the penicillin. A number of alternative treatment programs (tetracycline, ampicillin, or spectinomycin) are available for patients who prefer oral medication or who may be allergic to penicillin.

QUESTIONS

1. Where would one anticipate the swelling to occur when urine extravasation secondary to a urethral stricture has not eroded through Buck's fascia?
2. Three weeks after the diagnosis of epididymitis, an 18-year-old man still has an essentially unchanged, solid, confluent scrotal mass. What might be the most appropriate course of action?
3. What agent should be used for the treatment of gonococcal urethritis in a man with known penicillin allergy?
4. Thirty minutes after developing what appears to be septic shock, a 70-year-old man has a normal blood pressure restored through expansion of the extracellular space. However, he appears to be in respiratory distress with a respiratory rate of 42. What is the most probable cause?
5. Two days after an episode of right flank pain, a 28-year-old man develops the signs and symptoms of an acute urinary infection with frequency, straining to void, and small voidings. Urinalysis shows only 1 or 2 red cells per high-power field. What is the most probable cause?
6. What is one major disadvantage of treating ureteral colic with anticholinergic agents in the elderly man with moderate prostatism?
7. Six weeks after a myocardial infarct, a 54-year-old man is seen in the emergency room of a distant hospital with gross hematuria and left flank pain. What is the first question to ask the patient?
8. Why is it critical to establish the phase of voiding at which gross hematuria occurs?

CHAPTER 34

Acute blood loss

EARL J. WIPFLER, Jr.

Early one January morning several years ago, I was walking to the hospital from my home. A blanket of freshly fallen snow was on the ground. As I walked across the campus, I noticed on the snow a trail of blood that led all the way to the hospital entrance. In the emergency room I found that a student had accidentally lacerated his wrist. Bleeding occurred through a small tear in the radial artery. Obviously such massive blood loss was completely unnecessary. Had the injured student or one of his friends simply placed his thumb over the bleeding point of the radial artery, almost no blood loss would have occurred. Most copious blood loss at the time of accidents is caused by the inadequate application of pressure over the bleeding point.

A second and more massive bleeding episode comes to mind when I recall a case of a 15-year-old school boy who was practicing the "fast draw." Unfortunately he pulled the trigger on the gun much too soon and the bullet exploded into the right upper thigh, tearing the femoral artery and vein for a considerable length. He was alone with his mother in their home in the country, and his mother was unable to drive a car. Almost at that instant, however, a neighbor drove into the yard. Driving as fast as possible, they arrived at the University of Missouri Medical Center (approximately 5 miles away) and were immediately seen in the emergency room, where the victim was gradually losing consciousness and was without any palpable pulse or blood pressure. Immediate direct firm pressure was placed on the bleeding area in lieu of only partially occluding pressure that had been applied. Ringer's lactate solution and dextran were immediately started and the patient was rushed to the operating room where adequate control of the bleeding was accomplished, a saphenous graft was placed between the two torn ends of the femoral artery, and the femoral vein was reconstituted.

Bleeding from a laceration of a peripheral vessel is usually not a great control problem. On the other hand the problems presented in controlling hemorrhage from around the femoral or hip area, the shoulder, and the chest are not so simple. Intrathoracic hemorrhage and its control are described in more detail in Chapter 29. Major injuries to vessels of the trunk may occur without obvious signs of bleeding. It is important to realize that these occult injuries are usually associated with the absence of the pulse distal to site of injury, perhaps with a large hematoma, and even with a neurologic deficit. Several thousand milliliters of blood can be lost in the thigh alone.

The emergency transfusion of whole blood can, indeed, be lifesaving. Whether the use of the universal donor or unmatched whole blood is ever justified is open to argument because the instance of severe complications is high and because colloid as a blood substitute is especially effective as a volume expander. It is almost always desirable to use carefully cross-matched blood. Whole fresh blood also has the advantage of combating some of the coagulation abnormalities commonly present in cirrhotic patients.

Rapid transfusion of whole blood can be hazardous, particularly if it is cold blood that has not been rewarmed. Rapidly administered cold blood can have a decidedly adverse effect on myocardial contractility. Ideally blood should be warmed by allowing it to pass through tubing immersed in a warm water bath.

Arrest of hemorrhage is usually best accomplished by means of pressure dressings applied manually to the wound or by circumferential bandaging of the extremity. Deep wounds usually require broad pressure areas to arrest hemorrhage, whereas superficial wound hemorrhage can usually be controlled by more localized pressure. In most accident situations formal dressings and bandages are not readily available; therefore direct manual pressure applied over reasonably clean clothing material is most effective. When circumferential bandaging is used, care must be taken to avoid interference with the remaining arterial supply to, or venous drainage from, the distal extremity. Greater bleeding occurs from vessels that have been divided, as retraction and resultant narrowing of the opening are prevented.

A tourniquet should be used if direct wound pressure does not give satisfactory control of hemorrhage. A tourniquet is applied to the thigh or the arm; it is not applied to the leg or the forearm. The rationale involved in this application of tourniquets becomes obvious when one considers the fact that the two bones of the forearm or the leg act to prevent ordinary tourniquet pressure from compressing arteries that lie between the bones.

Easily available tourniquet material, such as ropes or belts, is usually too narrow. When tourniquets must be made from such materials, they should be applied over strips of clothing or other padding material in order to prevent tissue damage. Common mistakes in using tourniquets include the following:

1. Failure to try to control bleeding by application of pressure dressings before resorting to this more dangerous method
2. Loose application that results in increased venous bleeding from increased venous pressure during continuation of arterial flow to the wound and to the extremity
3. Failure to evaluate peripheral pulses and appearance of the extremity both prior to and during tourniquet application
4. Failure to record tourniquet time and to effect 5-minute periods of release at regular 45-minute intervals

Again it should be emphasized that tourniquets are to be used only when pressure, elevation, and immobilization are ineffective in controlling hemorrhage. Successful arterial reconstruction may be seriously handicapped by tourniquet application and amputation is an unfortunate sequel.

Careful arrest of hemorrhage and proper splinting of extremity fractures are the prime essentials of peripheral vascular first aid. Following institution of these measures and prior to the time that definitive care becomes available to the patient, observation is essential. Only careful observation can prevent detrimental results of first aid treatment. To enhance the chance of success, every effort should be made to provide reconstructive arterial surgery as soon as possible.

QUESTIONS

1. Comment on the desirability of administering unmatched whole blood in the emergency situation.

2. Does a completely severed vessel bleed more or less copiously than a partially divided one? Why?

3. Discuss at least three precautions that are applicable in the administration of whole blood as a part of the emergency care regimen.

4. Suspicion of occult injuries to thoracic vessels may be sustained by lack of or significant diminution in what?

CHAPTER 35

Dental emergencies

HUGH E. STEPHENSON, Sr.†

Of foremost importance in the consideration of dental emergencies is observation of the signal precaution that referral of the patient to the appropriate dental specialist should always be made in any case in which the mode of treatment is in any way debatable. It is frequently of particular significance to make far deeper considerations than those involved in the immediate medical emergency. In cases of fracture of the jaw, for instance, mere setting of the bony separation itself is relatively minor in comparison to other considerations.

The purpose of this section is to discuss several of the more common dental emergencies that may be encountered on a first-aid basis and to point out measures that may be used in the conservative handling of all except the most minor injuries until expert dental aid may become available. Injuries to the mouth are quite often involved in the general problem of today's accident victim. Emergency care of these injuries may present a real challenge to most practitioners who are relatively unfamiliar with dental problems.

CHIPPED OR BROKEN TEETH

The problem of chipped or broken teeth is one of the most frequently encountered dental emergencies and is particularly prevalent in the upper central and lateral incisors of children with mesioversion. Immediate handling of the emergency depends on the degree of involvement, particularly on whether the pulp is involved.

Examination should be made immediately for visibility of the pulp cavity at the broken edge of the tooth. The presence of bleeding is indicative of pulp-cavity involvement; however, bleeding from injury to the gum is not to be confused with bleeding from the pulp. Gentle removal of blood with a pledget of cotton may serve to distinguish bleeding of the gum from that of the pulp. Once the field is cleared, the severely chipped tooth may show a distinct cavity containing the artery, the vein, and the nerve in a sheath from which the tooth is fully calcified and sealed off at between 8 and 10 years of age. If the pulp is not involved, the dentist usually places on the immature tooth a thin stainless steel crown which eventually is replaced by a permanent porcelain jacket.

---

† Deceased.

Deciduous teeth, again the upper incisors in particular, may occasionally sustain a blow that literally drives them up into the gum line. In administration of first aid it is most important that this type of injury be carefully distinguished from that involving broken teeth. Again identification of the pulp cavity at the broken edge serves to identify a broken tooth.

In no case should any mechanical effort be made to bring such embedded teeth back into normal position. Such manipulation may easily injure the bud of the permanent tooth. Experience has shown that the embedded deciduous tooth gradually makes a spontaneous return to its original position within approximately 1 month's time.

MISSING TEETH

On administering first aid to a patient who has lost one or more teeth, the importance of their replacement should be made clear to him. Several points of dental hygiene dictate that any missing tooth should be replaced in some manner. Professional treatment should be urged for these reasons:

1. The remaining teeth can spread apart, leaving a space in which food may lodge, thereby causing a pyorrheatic condition.
2. Malocclusion of the opposing tooth can occur.
3. Constant attempts by the patient to force occlusion while chewing occasionally result in the even more serious matter of a misshapen jaw.

The use of bridges must, of course, be avoided in cases of missing teeth in developing mouths. The use of a partial plate until the mouth has matured preserves the alignment of adjoining teeth.

The accident victim (particularly if injuries are generalized) may tend to minimize the importance of losing a tooth unless the underlying dental principles are impressed on him as they are discussed here.

BROKEN JAW

When examining an emergency patient for a broken jaw, it is wise to remember that the break is almost always bilateral. This fact is particularly true as applied to the mandible, as is self-evident if one considers the physical principles involved in the application of a traumatic force to any part of an arch whose ends are relatively fixed.

The physician should not attempt to set the broken jaw. A dental surgeon should see the patient so that careful attention may be given to the occlusion of the teeth. Although apparently excellent setting of the fracture may be made in the physician's office—and occlusion may appear to be perfect—experience has shown that, on healing, jaws have had to be broken again and reset to proper occlusion. In many of these cases, it is difficult to properly evaluate relative anteroposterior occlusion, a problem that may well lead to the situation in which occlusion of only the back teeth is possible in the healed jaw. Severe attrition results, and only extensive dental surgery can save the back teeth.

Furthermore the dental surgeon uses currently available techniques that may make the jaw almost immediately usable, thereby adding greatly to the comfort and general well-being of the patient while knitting is taking place. For instance by making plaster cast models of the lower jaw, as broken, and by then cutting and setting the pieces of the model back to proper occlusion, an aluminum casting may be made for cementing onto the teeth as the bones are forced back into proper alignment. The aluminum casting acts not only as a splint but also provides a chewing surface that may be utilized almost at once. Hooks at the ends of the casting hold tissue in place.

Gauze wrappings should be applied to hold the fractured jaw closed while the patient is being transported for treatment by the dental surgeon. The possibility of severe hemorrhage is rare. Fracture of the upper jaw is considerably more rare but requires much more complicated treatment.

TOOTHACHE

The toothache is a not uncommon minor emergency for which first-aid treatment is requested. If a nerve is exposed or protruding, eugenol (active principle: oil of cloves) may be applied with cotton and gauze. Care should be used in such application to minimize the possibility of "burns" to adjacent oral tissues.

In case of any marked looseness of a tooth, it should be suspected that the pulp may be destroyed; professional dental aid should then be sought. When death of the pulp is suspected, the tooth is particularly susceptible to the application of heat in any form because of the simple physical principle of pressure from expanding gas volume.

Occasionally a patient may falsely describe the existence of pain in a tooth located adjacent to a maxillary sinus. Referred pain from a maxillary sinusitis is frequently elusive and may masquerade quite effectively as toothache. So-called pain in an apparently sound tooth in this area should occasion radiologic visualization for darkness of the maxillary sinus and referral to an otorhinolaryngologist.

Referred pain is a frequent problem in the entire oral area because of the neurologic implications involved in the union of the superior and inferior maxillary nerves with the ophthalmic nerve at the gasserian ganglion.

FOREIGN BODIES OF DENTAL ORIGIN

In the general picture of emergency care and first aid, it is important that the mouth of the injured patient be inspected not only because of the dental considerations previously emphasized but also because of the distinct possibility that a tooth, bridge, or plate—or a broken part thereof—may become a foreign body in the esophagus, trachea, or other part of the airway. Careful administration of first aid must include locating all the dental fragments.

A POINT OF MEDICODENTAL PHILOSOPHY

In urging that the accident victim be made aware of the extreme importance of seeking expert dental aid for any problems that may appear comparatively minor at the time, and in urging that the physician avoid all dental treatment except first aid, we are brought to the fundamental philosophy of this section. There is, today, a rapidly growing emphasis on dental rehabilitation rather than on mere immediate repair. An age-old tendency to ignore dental problems because they will not kill the patient is fortunately passing into oblivion. The dentist no longer simply fills one cavity at a time because it is causing toothache, he finds the cause by taking the mouth as an entity and seeking a balance. He sees the importance of properly functioning teeth in the picture of total health. He knows, for example, that malocclusion —as from an improperly set jaw fracture—may cause a condyle to wear down to the extent that the eustachian tube may be occluded, causing a serious hearing impairment. The dentist is interested not only in maintenance for today but also in looking toward a comfortable old age for the patient.

QUESTIONS

1. How can distinction be made between a bleeding gum and the bleeding pulp of the tooth?
2. Why should missing teeth be soon replaced in some manner?
3. Physicians should not attempt to set a broken jaw. True or false? Explain the reasoning involved.
4. Care should be used in applying eugenol (oil of cloves) to a toothache, to avoid what?

CHAPTER 36

Esoterica

There are a few well-known yet little-discussed emergency situations that challenge the writer of an emergency care textbook at least as much as they disturb the patient or those who are responsible for his initial—and in these cases perhaps definitive—care. They are ill adapted to fit comfortably into the usual chapters of either a topographically organized text or one oriented by emergency situations or by specialties. Therefore they are not frequently discussed, except by those who have suddenly found themselves solely responsible for their immediate care at inconvenient times and in "faraway" places. Then these situations rapidly cease to appear esoteric, merely lacking the aura of drama that characterizes many major emergencies.

HICCUPS

Hiccups, hiccoughs, or singultus may appear ludicrous or unimportant, at best, to one who has never experienced a protracted or even an intractable episode. The treatment, however, has taxed the ingenuity of the medical, paramedical, and non-medical practitioner for as long as one man has tried to help another.

Hiccups are defined as abrupt, intermittent, involuntary, purposeless, jerky diaphragmatic contractions resulting in sudden inspiration opposed by abrupt closure of the glottis. The phenomenon is frequently unilateral, the left side being most commonly involved. Most persons experience transitory episodes of hiccups at some time or other with little inconvenience; however, cases lasting as long as several years have been reported. Such cases prevent adequate eating and sleeping and may be accompanied by severe weight loss and extreme discomfort. At least one patient has been described in the literature in whom transient heart block was triggered through the vagal nerve stimulation involved in hiccups. Remedies have ranged all the way from quite colorful examples of folk medicine, through the perhaps physiologically and psychologically sound techniques of scaring or startling, to the ultimate expedient of crushing either one (usually the left) or both phrenic nerves for permanent relief. (The efferent limb of the hiccup reflex arc is apparently the phrenic nerve. The center is located at cervical cord levels between the third and fifth cervical segments. The afferent limb is the vagus nerve, phrenic nerve, and the sympathetic chain from the sixth to twelfth thoracic segments.)

Several recently published aids to hiccup control stop short of this rather drastic nerve-crushing procedure, however, and they appear worthy of brief consideration here.

Stimulation of the pharynx. Stimulation of the proper area of the pharynx by means of a nasally introduced catheter may stop hiccups. A plastic or rubber suction catheter is introduced through the naris to a distance varying from 3 to 4½ inches, and stimulation by a "jerky, to-and-fro movement" interrupts the reflex and effectively abolishes the hiccuping. Occasionally suction may be needed simultaneously to clear mucus from the pharynx. Orally introduced catheter stimulation, although found to be equally effective, is less well tolerated by the conscious patient. The catheter may be left in place for restimulation if needed.

The area of the pharynx to be stimulated is that just behind the uvula and opposite the body of the second cervical vertebra.

Use of methylphenidate. Various drugs, including amyl nitrite, inhaled ether, intravenous atropine, sedation with narcotics, barbiturates, chlorpromazine and other central nervous system depressants, quinidine, procaine given intravenously or instilled into the abdominal or thoracic cavity, methamphetamine hydrochloride, and large doses of edrophonium chloride (Tensilon) have all been variously recommended in suppressing singultus. Currently, however, more favorable results are being reported with the use of methylphenidate (Ritalin), administered intravenously in the amount of 20 mg. Considerably smaller doses may be effective in certain patients, and as much as 30 mg has been used in one patient. The method is apparently more effective with the conscious patient than in the unconscious or anesthetized patient, and its success—like other modalities in this area of treatment—is not universally endorsed.

Pulmonary inflation. Although its successful use has been reported primarily in the surgical patient whose hiccuping may have been occasioned by visceral manipulations (particularly if the anesthetic used was either nitrous oxide or tubocurarine), brief hyperinflation of the lungs bears an obvious relation to one of the favorite folklore remedies—holding the breath. Increasing airway pressure by manual compression of the reservoir bag for 10 to 20 seconds is effective; the apparent threshold pressure required ranges from 30 to 40 cm H_2O.

Regardless of the approach used, it should be emphasized that all of the suggested methods are actually the treating of a symptom rather than a cause; the multiplicity of the suggested forms of treatment is exceeded only by the variety of possible etiologies.

REMOVAL OF FISHHOOKS

A common minor emergency in coastal areas or those adjacent to the large lakes is the problem of the accidentally embedded fishhook. In addition to the usual precautions of wound treatment and tetanus prophylaxis, there is the problem of removing the hook from the skin with minimal tissue damage.

The usual method of choice has been the simple push-through technique. Under local anesthesia, the shank of the hook is grasped firmly and held at such an angle that the point with its barb can be forced out through the skin by the most direct route. Care should be taken that the direction of movement is, as much as possible, at right angles to the plane of the skin because any needless motion parallel to the plane of the skin causes unnecessary tissue damage. After the barb has been brought through the skin, it is cut off and the hook can be easily withdrawn. The method is particularly applicable when the point of the hook is nearly through the skin.

When the point is rather deeply embedded, a recently reported technique may best be used: After proper cleansing, a local anesthetic in relatively small amount is introduced into the entrance wound itself. Remembering that a fishhook barb is unilateral and located to point across the U of the hook toward the shaft, one grasps the hook and moves it in such a manner as to disengage the barb. The first motion is a slight one in the direction of the point; then pressing sidewise so that the unbarbed outside of the hook bears upon the subcutaneous tissue, the hook is backed out as far as possible. This maneuver, perhaps repeated a time or so, usually brings the barb out to just below the dermis.

A No. 11 Bard-Parker blade is then introduced alongside the shaft of the hook and carefully made to contact the point of the barb. The blade is used to incise the few fibers engaging the barb, and the blade is then rolled over and held firmly against the point of the barb. With the point thus covered, the hook can be brought through the skin without further enlarging the entrance wound.

Alternately an 18-gauge disposable needle may be introduced along the barbed side of the hook with the bevel toward the inside of the hook curve. Slight pressure upward on the hook shank disengages the barb from the flesh; the needle is pushed gently inward and rotated until the lumen locks firmly over the barb. Both the hook and the needle can then be maneuvered out through the entrance wound.

Another technique, described as having originated with native fisherman of Australia, involves the use of only 3 or 4 feet of string or fishline. A loop of the line is made around the curve of the embedded hook, and both ends are wound several times around an index finger in preparation for pulling it out. First, however, gentle pressure is applied to the hook in such a direction as to disengage the barb. Then holding the hook in this alignment with the free hand, the string is carefully aligned in the plane of the hook's long axis—and a quick yank brings it out.

Some time spent in the consideration needed to master one or more of these techniques may well be worthwhile for several reasons: simplicity, minimal distraction of tissue, less discomfort to the patient, small area of anesthesia needed, no need for cutting the shank of the hook, absence of a second wound and resulting scar, and possibility in some cases for handling situations where the shank has multiple hooks. The methods are not, of course, applicable where the point of the hook is already through or nearly through the skin.

THE RING-STRANGULATED FINGER

One can, of course, merely cut the ring off the finger with any one of several implements that may be handy, including—surprisingly enough until we reflect on the relative softness of the gold and silver alloys usually involved—a sturdy pair of ordinary scissors. But one not infrequently meets deeply emotional entreaties regarding the sentimental import attached to the ring. Such considerations may not be unimportant in the overall patient evaluation, particularly in the aged person who frequently presents this problem as a seemingly minor manifestation of a serious problem that may be causing the edema.

If there is time—and one must remember that gangrene may result within 4 or 5 hours, certainly within 10 to 12 hours if there is complete obstruction of the circulation—the following maneuver with a piece of string or suture may easily preserve the ring and make a significant emotional contribution to the patient's stability.

Starting at approximately the most distal joint, string is wound smoothly around the finger, with one strand touching the next, and tightly enough to compress the swollen tissues as much as possible. One should not skip areas that leave edematous projections between the rounds of string. One continues winding smoothly and tightly right up to the margin of the ring. (It has been recommended by some that winding start at the ring and proceed distally, but this procedure has a "milking" acting that tends to merely push the swelling further along the finger rather than compressing it.) The end of the string is slipped under and through the ring. If this proves to be difficult, any small, rounded object, such as a matchstick or the end of a clamp, may be slipped beneath the ring and then the string run through beside it. The string is then slowly unwound on the proximal side of the ring. The ring is gently twisted downward over the spiraled string as it is unwound from beneath the ring, thus providing a sort of leverage to help move the ring along the finger.

HEMATOMA BENEATH THE FINGERNAIL (SUBUNGAL HEMATOMA)

Bruised fingers can be excruciatingly painful. Mere analgesic treatment of the pain is unsatisfactory. Drainage of the hematoma is usually done by either making an incision from underneath the distal end of the nail or by drilling through the nail. Either of these procedures is usually traumatic in an already painful situation.

An alternative method of draining the hematoma involves the use of a straightened end of an ordinary paper clip. The clip is held in a hemostat, the straightened end is heated red-hot in any suitable flame, and it is used to melt through the nail. Immediate relief of pain occurs. The nailbed is protected from injury by the hematoma itself, and almost none of the pressure required for drilling need be applied to the painful area. The nail should be painted with an antiseptic solution before burning through. Any remaining blood may be easily expressed after penetration, and a light dressing should be applied to absorb further drainage.

ACUTE ARTERIAL OCCLUSION

The sudden onset of an acute arterial occlusion may present a dramatic sort of an emergency. For some reason an acute arterial occlusion frequently goes unrecognized. The sudden onset of an excruciating pain in the extremity associated with numbness and inability to move the limb should certainly point toward the possibility. The six P's of acute arterial occlusion may well be kept in mind: pain, pulselessness, paresthesia, paralysis, pallor, and prostration.

In most instances the immediate or emergency management of such a lesion prior to hospitalization is primarily to recognize that an urgent situation is present and that probable surgery is indicated. The rapidity with which the embolus is removed often determines the eventual outcome. Initial treatment should include protection of the limb from injury and avoidance of local application of heat.

QUESTIONS

1. What exactly is hiccups? What are some treatments of the symptoms?
2. How are fishhooks removed from skin with the least damage to the dermis?
3. What is the least painful way in which drainage of hematoma of a nail may take place?

PART NINE

Psychiatric emergencies

CHAPTER 37

Disordered behavior

JAMES M. A. WEISS

Psychiatric emergencies are those in which the patient demonstrates a disorder of thought, mood, or action that is likely to result in dangerous, self-destructive, or socially disturbing behavior.

Often in psychiatric emergencies either the patient, his family, or even casual onlookers demand immediate action. This insistent pressure probably results in more mistakes than any other single factor since hasty action generally makes the situation worse. In very few so-called psychiatric emergencies is there actual immediate danger to the life or health of the patient or those around him. The main factor that makes a psychiatric emergency an "emergency" is usually anxiety or fear on the part of the patient, his family, or both.

Almost all disordered behavior, no matter how disorganized or noneffective it may seem, represents an effort to adapt to internal ("psychologic") or external ("environmental") stress. The type and severity of a person's reaction to external stress depend on his personality and the internal tensions that already exist. For example, in wartime some soldiers react even to the mention of combat with panic, whereas other soldiers withstand many days of combat without demonstrating deviant behavior.

All human beings have psychologic defense mechanisms that generally operate to produce emotional homeostasis. Therefore the emergency nature of most psychiatric disorders is transient and temporary and not infrequently self-limited. Even the most acute emergency may be transitory; even the most bizarre, grotesque, and socially disruptive behavior may be short-lived. The important point is to recognize that most patients with such disorders—even violent patients—are usually frightened, anxious, and uncertain and that the nature of change in these disorders is often toward improvement, self-control, and more socially acceptable behavior.

BASIC PRINCIPLES OF EVALUATION AND TREATMENT

In evaluating a patient with a psychiatric disorder, the first step is to uncover as rapidly as possible the answers to four questions: (1) *What* are the symptoms and signs? (2) How *severe* are the symptoms and signs? (3) To what problems or stresses do the symptoms and signs represent a reaction—*why* have they occurred? (4) What is the general nature of the *disorder* manifested by the symptoms and signs?

Only after determining at least tentative answers to these four questions should one ask the last question: "What should be *done?*" Rational treatment (even first aid) must be based on rational evaluation. In dealing with psychiatric emergencies, however, proper evaluation is in itself often therapeutic and is, in fact, the beginning of any more prolonged treatment. In this respect, there are three fundamental principles to remember.

1. Be as calm, confident, direct, and purposeful as possible. Panic is communicable, and often the patient's relatives are themselves anxious, fearful, agitated, or panicky. This is understandable, but unfortunately such attitudes and feelings are usually conveyed to the patient, who then himself becomes more disturbed, thereby producing a vicious circle of disorder. If you are calm, confident, direct, and purposeful, both the patient and the family often react with improvement. On the other hand, if you appear to be upset, tense, hurried, or in a dither, the patient reacts either with more anxiety or with more manipulation of those about him because he may then believe that his disorder must be a severe one.

2. Begin evaluation and, if possible, treatment at the home or wherever the emergency occurs. Do not rush the patient off to the hospital until you have made some initial attempt to evaluate the situation. Just as the surgeon tries to follow the precept "splint them where they lie," so in dealing with a psychiatric emergency one should attempt to evaluate the situation wherever it occurs. This gives the frightened, stunned, or confused patient the chance to recover some emotional balance in familiar surroundings. It often helps the patient and his family to realize that at least this emergency phase of the disorder may be transient and reversible. And finally it permits simple and brief methods of treatment to be effective before maladaptive behavior patterns have become fixed by time, repetition, or "secondary gain" (the superimposed and usually obvious advantage that the patient can derive from "being ill").

3. To be effective, emergency treatment must be based on brief and relatively simple methods. These methods do not remove fearful or traumatic experiences, alter basic personality traits, or provide magical solutions for all of the patient's problems. The more lengthy and complex procedures should be reserved for the psychiatrist. However, experience has indicated that a brief, sympathetic, noncritical interview, with measures to relieve hunger, pain, and minor physical symptoms in an atmosphere suggesting that recovery is expected, provides the most favorable condition for rapid improvement. Such an interview serves both a diagnostic and a therapeutic purpose, providing psychologic support, alleviating the patient's basic anxiety or fear as well as his secondary symptoms and signs, and supplying an atmosphere in which more definitive treatment, if necessary, can be planned and arranged.

PRINCIPLES OF INTERVIEWING AND BRIEF PSYCHOTHERAPY IN EMERGENCY SITUATIONS

Size up the problem as accurately and as quickly as possible. Interview the patient *alone* if possible. Relatives can wait outside—you can obtain their stories later. Try to find out why the patient is behaving as he is. Frequently simply asking what happened to him may give you the answer. Let the patient reply in his own way. Let him "ventilate," tell *his* account of the problem and his feelings about it. This allows the patient to express anxiety, depression, anger, or other emotions and to feel better by just being able to talk about these emotions. Such a procedure helps the patient to reestablish communication and to feel that someone is trying to understand and to help him.

Do not attempt to direct the flow of conversation. Do not interrupt to ask routine "medical history" questions. You cannot let the patient ramble on endlessly, but you should allot 15 to 45 minutes for the interview. This time belongs to the patient and should not be shared with other distractions. Even 15 minutes in which the patient can talk freely often markedly relieves some of his feelings of helplessness and despair.

Be interested but not maudlin or oversympathetic. Treat the patient as a person you expect to improve. If you overwhelm him with pity, he will only feel more helpless because your attitude will confirm his worst fears about himself. Sometimes if the patient is excessively anxious or rather withdrawn or hostile, a cigarette or a drink of coffee, soup, or warm milk is enough to calm him and to establish rapport. Asking relatives to prepare coffee or soup may also divert *their* anxious fluttering about into purposeful activity.

Accept the patient's limitations and his right to have his own feelings. Do not blame, ridicule, judge, or criticize him for feeling as he does. Your job is to help him cope with his feelings, not to tell him how he *should* feel. Remember that each person has had certain unique experiences that can strongly affect his emotions in relation to subsequent events in his life. If a man's leg is shattered, no one expects him to stand up and walk. But if his ability to deal with his emotions is shattered, many (often including the patient himself) are inclined to expect him to function normally again almost immediately. It does not help to resent the patient's problems, to scold him, to tell him to "snap out of it," or to reassure him that he is "normal" when you yourself do not believe it.

Accept your own limitations in an emergency situation. Do not try to solve all the patient's or the family's problems. Many such problems require specialized psychiatric treatment, and your main job may be simply to calm the patient and his family so that you can get him to a psychiatric facility. The primary goal in psychiatric first aid is to establish effective contact with a disturbed, overwhelmed patient who has lost some degree of self-control or ability to communicate or capacity to evaluate the world as it is. Once this contact is made, it becomes relatively easy either to help him return to adaptive living or to arrange for more definitive professional care.

With some patients the simple ventilation of their feelings to you is sufficient treatment. When the problem seems to be situational ("environmental"), you may often be of most aid by serving as an objective auditor, one who is essentially not involved emotionally, in a discussion that helps the patient (or his relatives) to clarify the situation, to consider alternative courses for action, and to make a realistic decision. With more helpless patients direct advice or honest reassurance may be useful. Sometimes a patient insistently demands some article or action that has not been given him because it is inconvenient (but not dangerous) to do so. For example, a patient may want to telephone a distant relative in another city, but his family will not allow him to do so because they consider his request "silly" or "inappropriate." It is frequently reassuring if the patient is allowed his wish.

At some point before, during, or after the interview, it might become apparent that the patient's symptoms may be related to organic disorder, especially if the patient appears confused or disoriented, has memory loss, or is delirious. Emotional or behavioral disorders can be mimicked by or related to a variety of organic disorders ranging from cerebral abscess to thyroid dysfunction, from impending diabetic coma to heroin intoxication. A brief but reasonably comprehensive physical and neurologic examination most often rules out at least the most obvious organic disorders. Have someone (perhaps the calmest relative) stay with you and the patient during the physical examination. Explain what you are doing as you perform the examination, and reassure the patient in direct and simple language if the findings are negative (even if the patient does not seem to be attending to your words). Omit for the time being the more intimate portions of the physical examination, such as investigation of rectal, pelvic, and genital areas.

The course of the patient's behavior during this relatively brief period of evaluation usually soon clarifies whether he is having reasonable success in overcoming his initial internal turmoil or whether he requires more specialized care. Remember that most patients—even those who appear confused or disoriented—respond in some degree to the kind of communicative attempt outlined above. Do not assume that it is impossible to interview *any* patient until you have tried.

SPECIAL PROBLEMS IN PSYCHIATRIC EMERGENCIES

Psychiatric disorders are not clearly categorized as black or white but tend to range on a continuum from the least to the most severe disorganization of behavior. A simple classification system expresses disorganization as mild, moderate, or severe with symptoms or signs classified in one of six groups: *Affective* symptoms express mood disturbance (as elation, depression, or agitation). *Anxietal* symptoms express anxiety consciously perceived (as fright, fearfulness, or worry). *Behavioral* signs express disturbance manifested by overt action patterns (such as destructiveness or violence). *Mentational* symptoms express disturbance pertaining to intellectual functions, memory, orientation, or judgment. *Reality distortional* symptoms express gross failure in evaluating external reality ("seeing the world as it really is"), as evidenced by hallucinations, delusions, or bizarre or paranoid thinking. *Somatic* symptoms express a disturbance that the *patient* usually considers to be at least partly physical in origin. Within this classification certain syndromes stand out as common or especially important psychiatric emergencies.

Mild reactions

The *mild affective reaction (elated type)* is usually manifested by euphoria and overactivity of speech, thought, and movement. The patient may be restless, interfering, sleepless, and too distractable or too "busy" to pay much attention to food. He often seems rather similar to the man who becomes expansive after a few drinks. Although an interview is important to evaluate the situation, this reaction usually represents an early stage of a severe manic-depressive psychosis, and the biggest problem is to convince the patient and the family that prompt referral to a psychiatrist is of great importance.

The *mild affective reaction (depressed type)* is manifested by dejection, discouragement, self-accusation, tearfulness, and slowing of speech, thought, and movement. Such a depressive reaction may be hidden under a smiling "front," but the patient usually admits to "the blues" if he is asked. This reaction is perhaps less serious if the patient is reacting to an obvious external stress, such as the loss of a loved one. Unless suicide is a concern (see Chapter 38), brief psychotherapy will probably be adequate treatment.

The *mild affective reaction (agitated type)* is manifested by irritability, hyperactivity, and overdistractability. The basic mood is usually either elation or depression, and once this is determined in the interview, the patient can be treated as having a primary elated or depressive type of reaction.

The *mild anxiety reaction* may be manifested by apprehension, worry, increased muscular tension, gross trembling of any or all parts of the body but especially of the hands, temporary speech difficulties, sweating of the palms of the hands, poor appetite (sometimes with nausea or even vomiting), occasional abdominal discomfort, urinary frequency and urgency, diarrhea, rapid heartbeat, giddiness, or breathlessness. Such reactions are very common and are most often transitory, and the patient is helped by ventilation and reassurance in the interview situation.

The *mild behavioral and mentational reactions* only rarely occur as emergencies, and, if they do, can usually be easily treated on the basis of the principles already established.

Reality distortional symptoms are, in my opinion, always indicative of a serious disorder.

The *mild somatic reaction* may often involve symptoms that are "organized" so that they appear as part or parcel of a syndrome of organic disease (such as heart attack, stomach disorder, cerebral concussion, and many others). A supportive interview and a physical examination usually provide the solution to at least the emergency problem.

Moderate reactions

The person who has moderate to severe psychiatric reactions may demonstrate some impairment of verbal communication and usually appears sick or disabled to some degree. The *moderate affective reaction (elated type)* is manifested by a flurry of activity, rapid and often somewhat incoherent talk, inappropriate jokes, marked distractibility, and usually some grandiosity of plan or behavior. Because there is the danger of a sudden switch to assaultiveness or to suicidal depression, immediate hospitalization is indicated. Do not be taken in by the easy rapport one achieves with such persons—their high spirits may be contagious and their jokes may be funny, but they can rapidly become dangerous to themselves or to others.

The *moderate affective reaction (depressed type)* is manifested by marked dejection or apathy and retarded speech and action. A person suffering from this disorder often seems overwhelmed, with a vacant gaze, answering in monosyllables or not replying at all when spoken to, and perhaps suddenly breaking into tears. Unless this person responds rather well in the interview situation, and unless one is quite certain that this person is *not* suicidal, immediate hospitalization is generally required to avoid self-destruction.

The *moderate affective reaction (agitated type)* is usually manifested by tremulousness, choked speech, excessive sweating, a startled reaction to noise, wringing of hands and pacing up and down, and sometimes an appearance of great fearfulness. A brief interview not infrequently calms such a patient and allows you to determine whether the basic affect is one of elation, depression, or anxiety.

The *moderate anxiety reaction* usually has these same symptoms and can often be treated wth brief psychotherapy; but if elation or depression of this degree is suspected, it is important not to leave the patient alone (even for a moment while you step out to call the hospital) and to get the patient to a psychiatric facility. The *moderate anxiety reaction* may also be seen in the person who shows no evidence of depression, elation, or overt anxiety but who seems stunned, puzzled, or confused. The person may answer questions in monosyllables and make little or no effort to respond to any stimuli. The chances are that this syndrome represents a "stun reaction" to some sort of environmental catastrophe or to what the patient interprets as a catastrophe (which may not be obvious to the onlooker) or the syndrome may be a serious depressive reaction. If the patient does not respond rather rapidly to brief psychotherapy, treat him as having a serious depressive reaction until further evidence indicates otherwise.

The *moderate behavioral reaction* may be seen in the person who is angry, hostile, and threatening violence. If no alleviation of his behavior occurs after a psychotherapeutic interview, the emergency would appear to be more social and legal than medical and should probably be referred to the police or similar authority. However, if the interview reveals any bizarre thoughts or actions on the part of either the apathetic or the angry patient, a schizophrenic (reality distortional) break may be impending.

The *moderate reality distortional reaction* may be manifested by inappropriate apathy or anger, as well as by vague somatic symptoms, increasing withdrawal from occupational and social activities, eccentric or odd behavior or verbal expressions, feelings of outside control of thoughts or emotions, attributing special significance to irrelevant events, silly mannerisms and laughter, or excessive jealousy or suspiciousness. It is often difficult to empathize with such a patient, that is, to "put yourself in his shoes." A person with such symptoms is frequently aware that something is very wrong and accepts hospitalization voluntarily, but in any event immediate psychiatric treatment is necessary.

The *moderate* (or even *severe*) *mentational reaction* is manifested by confusion, disorientation, memory defects, and anxiety, fear, or shallow or quickly changeable emotions. This patient may be frankly delirious and may hallucinate. (Remember that all patients who hallucinate are not necessarily schizophrenic.) The condition tends to be exaggerated at night. Technically termed the organic brain syndrome, this reaction is commonly associated with an organic disease process. The first step in treating the patient in such an acute delirious or confused state, then, is to ascertain the cause, which may be uremia, coronary thrombosis, fluid or electrolyte imbalance (especially after trauma or surgical operation), cerebral neoplasm, pneumonia, drug intoxication, or a variety of other disorders. Basic treatment in this condition must be directed to this underlying cause.

The patient should have continuous nursing attendance in a room with a night light (which decreases liability to hallucinations and helps the patient orient to his surroundings). Friends or relatives of the patient should be about. If fluid, salt, or vitamin balances are disturbed, they should be corrected. Drugs should be avoided until the cause of the reaction is known; then if there are no contraindications, thioridazine hydrochloride or chlorpromazine may be administered. If the patient is quite disturbed, hospitalization may be necessary. The patient should be prevented from harming himself, and the possibility of suicide should be kept in mind.

The *moderate somatic reaction* is usually manifested as psychologic blindness, deafness, loss of voice, or weakness or paralysis of one or more extremities. Multiple aches and pains or loss of touch sensation in an unusual distribution may be present. Such symptoms usually involve the sensory or voluntary motor system and may include a sudden collapse, convulsive like seizures, or attacks of extreme pain. The patient is usually not agitated but rather presents a characteristic bland indifference.

A thorough physical examination to rule out organic disorder is a must, of course; however, if the examination is negative, one is sometimes tempted to believe that the patient is malingering or "faking." Most of these patients, however, are completely unaware that no physical basis for their symptoms exists, and they are just as disabled as if they had a physical injury. Furthermore the person who *is* malingering is emotionally ill in another way. Such patients, as well as those who have the psychologically related symptoms of amnesia, should be referred for thorough psychiatric evaluation and treatment.

Severe reactions

The *severe reactions* are generally manifested by symptoms and signs that are similar to but exaggerated forms of those in the moderate reactions. These tend to involve either marked overactivity or marked underactivity. Such persons are more or less out of contact with or dissociated from reality. For all practical purposes they have lost much of their ability to communicate rationally with others.

The *severe affective reaction (elated type)* is manifested by extreme euphoria, excitement, and even manic delirium, which may closely resemble the *severe mentational reaction*. Schizophrenic excitement, on the other hand, usually involves random impulsive activity or continuous unorganized hyperactivity, as well as rage, uncontrolled and seemingly purposeless destructiveness, sometimes incontinence or smearing of excretory material, and often response to hallucinations ("listening to" or "answering" an unseen person). Speech, if present, is incoherent, bizarre, or wild.

The *dissociated reaction* ("panic" or "blind flight") is somewhat similar, manifested by purposeless, undirected, uncontrolled motor behavior that may lead to self-destruction. This person runs about wildly and may weep or laugh uncontrollably. A severe dissociated or panic reaction can result when a person with obsessive or phobic thoughts is forced into an untenable situation—for example, the mother who has obsessive thoughts about killing her child and is left alone with that child, or the patient who has a phobia about being in small rooms and is trapped in an elevator.

When dealing with the excited, panicky, hyperactive patient, it is worthwhile to first try a calm, yet firm, interview approach. If this fails or if you cannot even get the attention of the patient to begin communication, tranquilizing drugs may be most helpful. If they are used, however, explain to the patient why you are using them, even if he does not seem to understand. Otherwise on awakening in a strange hospital, the patient may suffer increased confusion, anger, or even a paranoid hatred for you.

Such a patient must, of course, be taken to the nearest psychiatric inpatient facility as quickly as possible. You will need two or three others to help get the patient there, even if he is sedated (for he may suddenly become violent). If only one or two persons attempt to transport such a person, even by force, the patient will probably break away and become even more disturbed. For the same reason, mechanical restraints (such as leather cuffs) should be used only in a dire emergency, for patients so restrained often become more excited or combative or develop extreme physical exhaustion and sometimes cardiovascular collapse. It is better to "crowd" the patient with three or four people. It should go without saying that, contrary to popular belief, slapping an emotionally disorganized patient or dousing him with cold water usually makes things worse and may indeed provoke extreme assaultiveness.

The *severe apathetic reaction* ("stupor") is manifested by marked retardation in thinking, speech, and motor activity. A patient suffering from this reaction may be, in fact, mute and immobile. He may appear completely withdrawn and may not react at all to external stimuli. He may be incontinent or dribble saliva. He may seem very depressed or without any apparent overt emotion at all. Sometimes such a patient can be led like a small child. In *schizophrenic apathy*, the posture may be fixed with muscle rigidity; the patient sometimes demonstrates repetitious movements or mannerisms or appears negativistic, and he may act as if he is responding to hallucinations. Often such patients do not eat and refuse food when it is offered to them.

The severe apathetic reaction may also be a variant of the "stun" reaction or may involve an organic etiology. In any case, prompt hospitalization is necessary. Precautions should be taken, for as such patients begin to recover from their apathy they may become suicidal; or if the basic process is a schizophrenic one, the patient may suddenly switch to a state of homicidal excitement.

Finally the *severe delusional reaction* is characterized by false and bizarre beliefs that often relate to sinfulness, worthlessness, persecution by God or by a certain person or group (often by organizations such as the Federal Bureau of Investigation), and sometimes to grandiosity. Such distortions of reality always indicate severe psychiatric disorder and are best treated with immediate psychiatric hospitalization.

FINAL NOTE

Frequently a well-trained psychiatrist takes a calculated risk designed to benefit both the patient and society and, for example, follows someone who might conceivably be dangerous to himself or others on an outpatient basis. The psychiatrist takes this chance, however, on the basis of his special knowledge, knowledge of the probabilities and prognoses in similar cases, and knowledge of this particular patient based on intensive interviews, psychologic tests, social histories, and similar data.

The person who, without specialized training, attempts to take similar risks in dealing with psychiatric emergencies is providing only irresponsible disservice to the patient and to those around him. Thus the rule for the person who would render first aid in psychiatric emergencies should be: In case of doubt, get the patient to a psychiatrist or to a hospital. If possible, ascertain in advance which psychiatric facilities are available. Many general hospitals now provide psychiatric service. Even when such a service is not available, many psychiatrically disordered patients can be treated with brief psychotherapy and drugs, as well as with good nursing care, on the nonpsychiatric services of such a hospital. Finally remember that the local or state police or sheriff may be called on for assistance in an emergency; these officers are legally responsible for, and often equipped to deal with, the psychiatrically disturbed patient who may be dangerous to himself and others.

In psychiatric emergencies, however, the *attitude* of the person providing aid is likely to be the most important factor in the original contact with the patient and often makes the difference between success or failure in handling the situation. The basic features of this attitude include calmness, confidence, empathy, and the willingness to listen to the patient's problems. In these cases perhaps the best medicine the helper has is himself.

QUESTIONS

1. What are the four initial questions to consider in the evaluation of a patient with a psychiatric disorder?
2. What are the three fundamental principles in dealing with psychiatric emergencies?
3. A simple classification system expresses disorganization of behavior as mild, moderate, or severe. How are the symptoms or signs classified? List all six types of symptoms and give a brief description of each.

CHAPTER 38

The suicidal patient

JAMES M. A. WEISS

The suicide of a patient, because of its finality, is perhaps the most devastating experience that can occur when one is dealing with psychiatric emergencies. Furthermore suicide is the prime cause of death among psychiatric patients. Whether any individual human being will commit suicide appears to depend on the group attitudes in his particular society, the adverse environmental pressures that he must meet, and the interaction of these with the character and personality of that person.

The clinical problem is to determine which patients are actually suicidal. In evaluating suicidal danger one must remember that suicidal thoughts or ideas, considered in more than a passing manner, have been found in as many as half of so-called normal persons by some investigators. Some apparently suicidal persons make attempts that are simply suicidal gestures because persons in this group do not intend to end life and are certain that they will *not* die as a result of their actions, although the action is performed in a manner that other persons might interpret as suicidal in purpose. Such attempts seem to be made in many or most cases to gain attention or to influence other persons, and the individual often takes considerable precaution to ensure remaining alive by making the attempt with other persons present, informing someone of the attempt, or initiating his own rescue. Other persons who attempt suicide are quite sincere in their intention to end life, expect to die, and, indeed, are often sucessful in achieving their aim. Finally there are many persons who attempt suicide in such a way that death *might* result from their action but, again, might not—their action, in fact, has the nature of a gamble with death.

One study indicates that suicidal attempts are most likely to be serious or sucessful if the individual is older than 40 years, if he attributes his difficulty to "mental illness" or the fear of same, if he himself describes or admits his intent as serious, or if he appears to be clinically psychotic. Suicidal attempts are much less likely to be serious or successful if the individual is younger than 30 years, if he attributes his difficulty to family troubles, if he does not appear to be severely disturbed psychiatrically, and if his admitted intent is anything other than certain death. Serious or successful suicidal attempts are more likely to occur among older persons than among younger persons, among men rather than women, among whites rather than blacks, among persons isolated socially, among those who appear depressed, and among persons who have made prior suicidal attempts.

Such information only provides a guide to probabilities; the fact remains that any emotionally disturbed person who indicates suicidal intent should be evaluated by a competent psychiatrist. Every depressive reaction carries with it some danger of suicide, and no suicidal talk should be considered lightly. Several studies have indicated that a large majority of persons who successfully commit suicide communicate their intent to someone prior to the act. A depressive reaction involving feelings of futility, loss of appetite or loss of weight, insomnia (especially early waking with inability to fall asleep again), or distortions of reality must be considered as particularly dangerous. It is important to gauge the intensity of the patient's distress, but it should be kept in mind that people who talk about suicide often *do* kill themselves.

If there is any suspicion at all of suicidal intent, one should not be afraid to question a patient about it. When the patient makes some mention of his distress, one might ask: "Do you feel so depressed (upset, disturbed) that life does not seem to be worth living?" If the patient answers "Yes," one should then ask, "Have you thought about suicide (or about killing yourself)?" Such a procedure does *not* give the patient any ideas of suicide that he did not already have, and his response often helps you to determine his intent. If his response is bizarre or illogical or delusional, includes ideas of worthlessness, or indicates a preoccupation with thoughts of suicide and with actual concrete procedures for carrying out the act, one should consider that the danger of a serious or successful suicidal attempt is great. It should be remembered also, however, that suicidal desire may hide behind the reassuring words of the patient apparently recovering from a severe depression.

If suicidal intent is suspected, immediate hospitalization of a patient on a psychiatric inpatient service is indicated. It is most important that these patients not be left alone, even to go to the bathroom. A careful vigilance must be maintained until the patient is transferred to definitive professional care and treatment.

QUESTIONS

1. After what age are most suicidal attempts likely to be serious or successful? Before what age are they less likely to be serious?

2. If there is any suspicion at all of suicidal intent, one should not be reluctant to question a patient about it. True or false? Explain.

CHAPTER 39

Chemotherapy in psychiatric emergencies

JAMES M. A. WEISS

Because many new psychoactive drugs have been introduced in the past decade and because new pharmacologic agents are continuously being made available, it is a great temptation in dealing with psychiatric emergencies to use chemotherapy as *the* first aid, even before any attempt at competent evaluation has been made. There are, however, many reasons why drugs should be used only after the most thorough possible evaluation has been obtained and after brief psychotherapy ("interviewing") has been attempted. The psychoactive drugs can be useful in alleviating undesirable symptoms and signs in certain patients, but they do not act against specific known etiologic agents. When sufficient doses are given to control a disordered patient, they may cloud his symptoms, making correct diagnosis difficult or impossible, may modify the disorder temporarily so that definitive treatment or disposition becomes more complicated, or may even be toxic in their effect.

The psychiatrically disordered patient is one who does not think clearly. However calming a sedative or tranquilizing drug may be, it often adds to his confusion and makes him even more inaccessible to evaluation and treatment. It does seem that chemotherapy is simpler than other techniques when dealing with a wild, panicky, or severely agitated patient. But a seriously disorganized person often requires very large and dangerous doses of even appropriate drugs. These drugs may, in fact, produce paradoxic responses in which an agitated patient becomes even more excited or sometimes becomes suicidal when he is given a drug that usually has a sedative or tranquilizing effect. Sometimes so-called antidepressant drugs precipitate an excited, violent panic.

Frequently the psychoactive drugs are prescribed in quite small doses that are especially liable to produce a paradoxic effect or to have little or no effect at all. In this situation, one is tempted to try another and yet another drug and may end up giving the patient a series of drugs, all of inadequate dose but cumulatively dangerous. Even in small doses the effects of these drugs cannot always be predicted. Except in special situations, it is therefore preferable to leave the chemotherapeutic approach in psychiatric emergencies to the qualified psychiatrist or to use such drugs only in the hospital situation. If you do administer drugs and then send the patient on to a psychiatrist or a hospital, remember to indicate clearly what drug was given, what the dosage was, and when it was administered. Otherwise the patient may be given additional amounts of the same drug or a similar drug that could be most harmful in combination with the first dose.

The administration of *chloral hydrate*, 0.5 to 2 gm, or *paraldehyde*, 3 to 15 ml in orange juice, is still used in the treatment of excitement, mania, delirium, and severe anxiety. These drugs often have the desired quieting effect on motor behavior but also produce an undesirable somnolence and lethargy and may have other side effects. Chloral hydrate must be given orally or rectally (in olive oil) and does not take effect as quickly as a drug that can be injected intravenously or intramuscularly. Chloral hydrate is also dangerous in patients with liver or kidney damage and should never be administered simultaneously with coumarin anticoagulants.

In mild or moderate agitation or anxiety, *phenobarbital* or some of the newer sedatives are sometimes used. Recent research involving extensive clinical studies with hypnotic, sedative, and minor tranquilizing drugs has indicated that in most cases the oral barbiturates and *glutethimide* (Doriden), *methyprylon* (Noludar), *ethchlorvynol* (Placidyl), *methaqualone* (Quaalude), and *meprobamate* (Equanil, Miltown) lack efficacy or interfere with REM sleep or tend to produce habituation or addiction or have dangerous side effects or high toxicity. The benzodiazepine derivatives appear to be superior in almost all ways. Orally administered *chlordiazepoxide* (Librium), 25 mg, and *diazepam* (Valium), 10 mg, are useful minor tranquilizers, and *flurazepam* (Dalmane), 30 mg, is the hypnotic drug of choice. However, none of these drugs is really appropriate for emergency treatment; their administration is usually not necessary (psychotherapy is generally more effective) and their use can lead to the masking of important symptoms or may produce unwanted psychologic and physiologic side effects.

In more severe agitation, *thiopental* (Pentothal Sodium), 0.5 gm in 20 ml at the rate of 1 ml per minute until sleep occurs, and *amobarbital* (Amytal), 0.05 to 0.2 gm, possess short-acting sedative action and can be administered intravenously, but these drugs may depress respiration and vascular tone, may precipitate laryngospasm, may produce a paradoxic response, and may increase an underlying depressive affect in an agitated person. Such drugs are also dangerous in the presence of undetected liver, kidney, respiratory, or cardiovascular disorders.

In the emergency treatment of severely agitated states, however, the more potent tranquilizing drugs can be of great help. The route of administration of any psychoactive drug must depend on the patient's state. Oral administration is probably best if you or a relative can persuade the patient to take the medication. Many emotionally disturbed patients are frightened by an injection or regard it as some sort of an attack, but if necessary, the injectable form of these drugs can be used.

Therefore adequate doses by mouth of some major tranquilizer—specifically chlorpromazine (Thorazine), 100 mg, repeated in 1 hour if necessary, trifluoperazine (Stelazine), 5 mg, haloperidol (Haldol), 5 mg, or thioridazine hydrochloride (Mellaril), 100 mg—are the most helpful in the severely agitated patient. If the patient is so disturbed that parenteral therapy is required, the same drugs (except thioridazine hydrochloride) may be administered intramuscularly, but the recommended oral dosage should be cut in half and should be repeated only after 2 hours for chlorpromazine and 4 hours for trifluoperazine and haloperidol. (When one is using chlorpromazine [Thorazine] the danger of a sudden drop in blood pressure should be kept in mind.) In cases of delirium tremens, chlordiazepoxide (Librium) given intramuscularly in doses up to 100 mg has been found very useful.

Of course, all the dosages recommended in this discussion are ranges or averages and must be varied in relation to the patient's size, general physical condition, and degree of behavioral disorder. It should be remembered that tranquilizing drugs are neither specific nor curative, that their effects vary from patient to patient, and that their *continued* use should generally be under the direction of a psychiatrist, who is specifically trained to evaluate the indications for and the effects of these medicines.

A comparatively new group of drugs is the antidepressants (sometimes called "psychic energizers"). Currently, however, the action of these drugs is so variable, and undesirable side effects are so common, that they are *not* recommended for emergency use.

Other specialized somatic treatment (such as electroshock therapy) may also be very useful and even lifesaving in certain psychiatric emergencies; however, such treatment almost always requires a physician with advanced specialized training in psychiatry for administration and generally should be administered in a psychiatric inpatient setting.

QUESTIONS

1. What is most helpful in dealing with the severely agitated patient?

2. Tranquilizing drugs are neither specific nor curative for psychiatric patients in emergencies. True or false? Explain.

PART TEN

Prevention

CHAPTER 40

Tetanus

WESLEY FURSTE

Tetanus or lockjaw is a severe and dreaded infectious complication of wounds that is caused by the toxin-producing *Clostridium tetani*. This disease is characterized by tonic spasms of the voluntary muscles and by a tendency toward episodes of respiratory arrest. Throughout the entire world it has a mortality rate of about 50%.

Tetanus has been recognized as a terrifying disease for 2,300 years. Hippocrates referred as follows to the master of a large ship who smashed the index finger of his right hand with the anchor: "Seven days later a somewhat foul discharge appeared; then trouble with his tongue . . . on the third day opisthotonos occurred with sweating . . . 6 days later he died." In the second century, Aretaeus, the Cappadocian, called the disease an inhuman calamity, an unseemly sight, a spectacle painful even to the beholder. He wrote: "The wish of the physician that the patient should expire, otherwise irreverent and objectionable, is, in this case well taken."

Tetanus continues to occur as a complication of lacerations, open fractures, burns, abrasions, hypodermic injections, operations on the gastrointestinal tract, and birth (infection of the umbilical stump in the newborn).

The introduction of tetanus toxoid about four decades ago, which was followed in many parts of the world by programs of immunization of the population, contributed greatly to the control of tetanus. Nevertheless during the decade 1951-1960, tetanus remained an unsolved problem in many areas of the world. In August 1975, a World Health Organization official stated that tetanus was causing more than 1,000,000 deaths each year all over the world.

Relatively few cases of tetanus occur in the United States. In fact in 1975, only 94 cases were reported for the entire United States.

PROPHYLAXIS

The four bases on which the pyramid of tetanus prophylaxis for the wounded is founded are (1) tetanus toxoid, (2) surgical care, (3) antitoxin, and (4) emergency medical identification devices.

While every injury presents its own problems to the physician who is called on to treat it, active immunization with tetanus toxoid—as far as the risk of tetanus is concerned—has almost oversimplified tetanus prophylaxis in the majority of injured persons in that a small booster dose is usually given to those previously immunized and is most efficacious in preventing tetanus.

303

Table 40-1. Incidence of tetanus in the United States Army

	Admissions for wounds and injuries	Cases of tetanus	Cases per 100,000 wounds and injuries
Civil War	280,040	505	18.03
World War I	523,158	70	13.4
1920-1941*	580,283	14	2.4
World War II	2,734,819	12	0.44
Korean War		6-8	
1956-November 1971 (including Vietnam conflict)		0	

*Inclusive.

Sometimes a major problem, however, is the fact that neither the patient nor his physician can be completely certain of prior protection by toxoid unless the patient carries an emergency medical identification device indicating protection or sensitivity to toxoid.

In association with the ever-increasing use of tetanus toxoid and the steadily declining incidence of tetanus, there has possibly developed a decreasing awareness by physicians that tetanus can occur. The possibility of tetanus should at least be thought of in the individual with unexplained irritability or convulsions.

That tetanus can be prevented is amply documented. The incidence of tetanus in a group of wounded Manila civilians without tetanus toxoid immunization during World War II was 900,000% greater than in wounded United States Army personnel with such immunization (Table 40-1).

Wound prevention

For tetanus to occur, *Clostridium tetani* must gain entrance to the body by a wound, even though the wound may be so small that it is not recognized, and tetanus toxin, which is actually responsible for tetanus, must be produced. If wound prevention programs were completely efficacious everywhere, tetanus would not occur.

Individualization of wounded patients

Wounded patients are individuals. Some may not have had all the indicated tetanus toxoid injections, others may have had too many toxoid injections, and a small number may be hypersensitive to tetanus toxoid. A few may have insignificant wounds, others may have almost lethal wounds. Many may not have with them an up-to-date emergency medical identification device with significant tetanus toxoid injection information. Hence individualization of each patient for tetanus prophylaxis must be considered.

Toxoid

Prophylactic measures rendered at the time of injury to nonactively immunized persons cannot be guaranteed to offer protection, but with prior active immunization, a booster dose at the time of injury offers effective and prolonged protection. In the previously immunized person, a very small booster dose of toxoid produces

Table 40-2. Tetanus toxoid immunization status in 12 cases of tetanus
in 2,734,819 United States Army hospital admissions during World War II

	Fatal cases	Total cases
No active immunization	2	6
Initial immunization (three injections of fluid toxoid) accomplished but no emergency stimulating injection given	1	2
Initial immunization plus emergency stimulating injection given	2	4
TOTAL	5̄	1̄2̄

antibody levels in 3 weeks, which can be interpreted as equivalent to a 1,000 to 100,000 unit dose of heterologous or homologous passive antibody. In addition, it has been demonstrated in animal studies with toxin that an active booster response appears earlier than can be estimated by blood antitoxin levels. To give greater protection against severe, slight, and unrecognized wounds, to maintain this protection, and to avoid the extra care and cost entailed in active-passive immunization, every practicing physician, regardless of his specialty, should make every effort to actively immunize with tetanus toxoid—and to keep actively immunized—his patients, their families, his family, and himself.

United States Army experiences with tetanus toxoid. During World War II the almost 100% efficiency and safety of tetanus toxoid as a prophylactic agent were proved by the experience of the United States Army. Only 12 cases of tetanus occurred in a series of 2,734,819 hospital admissions for wounds and injuries. Five of these 12 patients (41.7%) died. As to immunization status, only 4 of these 12 patients had had both an initial immunization of fluid toxoid and a booster dose (Table 40-2).

Duration of effect of tetanus toxoid. The human body does not "forget" a dose of tetanus toxoid. The first injection sensitizes or triggers the body so that it responds to the second and reinforcing or booster doses of tetanus toxoid by producing circulation serum tetanus antitoxin and probably other protective mechanisms. A maximum period of time after which there is not an anamnestic response has not yet been determined. Antitoxin titers are frequently being determined for World War II veterans to determine whether there is such an interval.

A number of investigators have already shown an unexpectedly high incidence of long-lasting immunity; in their studies, 85% to 95% of individuals immunized against tetanus during World War II still carried protective antibody levels 15 to 21 years later. Furthermore with practically no exceptions these individuals responded well to a booster dose of toxoid.

No antitoxin if adequate tetanus toxoid immunization. It should be noted that in the United States armed forces in World War II, protection against tetanus by booster toxoid after wounding was achieved without the simultaneous use of antitoxin when there was adequate prior tetanus toxoid immunization. Credit is given to the United States military forces consultants who recommended that antitoxin is not necessary with adequate toxoid prophylaxis.

Reactions to tetanus toxoid. Significant reactions to tetanus toxoid continue to be rare but are occurring more frequently (Table 40-3).

Table 40-3. Reactions of a male to tetanus toxoid with repeated doses

Date; age	Type of toxoid given	Reason	Reaction
1949;2	DTP	Initial series	—
1949;2	DTP	Initial series	—
1951;4	Adsorbed T	Injury	—
1952;5	DTP	Booster	—
1953;6	Adsorbed T	Injury	—
1955;8	Adsorbed T	Injury	Redness and induration greater than anticipated
1963;16	Adsorbed T	Injury	Redness and induration of half of upper arm
1964;17	Adsorbed T	Injury	Redness and induration from elbow to shoulder; "almost double in size"

September 1965: serum tetanus antitoxin titer: 3 units per milliliter. The protective level is 0.01 units per milliliter.

From 1951 until 1970 more than 2.5 million injections of adsorbed tetanus toxoid had been given in Denmark with no reports of death and only a single case of neurologic complications with sequelae.

Because some individuals may be sensitive or become sensitive to tetanus toxoid, one main principle of active tetanus immunization must be to balance the dosage and administration of toxoid against the side reactions so as to obtain optimal protection with a minimal risk of complications.

Basic immunization; frequency of periodic nonwound tetanus toxoid boosters and of wound boosters. Since tetanus toxoid is a most effective antigen that may produce undesirable reactions, recommendations continue to be made for less frequent use and for smaller dosage of tetanus toxoid.

For *primary immunization* of children 2 months through 6 years, the manufacturer's recommended dose of diphtheria and tetanus toxoids and pertussis vaccine (DTP) is given intramuscularly on four occasions, three doses at 4- to 6-week intervals with a fourth dose approximately 1 year after the third injection. Ideally immunization should begin at 2 to 3 months of age or at the time of a 6-week checkup if that is an established routine. For schoolchildren and adults a series of three doses of tetanus and diphtheria toxoids, adult type (Td), is given intramuscularly, with the second dose 4 to 6 weeks after the first and the third dose 6 months to 1 year after the second.

For *routine nonwound booster doses* for children 3 through 6 years (preferably at time of school entrance, kindergarten or elementary school), one injection of the recommended dose of DTP is administered intramuscularly. Thereafter and for all other persons, the recommended dose of Td (adult) is given intramuscularly every 10 years. If a dose is administered sooner as part of wound management (see specific recommendations below), the next booster is not needed for another 10 years. More frequent booster doses are not indicated and may be associated with increased incidence and severity of reactions.

Table 40-4. Voluntary versus controlled tetanus prophylaxis

Category of cases	Number of cases
United States civilians: 1971	120
United States Army personnel: 1956–November 1971	0
United States Navy and Marine Corps personnel: 1946–April 1972	0

Table 40-5. Survey of use of emergency medical identification device (EMID)*

	Number	Percentage
Individuals surveyed	200	100%
EMID immediately available	14	7%
EMID with tetanus data	3	1.5%

*February 26, 1975 to April 23, 1975.

If an individual is wounded, the possibility of administration of a wound tetanus toxoid booster must be considered. Certain general principles that should be observed are given on p. 310 and then specific recommendations are made. This conservative guide to prophylaxis against tetanus in wound management has been developed in an endeavor to simultaneously eliminate unnecessary reactions to tetanus toxoid and absolutely prevent tetanus in the injured individual. A basic aspect of this guide is that for those with adequate prior active immunization, for the great majority of wounds, no booster dose of tetanus toxoid is needed unless more than 5 years have elapsed since the last tetanus toxoid injection. For severe, neglected, or old (more than 24 hours) wounds no booster dose is necessary unless more than 1 year has elapsed since the last booster dose. Such a conservative attitude is based on these concepts:

1. In general, surgeons see a more severe and a more unusual wound than the nonsurgical physician. The long intervals between wound boosters are for the "usual types" of wounds.
2. Tetanus may occur in individuals who have no demonstrable wound or who have very minor wounds; hence all individuals should have adequate serum tetanus antitoxin titers at all times.
3. Physicians want none of their patients—whether they have special problems or not—to develop tetanus.
4. The United States Army and Navy statistics are impressive: No cases of tetanus have been reported among active duty Army personnel from 1956 to November 1971 and among active duty Navy and Marine Corps personnel from 1946 to April 1972 (Table 40-4). In contrast to such statistics there were reported 120 civilian cases of tetanus in 1971 in the United States.
5. Patients do not have an immediately available emergency medical identification device with reliable tetanus data on it. In a survey of patients and their friends during a few months of 1975, only 3 of 200 (1.5%) had such data immediately available (Table 40-5). The recommendations of the U.S. Public Health Service are based on immediately available and accurate records with tetanus data.

6. For the particularly severe or contaminated, so-called tetanus-prone or unusual injuries, it has been stated that there is a need for additional booster doses.
7. In general, reactions to tetanus toxoid are minimal in contrast to the grim picture of a person with tetanus and to the average tetanus mortality rate of about 50%.
8. The drugstore cost of a booster dose of tetanus toxoid is small when compared to the hospital cost of a case of tetanus ($9,773.80 for a recent case).
9. There are still a number of individuals who do not have adequate tetanus toxoid immunization but who may erroneously be considered to have such immunization when they are seen as wounded patients. In 1970 it was stated that one third of a random group of children of all ages in Hamburg, Germany, did not have tetanus toxoid immunization. More recently the lagging immunity of our children in the United States is becoming a potentially serious problem (Fig. 1).
10. Cases of failure of booster tetanus toxoid injections to prevent tetanus many years after injections or cases of modified tetanus after such injections have been reported.
11. The professional liability responsibilities of the surgeon are greater than those of the nonsurgeon physician.

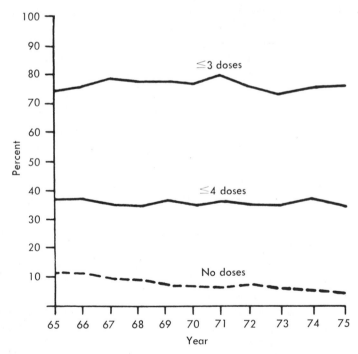

Fig. 1. Diphtheria-tetanus-pertusis immunization status of 1- to 4-year-old children in the United States, 1965-1975. (Data from United States Immunization Survey, 1975, Atlanta, Center for Disease Control.)

12. Surgeons—in respect to the prevention of tetanus—do not want to be like the poet, Ovid, who wrote: "Too late I grasp my shield after my wounds."

Rapid, active, basic immunization at the time of injury. Rapid active immunization, that is, three to five doses of tetanus toxoid approximately every other day, does not produce active immunity rapidly enough to protect an individual in whom such immunization is started just after a wound has been inflicted.

Prophylaxis against tetanus by the first injection of toxoid given at the time of injury. The initial injection of toxoid at the time of an injury does not provide immunity from tetanus for the injury. If an injured patient who has not previously been given tetanus toxoid is given it immediately after an injury, this first dose does not provide immunity for the injury.

No active immunity from tetanus. The amount of the very potent tetanus toxin necessary to produce clinical tetanus is so small that it does not incite an active antibody level high enough to prevent a second attack of tetanus. Consequently tetanus is a nonimmunizing disease; hence a history of tetanus does not rule out the possibility of a second attack of tetanus.

To prevent such a second attack, when a patient is recovering from tetanus and is about 4 weeks past the onset of tetanus, his attending physician should begin active immunization with tetanus toxoid.

Surgical wound care

Surgical prophylaxis consists of the removal of *Clostridium tetani* and nonviable tissues from wounds and of the best possible reconstruction of aerobic wounds. Optimal surgical care of wounds is provided when the following are observed:

1. The wounds are treated as soon as possible.
2. Aseptic technique is observed with the use of gloves, gowns, masks, and sterile instruments and the application of proper solutions to prepare the skin before the necessary operative procedures at the injured site.
3. During skin preparation, the wound is covered with gauze to prevent further contamination.
4. Proper lighting is employed so that the surgeon can exactly identify and protect vital structures such as nerves and vessels.
5. Adequate instruments and adequate help are at the surgeon's call to provide the best and gentlest possible retraction of structures in wounds.
6. Hemostasis is obtained with delicate instruments and with fine suture material so that there is a minimum of necrotic tissue left in wounds.
7. Gentle handling of tissues is emphasized at all times so that necrotic tissue is not produced.
8. Complete debridement with scalpel excision of necrotic tissue and with removal of foreign bodies is performed so that no pabulum is left on which any unremoved bacteria can propagate.
9. The wound is copiously irrigated with large amounts of physiologic salt solution to wash out minute avascular fragments of tissue and to eliminate foreign bodies.
10. If there is any doubt about producing anaerobic conditions in which the tetanus bacillus can grow and produce its lethal toxin, the wound is left wide open and drainage is instituted when necessary.

Guidelines for short-term prevention of tetanus in the injured*

I. General principles

    A. Both physician and nonphysician citizens are responsible for the prevention of tetanus.

    B. There are professional liability problems for physician and nonphysician citizens in regard to adequate prophylaxis against tetanus. To protect the medicolegal rights of the patient, of nonphysician personnel involved in the care of the patient, and of all physicians associated with the care of the patient, the complete care of the patient, including all skin or other sensitivity tests and all injections should be recorded on permanent and available records.

    C. The attending physician must determine individually for each patient with a wound what is required for adequate prophylaxis against tetanus.

    D. Each patient with a wound should be given adsorbed tetanus toxoid[1] intramuscularly at the time of injury, either as an initial immunizing dose or as a booster for previous immunization, unless he has received a booster or has completed his initial immunization series within the past 5 years. As the antigen concentration varies in different products, specific information on the volume of a single dose is provided on the label of the package.[2]

    E. Regardless of the active immunization status of the patient, for all wounds optimal surgical care should be rendered immediately, including removal of all devitalized tissue and foreign bodies. Such care is essential as part of the prophylaxis against tetanus.

    F. Whether or not to provide passive immunization with homologous tetanus immune globulin (human) must be decided individually for each patient.[3] The characteristics of the wound, conditions under which it was incurred, its treatment, its age, and the previous active immunization status of the patient must be considered.

    G. A written record of the immunization should be provided to every wounded patient and he should be instructed to carry the record at all times, and, if indicated, to complete active immunization. For precise tetanus prophylaxis, an accurate and immediately available history regarding previous active immunization against tetanus is required or a rapid reliable test to determine the patient's serum tetanus antitoxin level is required.

    H. Basic immunization with adsorbed tetanus toxoid requires three injections with the first two being given 4 to 6 weeks apart and the third being given 6 to 12 months after the second injection. A booster of adsorbed tetanus toxoid is indicated 10 years after the third injection or 10 years after an intervening wound booster. All individuals, including pregnant women, should have basic immunization and indicated booster injections. Neonatal tetanus is preventable by active immunization of the mother before or during the first 6 months of pregnancy. This immunization can be achieved by two intramuscular injections of adsorbed toxoid given 6 weeks apart.

---

*From Furste, W.: Guidelines for short-term prevention of tetanus in the injured. In Comptes rendus de la quatrième conférénce internationale sur le tétanos, Lyon, France, 1975, Foundation Mérieux.

II. Specific measures for patients with wounds

A. Previously immunized individuals

1. When the patient has been actively immunized within the past 10 years:

   a. To the great majority, 0.5 ml[2] of adsorbed tetanus toxoid[1] should be given as a booster unless it is certain that the patient has received a booster within the previous 5 years.

   b. To those with severe, neglected, or old (more than 24 hours) tetanus-prone wounds, 0.5 ml[2] of adsorbed tetanus toxoid[1] should be given unless it is certain that the patient has received a booster within the previous year.

2. When the patient has been actively immunized more than 10 years previously:

   a. To the great majority, 0.5 ml[2] of adsorbed tetanus toxoid[1] should be given.

   b. To those with severe, neglected, or old (more than 24 hours) tetanus-prone wounds:

      (1) 0.5 ml[2] of adsorbed tetanus toxoid[1,4] should be given.

      (2) 250 units[5] of tetanus immune globulin (human)[4] should be given.

      (3) The administration of oxytetracycline or penicillin should be considered.

B. Individuals *not* previously immunized

1. With clean minor wounds in which tetanus is most unlikely, 0.5 ml[2] of adsorbed tetanus toxoid[1] (initial immunizing dose) should be administered.

2. With all other wounds:

   a. 0.5 ml[2] of adsorbed tetanus toxoid[1,4] (initial immunizing dose) should be administered.

   b. 250 units[5] of tetanus immune globulin (human)[4] should be administered.

   c. The administration of oxytetracycline or penicillin should be considered.

---

1. DTP (diphtheria and tetanus toxoids combined with pertussis vaccine) is recommended for basic immunization in infants and children from 2 months through 6 years of age, and Td (combined tetanus and diphtheria toxoids: adult type) for basic immunization of those older than 6 years. For the latter group, Td toxoid is recommended for routine or wound boosters, but if there is any reason to suspect hypersensitivity to the diphtheria component, tetanus toxoid (T) should be substituted for Td.

2. With different preparations of toxoid, the volume of a single booster dose should be modified as stated on the package label.

3. The following precautions should be considered regarding passive immunization with heterologous tetanus antitoxin (equine):

   a. If the patient is not sensitive to heterologous tetanus antitoxin (equine) and if the decision is made to administer it for passive immunization, at least 3,000 units should be given intramuscularly.

   b. Heterologous tetanus antitoxin (equine) should not be administered except when tetanus immune globulin (human) is not available within 24 hours and only if the possibility of tetanus outweighs the danger of reaction to heterologous tetanus antitoxin (equine).

   c. Before heterologous tetanus antitoxin (equine) is used, the patient should be questioned for a history of allergy and tested for sensitivity. If the patient is sensitive to heterologous tetanus antitoxin (equine) it should not be used, as the danger of anaphylaxis probably outweighs the danger of tetanus; penicillin or oxytetracycline should be relied on. Desensitization should not be attempted, as it is not worthwhile.

4. Different syringes, needles, and sites of injection should be utilized.

5. In severe, neglected, or old (more than 24 hours) tetanus-prone wounds, a dose of 500 units of tetanus immune globulin (human) is advisable.

Table 40-6. Trade, commercial, or proprietary names for tetanus immune globulin (human)

United States	Europe
Hyper-Tet	Tetabullin (Austria)
Hu-Tet	Tetagam (West Germany)
Homo-Tet	Tetuman Berna (Switzerland)
Gamatet	Tetaglobuline (France)
Immu-Tetanus	Humotet (England)
T-I-Gammagee	
Pro-Tet	
Gamulin-T	
Artet	

Antitoxins

Heterologous antitoxins. In 1890, von Behring and Kitasato demonstrated the formation of tetanus antitoxin in the blood of mice and rabbits following active immunization. When injected into unvaccinated mice and rabbits, this antitoxin protected them against a subsequent tetanus infection. Other animals could also be treated with these sera with good results. Thus the practical value of both homologous and heterologous antisera was proved.

Few discoveries in the history of medicine have excited both scientists and laymen as much as this one did, for the ever-present threat of tetanus could now be banished. By the end of the nineteenth century, in spite of some skepticism, antitoxin therapy and particularly prophylaxis were widely adopted and approved.

Homologous antitoxin: tetanus immune globulin (human). Tetanus immune globulin (human) or TIG(H) has been referred to by numerous scientific and trade names (Table 40-6).

TIG(H), a sterile solution containing 165 ± 15 mg of gamma globulin per milliliter, is prepared from human blood plasma having a high titer of tetanus antitoxin. Such plasma is obtained from blood of hyperimmunized volunteers, from blood for gamma globulin manufacture that has been screened for tetanus antitoxin titers, or from placentas from mothers who received tetanus toxoid booster inoculations a few weeks preceding delivery.

TIG(H) is effective prophylactically in patients with wounds that may be contaminated with *Clostridium tetani*. Because it is of human origin, it is virtually free from the risk of inducing hypersensitivity. Its use is advised particularly when a history of active immunization with tetanus toxoid cannot be established with reasonable certainty and when the risk of immediate or delayed reactions to equine antitoxin must be avoided (patients known to be sensitive to horse serum, those who have had prior injections of horse serum, or those who have a history of allergy). When a history of previous active immunization can be established, the administration of a booster dose of tetanus toxoid is preferable.

Passive immunization with TIG(H) is neither a substitute for active immunization with tetanus toxoid nor a substitute for adequate surgical care of contaminated or potentially contaminated wounds. The half-life of passively acquired TIG(H) is

Table 40-7. Prophylactic doses of tetanus immune globulin (human) for infants and children

Age	Dose
10 years or older	250 units
5 to 10 years	125 units
Younger than 5 years	75 units

thought to be at least 3 weeks and possibly more than 4 weeks. By contrast, tetanus toxin antibodies from heterologous sources (equine or bovine antitoxins) have a relatively brief half-life, which may be as short as 2 or 3 days.

Studies on the absorption and persistence of TIG(H) indicate that about one half of an intramuscular dose appears in the plasma. The injection of 4 to 5 units per kilogram of body weight ensures a plasma level of 0.02 units per milliliter for as long as 4 weeks; this level is probably adequate to protect against any but a fulminating tetanus infection.

Unless extraneous contamination occurs, there is virtually no likelihood of transmitting viral hepatitis by the administration of this agent. The possibility that allergic reactions may occur is very remote. As with other gamma globulin preparations, however, pain and redness at the site of injection may rarely occur.

At the time of intramuscular administration, skin sensitivity testing need not be done, but care should be taken to draw back on the plunger of the syringe to be certain that the needle is not in a blood vessel. Under no circumstances should the globulin be given intravenously.

When TIG(H) is given, adsorbed tetanus toxoid should also be administered. A different sterile syringe and needle are used to inject the toxoid to lessen the possibility that some of the antitoxin and some of the toxoid may neutralize each other. Doses of 250 to 400 units of TIG(H) for adults and 75 to 250 units for infants and children do not appear to interfere appreciably with primary active immunization (Table 40-7). Thus simultaneous active-passive immunization, in which the adsorbed toxoid is injected into one deltoid muscle and the TIG(H) is injected into the contralateral gluteal muscles, can be accomplished. By such simultaneous immunization immediate passive protection is conferred and active protection is initiated.

Antibiotics

Antibiotics such as penicillin have been shown to be effective against vegetative tetanus bacilli both in vitro and in experimental animals. They have no effect against toxin. The effectiveness of antibiotics for prophylaxis remains unproved; if used, they should be given over a period of at least 5 days.

Antibiotics should not be used as a substitute for active or passive immunization or as a substitute for proper surgical care of the wound or both, and antibiotics are not necessary to prevent tetanus in the actively immunized.

Emergency medical identification devices

In the present era of sophisticated chemical and electronic equipment and complicated and heroic operative procedures, proper consideration should still be given generally to the patient's history and more specifically to the emergency medical identification device (EMID).

As much as possible should be known about the victim of trauma. Information vital for the care of such a patient can be immediately available by the use of the EMID. In the United States of America, where many individuals now are actively immunized for tetanus, such devices are becoming more, rather than less, important. Clinicians in active practice are constantly faced with these questions in the management of the wounded:

1. Has the patient been actively immunized for tetanus?
2. If the patient has been actively immunized for tetanus, when?
3. Have there been reactions to tetanus toxoid?
4. Should TIG(H) be given?

Such questions can be immediately answered if each individual has on his person an up-to-date EMID.

It is most distressing, considering the large population in the United States, to be called to take care of patients who have little or no knowledge of their immunization status and whose tetanus prophylaxis cannot therefore be scientifically planned. If their status is in doubt, simultaneous active-passive immunization can be effected, but in doing so TIG(H) may be wasted. If the history is vague and poorly documented, the patient should be given tetanus toxoid as though the dose or doses of toxoid in question had not been given.

Physicians have had patients tell them that they have been given tetanus toxoid injections, but, after a closer search of the history, they have learned that tetanus antitoxin, diphtheria toxoid, or perhaps typhoid vaccine had been given—but not tetanus toxoid.

In the United States at the present time, very few people have an EMID with tetanus data in their immediate possession (Table 40-5).

If every person carried some type of an EMID, history taking after injury could be greatly simplified and expedited, tetanus toxoid immunization could be accurately and scientifically performed, overdosage and unnecessary injections of tetanus toxoid could be avoided, and injections could be avoided in the rare individual who is sensitive to tetanus toxoid.

The American Medical Association has prepared for physicians at low cost an emergency medical identification card. On this card there is a reproduction of the American Medical Association identification symbol, which was adopted by the World Medical Association and was recommended for use in the countries represented by the World Medical Association members. Similar cards or records are also available from the World Health Organization, the United States Government Printing Office, the American Academy of Pediatrics, the American Academy of General Practice, and the Michigan State Medical Society.

At the 1967 World Congress of Motoring Medicine in Vienna, an asbestos, noninflammable card used in Austria was described in a discussion of EMIDs for motorists.

A button may be attached to underclothing, to a billfold, or to a purse. Metal tags are available in attractive configuration such as a heart. Tattoo marks, of course, are always on the patient, and are readily apparent if not destroyed by local trauma such as a burn. The use of such marks, however, has been questioned. Some years ago, the Committee on Emergency Medical Identification of the American Medical Association considered tattoos at some length, and decided that they are not suitable for several reasons. The primary reason is that many groups are antagonistic toward permanent markings as a result of the experiences they suffered during World Wars I and II. Also it is difficult to provide a tattoo in a place where it is accessible and—at the same time—inconspicuous.

Medicolegal aspects

The legal aspects of medical practice in the United States are receiving more consideration. To emphasize the problem, the following statement was mailed, in the form of a news release, to science writers, general and specialty medical publications, and the wire services on November 12, 1970:

> The Regents of the American College of Surgeons feel obligated to inform the public that the rising number of lawsuits against physicians is seriously threatening the quality of surgical care and increasing its cost to patients.

The following cases are examples of the types of problems that may occur. In these particular cases, some aspect or aspects of tetanus prophylaxis were of importance.

Dental extraction. According to hospital records submitted for medicolegal evaluation, a dentist extracted nine upper teeth from a 40-year-old woman. Seven days later the patient developed tetanus, and 9 days after the extraction she died. The dentist was sued for malpractice.

Heterologous tetanus antitoxin. In another lawsuit the responsible physician was being sued because his patient (an adult woman)—after a negative skin test—presumably developed a reaction to a dose of heterologous horse antitoxin.

Wringer injury of hand. In 1952, a 2-year-old boy suffered a wringer injury of his hand and developed tetanus. In 1968 the attending surgeon was sued for a high six-figure amount.

Departure from hospital against advice. In another case, a physician was to be tried before a court in East Germany for a case of tetanus. Apparently an injured patient had refused to stay in the hospital for indicated care, he went home, developed tetanus, was readmitted, and died.

Cost

Effective tetanus prophylaxis is one of the least expensive types of prophylaxis. As has been discussed in the prophylaxis section, a few injections of tetanus toxoid will prevent tetanus.

According to the amount of toxoid purchased and to the vial or ready-for-injection syringe in which tetanus toxoid is sold, the pharmacy cost for the patient of one dose of tetanus toxoid is somewhat less or somewhat more than a dollar. The hospital cost of one case of tetanus in the United States in 1971 was $9,773.80. The treatment of a dangerously ill patient, such as one with tetanus, in West Germany in 1967 was estimated to be up to 20,000 DM.

In view of the cost of tetanus toxoid and of the cost of the treatment of a case of tetanus, should any more be said about tetanus toxoid prophylaxis being an economic triumph?

Political considerations

In 1971, the following note was received from a physician in a country many centuries old:

> In our country we have no good documentations of previous tetanus toxoid injections in individuals. For this reason we are injecting 3000 u. TAT and tetanus toxoid. Sometimes we do not have tetanus toxoid, and then we are giving only TAT. We have no TIG (human) in our country.

Millions of American dollars are being spent to develop a perpetual peace. Should a minute fraction of such expenditures be diverted for the purchase and distribution of tetanus toxoid, TIG(H), and EMIDs to other countries of the world to prove that the United States is really interested in citizens of other countries and in their health?

CONCLUSION

The four bases of tetanus prophylaxis for the wounded are (1) tetanus toxoid, (2) surgical care, (3) antitoxin, and (4) EMIDs.

Approximately one and one-half decades ago, President Kennedy predicted that man would land on the moon; his prediction was confirmed. Hopefully by 1980 tetanus will no longer occur in the United States and will have become a disease of only historical significance.

QUESTIONS

1. Is it possible to eliminate tetanus?
2. If so, how?
3. Does the human body forget a dose of tetanus toxoid?
4. Is tetanus antitoxin necessary if tetanus toxoid immunization is properly planned and completed?
5. Is the first dose of tetanus toxoid given at the time of an injury effective in preventing tetanus as a result of the injury?
6. Is there active immunity from tetanus?
7. Describe optimal surgical care of wounds to prevent tetanus.
8. In the United States when should heterologous tetanus antitoxin be given.
9. List trade, commercial, or proprietary names for tetanus immune globulin (human).
10. Describe simultaneous active-passive tetanus immunization.
11. What are the advantages of simultaneous active-passive tetanus immunization?
12. Describe the types of emergency medical identification devices that are now available.

SUGGESTED READINGS

Bytchenko, B.: Letter (Each year, . . . one million deaths as a result of tetanus), World Health Organization, 8 Aug. 1975.

Committee on Trauma, American College of Surgeons (Artz, C., chairman): A guide to prophylaxis against tetanus in wound management, Bull. Am. Coll. Surg. **57**:32, 1972.

Furste, W.: Compost-contaminated wound hazards: gas gangrene and tetanus, J.A.M.A. **207**: 1923, 1969.

Furste, W.: Tetanus: the continuing problem of physicians and nonphysicians, J. Trauma **15**:549, 1975.

Furste, W.: Guidelines for short-term prevention of tetanus in the injured. In Comptes rendus de la quatrième conférence internationale sur le tétanos, Lyon, France, 1975, Foundation Mérieux.

Furste, W., Veronesi, R., del Rey, J., and Román, G.: Tetanos, Bogotá, 1974, Ediciones Lerner Ltda. (Monograph for Federación Panamericana de Asociaciones de Facultades (Escuelas) de Medicina, Bogotá.)

Furste, W., and Wheeler, W.: Tetanus: a team disease, Curr. Probl. Surg. **3**:72, 1972.

CHAPTER 41

Rabies

JEAN-RENÉ DUPONT

TREATMENT

For many years we have believed that, once clinically manifest, rabies seems incurable. However, poorly documented reports of nonfatal human rabies have appeared, and recovery from rabies in several animal species is accepted. In 1972 a well-substantiated recovery of a child from rabies was published. This has added a ray of hope in the clinical management of rabies encephalitis. Aggressive care can cure!

Rabies treatment may be viewed as

1. Preexposure vaccination
2. Postexposure prophylaxis
3. Supportive measures

Preexposure vaccination may be indicated in high-risk individuals, such as laboratory workers, humane officers, foresters, and veterinarians. Two 1 ml injections 1 month apart followed by a booster 6 months after the second dose usually produces neutralizing antibodies in 80% to 90% of cases. (Another satisfactory schedule is three doses at weekly intervals followed by a booster 3 months later.)

"To treat or not to treat?" That is the tantalizing question often confronting the physician who attempts to manage persons exposed to rabies: The significance of the exposure, the risk of infection, and the risk of a serious reaction to postexposure prophylaxis must each be weighed one against the other.

Management of the wound is important. The wound should be carefully flushed under running water and scrubbed with a brush and a cleansing compound, such as soap. It is not necessary to use silver nitrate or electocautery on these wounds. Mechanical cleansing is thought to be the most salutary. Depending on the severity of the wound and the history of the offending animal, antirabies serum or vaccine (or both) may be administered. Tetanus prophylaxis is also given, and if the wound is large with a considerable amount of soft tissue destruction, antibiotics can be added to the regimen.

If the offending animal is domestic, and if no lesions are present, antirabies serum or vaccine need not be administered. If the exposure is severe, if the biting animal is rabid or has disappeared or is a wild carnivore, bat, or squirrel, both serum and vaccine may be indicated. The administration of vaccine within 24 hours following the initial dose of antirabies serum is thought to be of value. Two preparations of

Table 41-1. Management of rabies

Animal bite treatment checklist
1. Flush wound immediately (first aid).
2. Cleanse wound thoroughly under medical supervision.
3. Give antirabies serum and/or vaccine as indicated.
4. Give tetanus prophylaxis and antibacterial regimen when required.

Postexposure antirabies prophylaxis guide

Animal bite		Treatment per degree of exposure*		
Species	Status at time of attack	No lesion	Mild	Severe
Dog or cat	Healthy	None	None	Serum
	Signs suggestive of rabies	None	Vaccine	Serum/vaccine
	Escaped or unknown	None	Vaccine	Serum/vaccine
	Rabid	None	Serum/vaccine	Serum/vaccine
Skunk, fox, raccoon, coyote, bat	Regard as rabid in unprovoked attack	None	Serum/vaccine	Serum/vaccine

*Vaccine refers to duck embryo high egg passage vaccine. (Serum used for hyperimmune antirabies serum.) The vaccine is given in 21 injections of 1 ml of a 10% tissue emulsion or 2 ml of a 5% emulsion, depending on the manufacturing process. Hyperimmune serum may be administered in doses of 40 to 100 IU per kilogram of body weight, depending on the severity of exposure. Human globulin is given in 20 IU per kilogram of body weight.

hyperimmune serum are available—antirabies serum (ARS) of equine origin and hyperimmune rabies immunoglobulin (HRIG) obtained from human volunteers. The former should be administered in a dose of 40 international units per kilogram, the latter in half that dose (20 IU per kilogram). Fifty percent of the antiserum should be infiltrated about the wound; the rest is given intramuscularly. Horse serum produces serum sickness in 15% to 40% of the recipients, while HRIG eliminates that problem. However, the human globulin is expensive and in short supply.

The administration of HRIG results in the early appearance of antibodies but inhibits the development of active antibodies in patients who also receive duck embryo vaccine (DEV). The immunosuppression is overcome by 23 doses of DEV, which is now the recommended postexposure prophylaxis when used with HRIG.* Otherwise the primary series is 21 doses of DEV. This is followed by two booster doses on the tenth and twentieth days after the primary series. In cases of severe

*It is my opinion that recent developments in the postexposure treatment of rabies will cause the Food and Drug Administration to approve the new human diploid cell vaccine (HDCV) for use in this country within the next year. It is expected that the new recommendations for postexposure treatment will read as follows: Human rabies immune globulin (HRIG, Cutter Laboratories), one dose of 20 IU per kilogram of body weight with one-half injected at the site of the bite or scratch as soon after exposure as possible, then 1 ml intramuscularly of HDCV administered in five doses on days 0, 3, 7, 14, and 30, following exposure. This will replace the DEV.

exposure the dose may be doubled or given in half the time. It is safe to modify the treatment when rendered according to knowledge of wildlife rabies in the area and the status of the offending animal.

An animal with clinical rabies will be dead from 5 to 7 days following the onset of symptoms. If a biting dog is observed for this period of time and remains well, he is quite unlikely to be shedding rabies virus in the saliva. Any captured wild animal that bites or scratches should be killed, and the head should be sent to the appropriate laboratory for examination. If the brain tissue is negative for rabies when tested by the fluorescent antibody technique, it may be assumed that the saliva contains no virus and the exposed person need not be treated.

It is not unlikely that the future development of a potent rabies vaccine will be based on the use of virus grown in human tissue culture. At the present time the duck embryo (DEV) high egg passage (HEP) vaccine has largely replaced the older spinal cord vaccines of Semple, Pasteur, and Fermi.* The low egg passage vaccine (LEP) is generally used for immunization of animals but may at times prove virulent to cats.

Vaccination has been found to be helpful only when the incubation period of rabies is shorter than 30 days. All persons receiving vaccine for rabies exposure should also be given a booster injection 10, 20, and 30 days after the series has been completed. If central nervous system symptoms should appear during the course of vaccination, the injections should be stopped immediately for fear of precipitating an irreversible demyelinating disease. The common side effects caused by the duck embryo vaccine are pruritus, pain, and erythema at the site of inoculation. Adrenocortical steroids and epinephrine are helpful in combating the immediate reactions.

A number of treatment failures have been observed. However, in recent years, with the use of hyperimmune serum and modern vaccines in increasing dosages, the incidence of treatment failures has been reduced to an absolute minmum whenever treatment with the serum commences within 24 hours after exposure.

Once clinical rabies appears, supportive measures similar to those employed in tetanus may be efficacious. This entails prevention of fatal complications such as seizures, cardiac arrythmias, aspiration, or asphyxiation. It is of some comfort to the physician attending a rabies victim to know that transmission from man to man has not been described in the modern literature.

PREVENTION

Prevention, of course, is of paramount importance in a disease such as rabies, which has no cure for the clinical illness. The following measures are effective and reasonable:

1. Wild animal reservoirs should be reduced or exterminated if the risk of infection outweighs economic and ecologic considerations. It appears that the rabies virus has an epizootic cycle of about 100 years.

---

*The following are the more common spinal cord or brain vaccines: Pasteur, Hogyes, Fermi, and Semple. Avian vaccines include the duck embryo or the chick embryo HEP or LEP (high, 180, and low, 40 to 50 egg passages). The names Flury and Kelev imply a certain strain of the virus, the former being named after a young rabies victim from whom it was isolated in 1939.

2. Stray dogs ought to be quarantined, vaccinated, and domesticated. If this is impossible, they should be eradicated.

3. Domestic dogs, cats, and other animals must be vaccinated if exposure to rabies is possible or probable.

4. Persons should avoid wild animals that appear to have lost their natural shyness when approached (skunks, coyotes, foxes, etc.). All animals displaying an abnormal behavior or odd patterns of movements are best left alone (bats flying in daytime or biting, groggy canines).

5. Domestic dogs and cats biting without cause or provocation should be suspected of having rabies. They should be quarantined for no less than 7 days, at which time they may be returned to the owner if showing no symptoms of rabies.

6. Animal handlers and high-risk personnel should be vaccinated against rabies and should receive a booster injection every year. Booster injections administered every 6 months induce earlier antibody formation.

7. Animals entering a country should be kept in quarantine for at least 45 days and should receive vaccination on entry.

8. The virus does not penetrate intact skin but may enter through mucous membranes. Postexposure prophylactic vaccination should be undertaken when any person is bitten by wild animals, including bats or domestic animals showing signs of rabies.

PHYSICAL EXAMINATION

During the prodromal phase of the disease the physical examination is often unremarkable. One may find a healed scar from a previous bite or scratch, or there may be no history of previous animal exposure. Neuritic pain referred to the site of the original bite is a frequent complaint. The patient is agitated, excitable, and restless. He has a mild coryza. Bradycardia out of proportion to the fever has been stressed as an important physical finding, but it is not invariably present. These vague findings during the early stages of the disease have often resulted in an initial diagnosis of "psychoneurotic disorder."

During the late stages of the illness paralysis appears, but most victims die before total paralysis has time to set in. It is during this time that the classic autonomic manifestations of pharyngeal spasms, hydrophobia, vomiting, retching, convulsions, tremor, cutis anserina, and excessive salivation are seen.

LABORATORY DIAGNOSIS

The laboratory diagnosis of rabies centers around two avenues of approach: (1) the histopathologic examination of the rabies victim at postmortem and (2) the serologic diagnosis of the disease.

Neutralizing antibodies to rabies can be demonstrated in the serum, and with the advent of the fluorescent antibody technique, a sensitive tool has been furnished the clinician. These same two methods of diagnosis are available to the public health officer. It must be borne in mind that tissue examination of the brain of rabies victims should be carried out on fixed tissue, whereas serologic testing is limited to the fresh frozen specimen.

The routine laboratory tests are normal, including the spinal fluid. Both albuminuria and a relative polymorphonuclear neutrophilia occur with regularity.

HISTOPATHOLOGY

Rabies encephalitis is an acute viral infection of the central nervous system predominantly affecting the gray matter of the brainstem. It is therefore a viral polioencephalitis. Present-day knowledge holds that the disease is caused by a single serologically distinct, rather large virus (100 to 150 nm by filtration) that has some of the characteristics of a myxovirus.

PUBLIC HEALTH DATA

Rabies is a disease that may occur from Greenland to Cape Horn. South Central Asia and Southeast Asia, with 50% of the cases in recent years, appear to harbor the largest source of human exposures. New Zealand, Australia, and the Scandinavian countries reportedly have been free of rabies for several decades.

Because of rapid transportation today, unsuspected cases of rabies may crop up in the western hemisphere at odd times. Rabies has been diagnosed in patients visiting London and Western Europe from the Orient. In the United States the largest reservoir seems to be in the South and Southwest, as far as human case material is concerned. However, wildlife rabies is rampant throughout most of the central United States as far east as Maryland, as far north as the Dakotas, and south to the Mexican border and the Florida peninsula. A definite concentration of rabies in skunks and foxes appears to be found in Kentucky, Tennessee, and the neighboring states.

Prior to 1940 the domestic dog was by far the most important carrier as far as human exposure was concerned. Over the past two decades this has changed. The important carrier today is the wild animal, particularly the skunk, fox, and bat. Furthermore it has been demonstrated that the skunk sheds the virus in extremely high concentrations in the saliva. Skunk bites should therefore always be considered dangerous.

INCIDENCE

As with any viral encephalitis, the very young have an affinity for rabies. The female of the species seems to be more resistant to the virus than is the male, and the black individual is overwhelmingly more resistant to rabies infection than is the white one. In most series the ratio of male to female affinity is generally three to one. In experimental animals it may go as high as seven males to one female.

TRANSMISSION

Rabies encephalitis is generally thought to be transmitted by the bite of a rabid animal. The virus is harbored in quantity in the saliva of clinically rabid animals, but it may be demonstrated in other parts of the body of these animals by special methods, such as fluorescent antibody technique. Apparently a certain number of wild animals can develop serum neutralizing antibodies to rabies without showing the clinically apparent disease. Today more than 50% of human cases are accounted for by wildlife exposure. In any study of rabies it is important to note that one third to one fourth of the patients yield no history of an actual animal bite or scratch. It has been believed that droplet and fomite transmission may be important. At the same time, however, one must consider that rabies virus does not appear to be an extremely infectious agent. It has been estimated that less than 10% of human exposures to actually known rabid animals will result in encephalitis and death. Most bites are on the hand; it is believed by some that bites on the extremities are less likely to result in clinical rabies than are bites on the face.

The average incubation period is approximately 57 days, with a range of 20 to 150 days. After the prodrome appears, the clinical course usually averages 7 to 8 days. If a very short clinical course is encountered in a patient who has received rabies vaccination, the physician should suspect an allergic reaction to the rabies vaccine rather than rabies encephalitis itself. It is an accepted fact that the incubation period is entirely unpredictable and has no relationship to the virulence of the clinical course. However, it is our belief that the most virulent form of the disease is encountered when the amount of local tissue destruction is great and the size of the inoculum is large, such as is seen in facial bites from rabid wolves. The overt manifestations of the disease are completely unrelated to the site of the initial bite.

QUESTIONS

1. What sort of individuals may be considered likely candidates for preexposure vaccination?
2. List the factors to be considered in deciding whether "to treat or not to treat" the person exposed to possible rabies infection.
3. Discuss wound management as related to control of rabies.
4. What period of observation of the suspected animal is indicated in rabies control?
5. Explain the salient factors of rabies prevention, and indicate why they are of paramount importance.
6. What particular avenues of approach are most helpful in laboratory diagnosis of rabies?
7. Discuss the change that has occurred during the past few years in the relative frequency of the various animal species as rabies vectors.
8. What is the importance of droplet and fomite transmission of rabies?
9. Contrast the two preparations of hyperimmune serum.
10. Discuss modification of rabies treatment according to various factors, such as the status of the offending animal or knowledge of wildlife rabies in the area.
11. What is the importance of the physical examination in the total picture of rabies management?

SUGGESTED READINGS

Corey, L., and Hattwick, M.: Special communication: treatment of persons exposed to rabies, J.A.M.A. **232**:272-276, 1975.

Hattwick, M., Weis, T. T., Stechschulte, C. J., Baer, G. M., and Gregg, M. B.: Recovery from rabies: a case report, Ann. Med. **76**:931-942, 1972.

Hattwick, M., Rubin, R. H., Music, S., Sikes, R. K., Smith, J. S., and Gregg, M. B.: Postexposure rabies prophylaxis with human rabies immune globulin, J.A.M.A. **227**:407-410, 1974.

Kelly, P. C.: Rabies—A brief review of current management, Ariz. Med. **31**:27-35, 1975.

PART ELEVEN

Medicolegal considerations

ELWYN E. CADY, Jr.

Lawsuits against physicians who gratuitously render immediate aid are extremely rare. Medicolegal interest is heightened nevertheless by passage of "Good Samaritan" legislation in a number of states and by re-examination of legal rules of conduct imposed in emergency situations. An immediate goal is the prevention of legal entanglements.

EMERGENCY DEFINED

Although the law does not slavishly follow lexicographers in defining words, *Webster's Third New International Dictionary,* Unabridged (1961), notes three shades of meaning for "emergency":
1. An unforeseen combination of circumstances or the resulting state that calls for immediate action.
2. A sudden bodily illness such as is likely to require immediate medical attention.
3. A distressing event or condition that can often be anticipated or prepared for but that is seldom foreseen.

Likewise the definition of "first aid" is helpful: emergency and sometimes makeshift treatment given to someone (as the victim of an accident) requiring immediate attention where regular medical or surgical care is not available.

With these generalizations as background, we should consider the obligations of a physician to undertake immediate care, the measure of his proper conduct toward the patient, and special medicolegal problems in which the concept of "emergency" figures.

ETHICAL DUTY

Although it is true that a physician is ordinarily under no legal obligation to undertake immediate care, Section 5 of the *Principles of Medical Ethics* (1957 edition of the American Medical Association) places a rather strict moral burden on the AMA-guided practitioner: "In an emergency . . . he should undertake to render service to the best of his ability."

The 1955 edition of the *Principles,* still used as an authoritative source by the AMA Judicial Council, was more detailed:

323

He should . . . respond to any request for his assistance in an emergency or whenever temperate public opinion expects the service . . . (Sec. 4). When a physician is called in an emergency because the personal or family physician is not at hand, he should provide only for the patient's immediate need and should withdraw from the case on arrival of the personal or family physician. However, he should first report to the personal or family physician the condition found and treatment administered (Sec. 5).

Thus the ethical practitioner is bound to engage in emergency treatment from time to time.

LEGAL STANDARDS OF CONDUCT

Once the physician undertakes to treat a victim of an accident, he then becomes subject to legal rules that measure the quality of his conduct. The basic rules are comprehended in the concept of "legal duty," the breach of which amounts to negligence in the basic liability formula (see Fig. 2).

Specifically a physician is required to exercise the following qualities to avoid liability:

Knowledge or learning based on advanced training, degree, and license. Whether undertaking treatment without "paper qualifications" constitutes negligence has been debated in law reports. In emergency care and first aid, however, the necessity

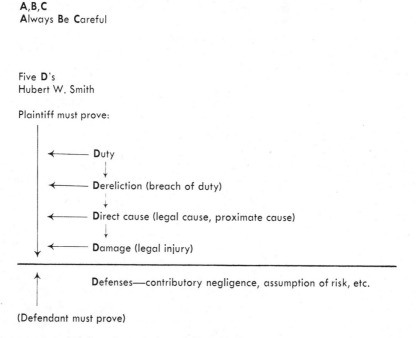

A,B,C
Always Be Careful

Five **D**'s
Hubert W. Smith

Plaintiff must prove:

← Duty

← Dereliction (breach of duty)

← Direct cause (legal cause, proximate cause)

← Damage (legal injury)

Defenses—contributory negligence, assumption of risk, etc.

(Defendant must prove)

Fig. 2. Mnemonic liability chart. (Adapted from Cady, E. L., Jr.: Law relating to medical practice: the doctor's diagnosis and treatment of patients. In Gradwohl, R. B. H.: Legal medicine, St. Louis, 1954, The C. V. Mosby Co.)

for immediate action is intrinsic. "The emergency begets the man"; he is not selected on the basis of prior qualifications or training. Consequently the law is not inclined to penalize him for proceeding even though his background is deficient. He would not be relieved from the obligation of exercising ordinary care, the proper inquiry being whether he acted prudently in the context of the facts of the emergency.

Reasonable skill. This duty is the possession and exercise of that reasonable degree of skill ordinarily possessed by others of his profession practicing in similar circumstances. Although a direct test in court as to requisite skill in an emergency has not been denoted, the cases justify certain generalizations:

1. A specialist in fact, who also holds himself out as a specialist, would be held to the skill of the up-to-date specialist in his particular field.

2. A general practitioner would be held to the standard of a general practitioner. Perhaps a specialist in fact who did not hold himself out as anything but "a doctor" when responding to an emergency call would need only meet this standard.

3. Residents, interns, externs, medical students, nurses, and nursing students would all be held to the standard commensurate with their particular level of training and experience.

4. Persons having particular training in first aid would presumably have this considered when a judge or jury weighed their conduct. A myocardial infarction case turned on the negligence of a purser, also serving as pharmacist's mate, aboard a ship docked in London who permitted the patient to walk about the ship and to go ashore to a hospital. Judge Kraft held that it was not legal error to admit statements contained in a volume entitled *The Ship's Medicine Chest and First Aid at Sea:*

> This book was required to be aboard the United States Lines' ships, and was, in fact, aboard the vessel here involved and available to the purser. The purser admitted that he did not refer to the book when plaintiff consulted him on the morning of his heart attack. Briefly, the statements admitted described the symptoms of coronary heart disease and emphasized the importance of "strict bed rest." The statements were offered and received for the limited purpose of showing the purser's knowledge, and the trial Judge carefully instructed the jury that the statements were not admitted as evidence of the truth of the matters asserted, or for any purpose other than to prove notice to the purser.
>
> The statements were clearly admissible as circumstantial evidence of the purser's knowledge of the facts, and of the acts or omissions on his part which might constitute negligence. Downie v. United States Lines Co., 231 F. Supp. 192 (1964).

Ordinary care. This represents a minimum objective standard. Although referred to as "average care," this does not mean that half of the professional group is automatically "below standard." Variability of this standard is illustrated by (1) the "proportionate to the character of injury" instruction and by (2) the "keeping abreast" rule:

1. Under a jury instruction that care and diligence used in attending an injured person should be proportionate to the character of the injury, an advocate can argue that actual performance in a life-threatening emergency should be superior to that expected in "minor emergencies." It is recognized, however, that to include the item of "skill" in such an instruction is wrong. "It can hardly be said that his skill should increase in proportion to the severity of the injury. One's skill is a matter

of slow growth and cannot be increased on short notice." Judge Sturgis in Fowler v. Burris, 180 Mo. App. 347, 171 S.W. 620 (1914). A Kentucky court phrased it: "The duty performed is according to the exigencies of the case and proportionate to the dangers to be apprehended and guarded against." Johnson v. Vaughan, 370 S.W. 2d 591 (1963).

2. Ordinary care must reflect action consistent with technical advances. Thus Judge Choate included the following findings of fact in a cardiac arrest case, Kolesar v. United States, 198 F. Supp. 517 (1961):

> A deprivation of an adequate supply of oxygen to the brain of a human being beyond the period of four minutes will most likely cause irreversible damage to the higher centers of the brain tissue and results in a neurological deficiency in a human being. The extent of brain damage has a direct relation to the passage of time. This period was generally accepted by the medical profession on January 21, 1958.
>
> Acceptable medical practice at Key West Naval Hospital on January 21, 1958, dictated a diagnosis of cardiac arrest and circulatory insufficiency as to Marrian Kolesar at the time her abdominal incision did not bleed and she had no obtainable pulse.
>
> No notice was taken, or record kept, of the passage of time during either the various resuscitative procedures adopted or in connection with the initiation of a thoracotomy so as to manually restore circulation within the four minute period.
>
> A period materially in excess of four minutes occurred between the time Marrian Kolesar's abdominal incision did not bleed, and her pulse became unobtainable until the time when resuscitative procedures were effective in that manual cardiac massage restored the flow of blood to the patient's brain. This constituted a departure from acceptable medical practice at Key West Naval Hospital on January 21, 1958.

Ordinary diligence. Emphasis on persistence characterizes this requirement. In evaluating a cardiac arrest situation, this diligence would imply a continuation of artificial respiration and massage through an extended period of time. (See Chapter 12.)

Best judgment. This element has particular application in emergency situations. It comprehends a subjective standard in contrast to the objective criteria for diligence and care. Thus presumably one could use his best judgment and, though it were far inferior to the judgment used by the average practitioner, he would still "pass muster." On the other hand, a particular physician actually possessing superior judgment would be bound to use it. So long as the physician used his best judgment at the particular time and under the particular circumstances, an error in his decision as to the proper course is excused.

Courts do not impose liability for "mere error of judgment" in this context. Furthermore courts applying the "emergency doctrine" suggest that something less than "best judgment" is the requirement (see Fig. 3.):

> [T]he emergency doctrine . . . is that where one is confronted with a sudden emergency, without sufficient time to determine with certainty the best course to pursue, he is not held to the same accuracy of judgment as would be required of him if he had time for deliberation. Justice Anderson in Mississippi Cent. R. Co. v. Aultman, 173 Miss. 622, 160 So. 737, 940 (1935).
>
> [E]mergency does not lessen the obligation to use care, but merely excuses errors

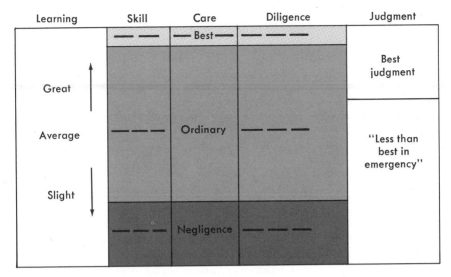

Fig. 3. Elements of legal duty.

of judgment due to the excitement and necessity for haste produced by the emergency. Judge Dobie in Lachman v. Pennsylvania Greyhound Lines, 160 F. 2d 496, 502 (4th Cir. 1947).

It must be emphasized that the "emergency doctrine" is applied primarily to automobile accident cases in the law reports. Its use was tried unsuccessfully in the defense of a surgeon who "left" a hemostat. Long v. Sledge, 209 So. 2d 814 (Mississippi, 1968). One might well argue that all practitioners, or even students, should be prepared to meet a medical or surgical emergency with their best judgment. This, of course, is on the basis that an integral part of medical education is training in proper handling of emergency situations "with a cool head."

GOOD SAMARITAN LEGISLATION

California, in 1959, and other states since then have enacted statutes that purport to exempt physicians from negligence liability in emergency cases.

Under the common law system, conclusions as to the validity of such legislation must await court tests. Serious doubts on the constitutionality of such legislation have been voiced.

The first significant case construing such legislation concerned a passing motorist, Mrs. Turner, giving a ride to a man who had wrecked his car on the highway. Judge Wood interpreted the statute as applied to the facts in these words (Dahl v. Turner, 80 N. Mex. 608, 458 P. 2d 860 [1969]):

The pertinent part of [the statute] reads: "No person who shall administer emergency care in good faith at or near the scene of an emergency, as defined herein, shall be held liable for any civil damages as a result of any action or omission by such person in administering said care, except for gross negligence; . . ."

[The statute] defines emergency to mean: " . . . an unexpected occurrence involving injury or illness to persons, including motor vehicle accidents and collisions, disasters, and other accidents and events of similar nature occurring in public or private places." . . .

If Mrs. Turner was administering "care" in providing transportation to plaintiff, such care was not emergency care within the meaning of the statute. There are no facts indicating a pressing necessity for such transportation; no facts indicating that the transportation was immediately called for.

After plaintiff wrecked his car he had a cut on his arm and appeared in a confused state. In such a situation, the State Police Officer would have tried to get plaintiff to go to the hospital but wouldn't have forced him to go. Plaintiff didn't want to go to a doctor. Plaintiff wanted to be taken to a friend at a motel in Silver City. That's what Mrs. Turner was doing. . . .

LIMITATIONS BY CONTRACT

Although agreements that purport to absolve physicians from negligence liability are frowned on, it is possible to limit the ambit of medical services by contract. In particular it is entirely proper to limit one's obligations to immediate care only, and indeed this should be the practice of the physician who treats an emergency case when the victim's own physician is unavailable. Oral statements are mostly employed, ideally with witnesses present, but written forms are available.

CONSENT IMPLIED

Any touching of the person without consent ordinarily constitutes an unlawful battery so that civil and perhaps criminal liability can attach. Bona fide immediate care, including heroic surgery, is permitted without the usual legal consent, however. As stated by Chief Justice Chavez: "It would indeed be most unusual for a doctor, with his patient who had just been bitten by a venomous snake, to calmly sit down and first fully discuss the various available methods of treating snakebite and the possible consequences, while the venom was being pumped through the patient's body." Crouch v. Most. 78 N. Mex. 406, 432 P. 2d 250 (1967).

Legal theorists say that consent is implied in fact or as a matter of law. Regardless of theory, the law does give a definite privilege for immediate care to proceed even though no actual consent is obtained. I will stand on this proposition even though contrary dictum is stated in some of the books authored by nurses or physicians who, it is submitted, fail to heed a basic view that the law represents "crystallized common sense." There has even been discussion as to whether or not there should be efforts made to gain consent from a victim's legal representative (such as parent, spouse, or guardian) before undertaking emergency surgery. The immediacy of surgery under principles of good practice as well as the impracticability of consulting such representatives should justify such surgery.

A related matter has been deviation from an original nonemergency procedure to one classed as an emergency based on "newly discovered evidence." The trend of decision has been toward the doctrine enunciated by Judge Clayton of the Municipal Court of Appeals for the District of Columbia in Barnett v. Bachrach, 34 A. 2d 626 (1943):

> We hold the law to be that in case of emergency a surgeon may lawfully perform, and it is his duty to perform, such operations as good surgery demands even when it means extending the operation further than was originally contemplated.

EMERGENCY INVOLUNTARY HOSPITALIZATION

The old common law evolved a doctrine permitting anyone to restrain a person who became dangerous to himself or to others because of mental disorder. The doctrine was designed for instances in which the urgency of the situation demands immediate intervention, that is, an emergency. Today this doctrine has been supplemented in many states by mental health acts that authorize an emergency hospitalization for a limited period on medical certification.

DUTY OF HOSPITAL TO PROVIDE IMMEDIATE CARE

It has become commonplace for hospitals to establish and maintain emergency rooms. A strong concurrent development in today's jurisprudence is a recognition that such hospitals have a positive duty to render immediate care.

Chief Justice Southerland of Delaware commented in Wilmington General Hospital v. Manlove, 174 A. 2d 135 (1961):

> It may be conceded that a private hospital is under no legal obligation to the public to maintain an emergency ward, or, for that matter, a public clinic. . . .
>
> But the maintenance of such a ward to render first-aid to injured persons has become a well-established adjunct to the main business of a hospital. If a person, seriously hurt, applies for such aid at an emergency ward, relying on the established custom to render it, is it still the right of the hospital to turn him away without any reason? In such a case, it seems to us, such a refusal might well result in worsening the condition of the injured person, because of the time lost in a useless attempt to obtain medical aid.
>
> Such a set of circumstances is analogous to the case of the negligent termination of gratuitious services, which creates a tort liability. . . . Liability on the part of a hospital may be predicated on the refusal of service to a patient in case of an unmistakable emergency. . . .

The case was remanded for the trial court to determine whether an actual emergency existed:

> What is the standard hospital practice when an applicant for aid seeks medical aid for sickness at the emergency ward? Is it the practice for the nurse to determine whether or not an emergency exists, or is it her duty to call the interne in every case? Assuming (as seems probable) that it is her duty to make such a determination, was her determination in this case within the reasonable limits of judgment of a graduate nurse, even though mistaken, or was she derelict in her duty, as a graduate nurse, in not recognizing an emergency from the symptoms related to her? To resolve these questions additional evidence, probably expert opinion, would seem to be required.

TOWARD PREVENTION

To forestall medicolegal complications, several prophylactic avenues have been championed:

1. Detailed advance instructions should be given for the handling of emergency situations. As an example, the Medical Defense Union in England has issued the following memorandum in hope that "the wrong patient or part" cases may be minimized:

The Medical Defense Union and the Royal College of Nursing have given consideration to the steps that might be taken to obviate the risk of an operation being performed on:

(a) the wrong patient,

(b) the wrong side,

(c) the wrong digit.

During the period October, 1959, to September, 1961, the Medical Defense Union dealt with no fewer than *twenty-eight such cases* and it is hardly necessary to say that *these avoidable mistakes are quite indefensible.*

The Councils of the Medical Defense Union and the Royal College of Nursing are firmly of the opinion that in order to minimize the risk of such occurrences it is eminently desirable that wherever practicable the suggested safeguards as outlined below should be taken. It is appreciated that in certain out-lying or "cottage" hospitals there is no resident medical staff and that in some hospitals it may not always be possible to adopt these safeguards in their entirety.

(a) Operating on the wrong patient

Causes predisposing to error.

    (i) In hospitals which undertake a vast amount of casualty work, where *emergency patients* are being admitted in quick succession, some of them unconscious, there is the possibility of the notes becoming attached to the wrong patient. Where it is the practice to attach the patient's name to the clothing which has been removed in the casualty department, this does not always provide an adequate check because the clothes may be detached from the patient before or on admission to the ward.

    (ii) In respect of patients for non-emergency operations who have been in the ward for a day or two prior to operation, mistakes may arise if on the day of operation the beds are changed round. This situation is exacerbated if the day of operation coincides with a change in several of the nursing staff and could lead to the wrong patient being sent to the theatre if the routine did not provide adequate safeguards against error.

    (iii) Mistakes may occur when changes are made in theatre lists following the commencement of the operating session, particularly if such changes have not been notified to the ward immediately they have been made.

Suggested safeguards.

(1) All unconscious patients admitted through the casualty department should be labelled before they are taken to the wards. The identity disc or label should bear the patient's name, initials and hospital number where possible. *The labelling of the patient* should be the responsibility of the casualty sister or her deputy, or by night, the nurse-in-charge or her deputy.

(2) Following the admission to the hospital of a patient who is to undergo an operation, he *should be seen in the ward by the surgeon* who is to perform the operation. Prior to the operation the surgeon should examine the patient's records and make sure that the notes do in fact relate to that particular patient and that the entries contained therein are correct.

(3) All patients going to the operating theatre should be labelled by means of an *identity disc or label attached to the wrist or ankle.* The identity disc or label should bear the patient's name, initials and hospital number. The labelling should be carried out in the ward at the time the patient is prepared for the operating theatre and should be the responsibility of the ward sister or her deputy.

In rare cases where the patient goes direct from the casualty department to the operating theatre, the onus of correct labelling should rest on the casualty sister or her deputy. In either instance the labelling would constitute an additional check that the correct patient received the prescribed premedication and that the correct patient was sent to the theatre.

(4) In addition to the nature of the operation, the patient's name, initials and hospital number should also appear on the operation list. A copy of the *operation list should be displayed in the anaesthetic room as well as in the operating theatre, thus enabling both the*

anaesthetist and the surgeon to check and ensure that the right patient is presented for operation. A copy of the operation list should also be made available to wards in which the patients who are to undergo operation are accommodated.

(5) Patients should be sent for from the operating theatre by name and number and never as "the patient from such and such a ward." Where it is the practice for a porter from the theatre to collect the patients from the ward he should bring with him a slip bearing the name of the patient and his hospital number. In hospitals where the procedure is to telephone the ward to ask that the patient concerned be sent to the theatre, the patient's hospital number, as well as the name, should be quoted. The *ward sister* or her deputy should be responsible for seeing that:

(a) the correct patient is sent to the operating theatre;

(b) the patient has already signed the appropriate consent to operation form;

(c) the patient has received the prescribed pre-operative preparation including premedication;

(d) where appropriate the side of operation has been marked (see Section [b] Clause [1]);

(e) the correct case papers, X-rays, etc., accompany the patient to the theatre.

(6) In the operating theatre one person should be made responsible for sending for patients. This should be the responsibility of the theatre superintendent but in large operating theatre suites it may be necessary for her to delegate this responsibility to some other person, e.g., the sister-in-charge of a particular theatre or the nurse taking the list in a particular theatre.

(7) When out-patients are admitted to the wards for the day for a minor operation, they should be labelled in the same way as the in-patients before they are taken to the operating theatre.

(8) Patients who are to be operated on in the out-patient theatre under a general anaesthetic should be labelled in the same way as the in-patients.

(9) Patients should have one hospital number which should be quoted on all papers concerning the patient. Where it is the practice to have departmental numbers these may be used additionally on the appropriate papers but never exclusively.

(10) In so far as children are concerned, the labelling should be carried out when they are admitted to the ward. As the case histories must be taken from the patient's relatives (who may not be present immediately prior to the operation) it is vital that no error should occur in these notes in reference to the side, limb or digit on which the operation is to be performed.

(b) Operating on the wrong side or limb

Causes predisposing to error.

(i) Wrong information on the case papers of the patient, i.e., "right" instead of "left."

(ii) Abbreviation of the words "right" and "left."

(iii) Illegible writing on the case papers.

(iv) Failure to check immediately prior to commencing to operate the entry on the operation list with the notes taken to the operating theatre.

(v) The wrong case papers accompanying the patient, combined with (iv) above.

(vi) The preparation of the wrong side or limb, combined with (iv) above.

(vii) No routine procedure for marking the operation side.

Suggested safeguards.

(1) The side on which the operation is to be performed should be indelibly marked before the patient reaches the theatre, and in order to denote the side a mark should be made with *an indelible skin pencil on the forehead* of the patient. This should normally be made the responsibility of the house surgeon. In the case of "listed" patients already in the ward, it is usual for the house surgeon or a house officer to see the patient on the evening before the

operation and this would give the practitioner concerned an opportunity of marking the operation side. In the case of emergency operations the surgeon generally sees the patient in the ward before he is taken to the operating theatre, thus providing him with an opportunity for marking the operation side. In the rare instance of a patient who is taken direct from the casualty department to the operating theatre, the practitioner who decides upon an immediate operation should be made responsible for marking the operation side.

In the event of the ward sister or her deputy, or exceptionally the casualty sister or her deputy, finding that the side of operation has not been marked when the patient is due to be sent to the operating theatre, she should see that the surgeon who is to operate is informed accordingly, but she should not herself undertake the marking.

(2) The words "right" and "left" should be written in full in the patient's notes and in the operation list.

(c) Operating on the wrong digit

Causes predisposing to error.

(i) Fingers referred to by numbers instead of by name.

(ii) Wrong information on the case papers of the patient, i.e., "right" instead of "left."

(iii) Illegible writing on the case papers.

(iv) Failure to check immediately prior to commencing to operate the entry on the operation list with the notes taken to the operating theatre.

(v) The wrong case papers accompanying the patient, combined with (iv) above.

(vi) The preparation of the wrong digit combined with (iv) above.

(vii) No routine procedure for marking the side on which the operation is to be performed.

Suggested safeguards.

(1) In order to avoid the possibility of any ambiguity concerning the finger(s) on which the operation is to be performed, the finger(s) should always be described as thumb, index, middle, ring and little fingers and not as first, second, third, fourth and fifth. In so far as the toes are concerned, the accepted practice is to describe them has hallux (big), second, third, fourth and fifth (little) toes and this should always be adhered to.

(2) The words "right" and "left" should be written in full in the patient's notes and on the operation list.

In order to reach agreement on a routine procedure, incorporating as far as possible the safeguards put forward in this memorandum, to be adopted in a particular hospital or group of hospitals, it is suggested that joint committees of medical and nursing staff should be set up on a local basis. The committees should include, inter alios, the matron and a representative of the consultant surgical staff.

2. Competent medicolegal consultation services should be made immediately available. Unusual situations may necessitate sound medicolegal guidance for the practitioner. As a rule, such advice should be secured promptly so that "hindsight headaches" can be avoided.

3. Emphasis should be given to the swiftness and thoroughness with which immediate concern for the patient proceeds. Indeed this represents the philosophy of this text as outlined in Chapter 1. There is no time for thoughts of "defensive medicine" (whether this be myth or reality)!

4. Above all, the practitioner should keep the anxiety-relieving thought in mind, grasping a few fundamentals mentioned here, that "pitching in" with first aid and immediate care is *not* legally hazardous. Statistically speaking, true Good Samaritans rarely lose lawsuits!

QUESTIONS

1. Define *first aid* and *emergency*.
2. What are the "five D's"?
3. Does bona fide emergency care require consent legally?
4. What steps can be taken to avoid operations on the wrong limb?
5. How can one limit responsibility for immediate care?

SUGGESTED READINGS

American Law Reports, Rochester, N.Y.; The Lawyer's Cooperative Publishing Co., Annotations:

1. Duty and liability of one who voluntarily undertakes to care for injured person, 64 ALR 2d 1179 (1959).
2. Violation of statute requiring one involved in an accident to stop and render aid as affecting civil liability, 80 ALR 2d 299 (1961).
3. Construction of "Good Samaritan" statutes excusing from civil liability one rendering care in emergencies, 39 ALR 3d 222 (1971).

Cahal, M. F. and Cady, E. L., Jr.: Medicolegal case studies: Assault and Battery, 26 GP **2:** 185 1962.

Cahal, M. F. and Cady, E. L., Jr.: Medicolegal trends: emergency aid, 29 GP **5:**207 1964.

Cady, E. L., Jr.: Law and contemporary nursing, Paterson, N.J., 1961, Littlefield, Adams & Co.

Cady, E. L., Jr.: Legal relations of the mentally ill. In Gradwohl, R. B. H., editor: Legal Medicine, St. Louis, 1954, The C. V. Mosby Co.

Cady, E. L., Jr.: Medicolegal aspects of cardiac arrest and resuscitation. In Stephenson, H. E., Jr.: Cardiac arrest and resuscitation, ed. 4, St. Louis, 1974, The C. V. Mosby Co.

Moore, J. L., Jr.: The Good Samaritan, J. Med. Assoc. Ga. **51:**554, 1962.

Report of the Secretary's Commission on Medical Malpractice: Appendix, Washington, D.C., 1973, U.S. Department of Health, Education and Welfare.

Smith, H. W.: Legal responsibility for medical malpractice. 5. Further information about duty and dereliction, J.A.M.A. **116:**2757, 1941.

Index